REDISCOVERING PIERRE JANET

Rediscovering Pierre Janet explores the legacy left by the pioneering French psychologist, philosopher and psychotherapist (1859–1947), from the relationship between Janet and Freud to the influence of his dissociation theory on contemporary psychotraumatology.

Divided into three parts, the first section places Janetian psychological analysis and psychoanalysis in the context of the foundational tenets of psychoanalysis, from Freud to relational theory, before the book explores Janet's work on trauma and dissociation and its influence on contemporary thinking. Part three presents several contemporary psychotherapy approaches directly influenced by Janetian theory, including the treatment of posttraumatic stress disorder and dissociative identity disorder.

Rediscovering Pierre Janet draws together eminent scholars from a variety of backgrounds, each of whom has developed Janetian constructs according to his or her own theoretical and clinical models. It provides an integrative approach that offers contemporary perspectives on Janet's work, and will be of significant interest to practicing psychoanalysts, psychiatrists, and psychotherapists, especially those treating trauma-related dissociative disorders, as well as researchers with an interest in psychological trauma.

Giuseppe Craparo, PhD, is a psychologist, psychoanalyst, and associate professor of clinical psychology at the Kore University of Enna, Italy. He is a member of the following associations: American Psychological Association, Italian Psychological Association, Association of Psychoanalytic Studies, and International Federation of Psychoanalytic Societies.

Francesca Ortu, PhD, is a psychologist and full professor at "La Sapienza" University of Rome, has investigated issues concerning the origin of psychoanalysis, emphasizing the points of contact with, and distance from, the theories that the French school, and particularly Pierre Janet, were elaborating. She has devoted a series of studies to the analysis of Janetian theory and its clinical importance.

Onno van der Hart, PhD, is a psychologist, retired psychotherapist, and emeritus professor at Utrecht University. A former president of the International Society for Traumatic Stress Studies and honorary president of L'Association Française Pierre Janet, he is also a member of the International Society for the Study of Trauma and Dissociation, and the European Society for Trauma and Dissociation.

THE HISTORY OF PSYCHOANALYSIS SERIES

Professor Brett Kahr and Professor Peter L. Rudnytsky (Series Editors)

This series seeks to present outstanding new books that illuminate any aspect of the history of psychoanalysis from its earliest days to the present, and to reintroduce classic texts to contemporary readers.

Other titles in the series:

What is this Professor Freud Like? A Diary of an Analysis with Historical Comments
Edited by Anna Koellreuter

Corresponding Lives
Mabel Dodge Luhan, A. A. Brill, and the Psychoanalytic Adventure in America
Patricia R. Everett

A Forgotten Freudian
The Passion of Karl Stern
Daniel Burston

The Skin-Ego
A New Translation by Naomi Segal
Didier Anzieu

Karl Abraham
Life and Work, a Biography
Anna Bentinck van Schoonheten

The Freudian Orient
Early Psychoanalysis, Anti-Semitic Challenge, and the Vicissitudes of Orientalist Discourse
Frank F. Scherer

For further information about this series please visit https://www.routledge.com/The-History-of-Psychoanalysis-Series/book-series/KARNHIPSY

REDISCOVERING PIERRE JANET

Trauma, Dissociation, and a New Context for Psychoanalysis

Edited by Giuseppe Craparo, Francesca Ortu, and Onno van der Hart

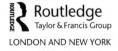

Routledge
Taylor & Francis Group

LONDON AND NEW YORK

First published 2019
by Routledge
2 Park Square, Milton Park, Abingdon, Oxon OX14 4RN

and by Routledge
52 Vanderbilt Avenue, New York, NY 10017

Routledge is an imprint of the Taylor & Francis Group, an informa business

British Library Cataloguing-in-Publication Data
A catalogue record for this book is available from the British Library

Library of Congress Cataloging-in-Publication Data
A catalog record has been requested for this book

ISBN: 978-0-367-19354-6 (hbk)
ISBN: 978-0-367-19356-0 (pbk)
ISBN: 978-0-429-20187-5 (ebk)

Typeset in Bembo
by Deanta Global Publishing Services, Chennai, India

CONTENTS

SERIES EDITOR'S FOREWORD

The history of psychoanalysis is frequently, and justifiably, told as a story of splits – of the ruptures, excommunications, and personal conflicts in which Freud became repeatedly embroiled and that allowed him to assert sovereignty over his domain by defining it in negative fashion in terms of what it was *not*. The names of the outcasts are legion. Breuer, Fliess, Adler, Stekel, Jung, Rank, even Ferenczi at the end – all these are part of the canonical narrative as it has been handed down by Freud himself and then consolidated by Jones in his authorized biography. The effect of these breakups, from the orthodox perspective, is that the later careers of the renegades have been effectively relegated to oblivion, their work deemed no longer worth reading once they parted ways with Freud, since, as he wrote dismissively of Jung in the *New Introductory Lectures* (1933), "This may be a school of wisdom; but it is no longer analysis" (p. 143).

But if at least the names of these heretics have been preserved in the collective psychoanalytic memory, the same cannot be said of the subject of this book. Pierre Janet (1859–1947) has been all but effaced from our history because the period in which he was regarded favourably by Freud was limited to the years of the collaboration with Breuer on *Studies on Hysteria* (1895), and thus belongs to the prehistory of the field. Since he never became part of the movement, Janet did not have to be excommunicated, but could simply be left behind and treated as a jealous rival who had missed the boat when it came to Freud's revolutionary discoveries about sexuality and the unconscious. The keynote of the received critique of Janet is struck in the second of the Clark lectures, where Freud (1910), after acknowledging that he and Breuer had "followed [Janet's] example when we took the splitting of the mind and dissociation of the personality as the centre of our position," went on to ridicule Janet by likening his view of the hysterical patient to a "feeble woman" laden with packages who "cannot contain the whole of heap of them with her two arms and ten fingers" (p. 21), so she keeps dropping one every time she bends over to pick up another.

Although Freud sought to belittle Janet, there can be no doubt that the Frenchman – like all his other banished adversaries – exerted a tenacious hold on Freud's psyche, as he again took up the cudgels against Janet not only in *On the History of the Psycho-Analytic Movement* (1914) but also in *An Autobiographical Study* (1925), where he claimed that "historically psycho-analysis is completely independent of Janet's discoveries, just as in its content it diverges from them and goes far beyond them" (p. 31). But if Janet has been consigned to the ash heap of psychoanalytic history, why should we seek to resurrect him today?

The answer, as I have set forth at greater length elsewhere (Rudnytsky, 2019, ch. 5), is that the return to trauma theory in psychoanalysis, which is inseparable from the rehabilitation of Ferenczi as an indispensable precursor of contemporary relational and interpersonal thinking, has as its corollary a view of the mind based not on the repression of endogenous instinctual drives, as Freud would have it, but rather on dissociation and multiple self-states result- ing from experiences of abuse and neglect beginning in childhood. In seek- ing to understand the origins of this alternative model of the mind, one can discern the outline, if not of a tradition then of a series of beacons who have lighted the way to where we are today. In addition to Ferenczi, the essential landmarks from the past include Breuer, Fairbairn, and Sullivan, while it is in the work of Donnel Stern and Philip Bromberg, both at the William Alanson White Institute in New York City, that the paradigm shift has been most fully consolidated in our own time.

It is this increasingly shared awareness among psychoanalysts of the crucial link between trauma theory and dissociation theory that leads us ineluctably back to Janet, who made it the cornerstone of his life's work. As Henri Ellenberger has written in his invaluable chapter, "Pierre Janet and psychological analysis," in *The Discovery of the Unconscious* (1970):

> Janet contended that certain hysterical symptoms can be related to the exist- ence of split parts of the personality (subconscious fixed ideas) endowed with autonomous life and development. He showed their origin in trau- matic events of the past and the possibility of a cure of hysterical symptoms through the discovery and subsequent dissolution of these subconscious psychological systems.
>
> *(p. 361)*

As Ellenberger elaborates, the process by which "subconscious fixed ideas" are replaced by symptoms is held by Janet to be connected with a "narrowing of the field of consciousness" that makes the fixed ideas at once "the cause and the effect of mental weakness" (p. 373). Here we see the gist of the conception mocked by Freud in his metaphor of the "feeble woman," as well as of Breuer's "hypnoid state" theory in *Studies on Hysteria* (1895).

Despite having been supposedly discredited by Freud's "defence" theory, Janet's conception warrants reappraisal in light of our renewed appreciation of how the psychic death and fracturing of a sense of self that are the consequences of trauma are more fundamental phenomena for severely disturbed patients than are the more visible conflicts and defences that are only their outcroppings. When we add to this Ellenberger's observations that "the word 'subconscious' was coined by Janet" and that the concept of "complexes," which was transmitted to Freud by Jung, who had attended Janet's lectures in Paris in 1902–1903, was "originally nothing but the equivalent of Janet's 'subconscious fixed ideas'" (p. 406), then we can see how truly seminal are Janet's contributions.

Rather than proscribe the term "subconscious" from our lexicon, as has been *de rigueur* in psychoanalysis ever since Freud (1915) proclaimed it be "incorrect and misleading," even as he argued that "the well-known cases of '*double conscience*' (splitting of consciousness) prove nothing against our view" (pp. 170–171), perhaps it should be rehabilitated, especially since it seems to fit with Stern's (1997) definition of the unconscious as "unformulated experience." As Janet himself wrote in 1893 in arguing that the "narrowing of the field of consciousness" was a defining feature of hysteria, "The hysterical personality cannot perceive all the phenomena; it definitively sacrifices some of them. It is a kind of autotomia [i.e. a self-severing], and the abandoned phenomena develop independently without the subject being aware of them" (qtd. in Ellenberger, 1970, p. 375). If we follow this line of reasoning to its logical conclusion, might we even entertain the possibility that Janet's report at the 1913 International Congress of Medicine in London, where, in Ellenberger's (1970) words, he "claimed priority in having discovered the cathartic cure of neurosis brought forth by the clarification of traumatic origins," but "sharply criticized Freud's method of symbolic interpretation of dreams and his theory of the sexual origin of neurosis" (p. 344), to which Freud (1914) took vehement exception as alleging "that everything good in psycho-analysis is a repetition of Janet's views, and that everything else in it is bad" (p. 32), has at least a kernel of truth to it, so that the Freudian school, rather than having superseded Janet, should be seen instead as one of the fertile tributaries that has its source in the broad river of "psychological analysis"?

From Ellenberger (1970), we learn that Janet shared with Freud the fate of being the eldest son of a remarried father in his forties who was more than twice the age of his new wife (p. 333), though his mother died at the age of 49, rather than, like Amalia Freud, at 95. But it would otherwise be difficult to find two more different men than the Parisian who was originally trained in philosophy before becoming the cautiously empirical "Doctor Pencil" who took meticulous notes on some 5,000 patients in the course of his career and the Viennese neurologist who paid his dues as a bench scientist in the laboratories of Claus and Brücke before becoming the speculative conquistador of the Dora and Wolf-Man cases. Could we imagine Freud attending the lectures of one of his former students, as Janet did for an entire academic year at the age of 83 (pp. 346–347)? It is telling that, when Janet went to Vienna in 1937 to visit Julius Wagner-Jauregg,

Freud declined to meet him (p. 346), just as he refused to shake Ferenczi's hand at their final parting in Vienna in 1932 (Fromm, 1959, p. 70), pretended not to see the elderly Breuer who had opened his arms when he chanced to run into Freud on a Vienna street (Breger, 2000, p. 125), and rebuffed Stekel's overtures of reconciliation both when Freud underwent surgery for his cancer of the jaw in 1923 and when he arrived in England as a refugee in 1938 (Rudnytsky, 2011, pp. 38–39). Janet, on the other hand, after having delivered his critical assessment of psychoanalysis at the 1913 London conference, came to Freud's defence when he was fiercely attacked at a meeting of the Société de Psychothérapie the following year (Ellenberger, 1970, p. 344).

At the age of 24, Janet gave an address in Le Havre, where he was teaching, in which he affirmed that the "true aim of philosophy is to teach man to beware of his own preconceived opinions and to respect the opinions of his fellowmen" (Ellenberger, 1970, p. 337). This excellent counsel is in keeping with Janet's unwillingness to assert a titular claim over psychological analysis as "his own method" (p. 374), believing it to be rather the common property of all workers in the field. Nor did he "ever belong to a group or team," he had "no disciples or school," and "any kind of proselytism was absolutely alien to him" (p. 408). In all these respects, of course, Janet is the antithesis of Freud. In contrast to Freud's "hermeneutics of suspicion," moreover, Janet told one of his visitors at the Salpêtrière – where he worked beginning in 1889 and then steadily from 1893 to 1902 – that he started from the premise, "I believe these people, until it is proven to me that what they say is untrue," so that seemingly incredible delusions reflect the reality that "these people are persecuted by something, and you must investigate carefully until you get at the root" (qtd. p. 351). Finally, Janet advocated an integrative approach to psychological treatment, welcoming in his final years the advent of both electroshock therapy for depressed patients and the use of medications as adjuncts to his version of an "experimental approach," which, he said, "consists above all in knowing one's patient well" in all the unique details of his life and at the same time in recognizing that "one never knows him enough" (qtd. p. 364; see p. 347).

To be sure, the diligent Anglophone student can find resources in the trauma literature that serve as stepping stones to Janet. These include Bessel van der Kolk's *The Body Keeps the Score* (2014), Elizabeth F. Howell's *The Dissociative Mind* (2005), and Onno van der Hart, Ellert Nijenhuis, and Kathy Steele's *The Haunted Self* (2006). But the present volume, with its distinguished roster of international contributors, offers the first comprehensive reassessment of Janet both as a theorist in his own right and in his complex relation to psychoanalysis. The editors of *Rediscovering Pierre Janet* are thus to be congratulated for having conceived and brought to fruition an exceptionally timely book, and it would be splendid if it were to be followed by a *Pierre Janet Reader* that would contain the essential texts by Janet himself which are still all but inaccessible to his vast prospective audience in the twenty-first century. Ellenberger (1970) concludes his chapter on Janet by comparing his work "to a vast buried city beneath ashes, like Pompeii," which may "perhaps be unearthed some day and brought back to life" (p. 409). Although Ellenberger's metaphor of the "buried city" is in one respect unfortunate, since it was employed by Freud to describe his concept of repression, and thus paradoxically effaces the distinctiveness of Janet in the very act of paying homage to him, it also has the virtue of foreshadowing the rectification of the historical amnesia and indeed autotomy of Janet's legacy by the psychoanalytic tradition that Giuseppe Craparo, Francesca Ortu, and Onno van der Hart have accomplished here.

Peter L. Rudnytsky
Gainesville, Florida

References

Breger, L. (2000). *Freud: Darkness in the Midst of Vision*. New York: Wiley.

Ellenberger, H. (1970). *The Discovery of the Unconscious: The History and Evolution of Dynamic Psychiatry*. New York: Basic Books.

Freud, S. (1910). *Five Lectures on Psycho-Analysis*. *S. E.*, 11: 9–55. London: Hogarth.

Freud, S. (1914). *On the History of the Psycho-Analytic Movement*. *S. E.*, 14: 7–66. London: Hogarth.

Freud, S. (1915). The Unconscious. *S. E.*, 14: 166–215. London: Hogarth.

Freud, S. (1925). *An Autobiographical Study*. *S. E.*, 20: 7–74. London: Hogarth.

Freud, S. (1933). *New Introductory Lectures on Psycho-Analysis*. *S. E.*, 5: 182.

Freud, S., & Breuer, J. (1895). *Studies on Hysteria*. *S. E.*, 2.

Fromm, E. (1959). *Sigmund Freud's Mission*. New York: Grove Press, 1963.

Howell, E. F. (2005). *The Dissociative Mind*. New York: Routledge.

Rudnytsky, P. L. (2011). *Rescuing Psychoanalysis from Freud and Other Essays in Re-Vision*. London: Karnac.

Rudnytsky, P. L. (2019). *Formulated Experiences: Hidden Realities and Emergent Meanings from Shakespeare to Fromm*. New York: Routledge.

Stern, D. (1997). *Unformulated Experience: From Dissociation to Imagination in Psychoanalysis*. Hillsdale, NJ: Analytic Press.

van der Hart, O., Nijenhuis, E. R. S., & Steele, K. (2006). *The Haunted Self: Structural Dissociation and the Treatment of Chronic Traumatization*. New York: Norton.

Van der Kolk, B. (2014). *The Body Keeps the Score: Brain, Mind, and Body in the Healing of Trauma*. New York: Penguin, 2015.

ABOUT THE EDITORS AND CONTRIBUTORS

Cécile Barral, PhD, is a psychotherapist in private practice in Sydney and Newcastle, NSW, Australia. She graduated from the ANZAP (Australia and New Zealand Association of Psychotherapy) training in the Conversational Model in 1996 and feels privileged to be part of the team of practitioners of the Conversational Model who are able to follow closely the evolution of Russell Meares' thinking. She has presented many papers at ANZAP conferences and is on the ANZAP faculty. She has just finished a three-year position as director of studies for the ANZAP three-year training course. She was born in Germany from French parents and educated mostly in France. She trained in somatic psychotherapy at the Boyesen Institute in London before emigrating to Australia, where she discovered first self-psychology and then the Conversational Model. She enjoys and appreciates being able to read Janet in the original text and translate some of his work, all the more as Janet has been such an influential person for Russell Meares and his development of the Conversational Model.

Vanessa Beavan, PhD, is a clinical psychologist, specializing in psychosis since 2006, and has held an academic position teaching clinical psychology at the Australian College of Applied Psychology, Sydney since 2012. She completed her Master's Degree in Clinical Psychology (Université de Bordeaux II, France) and a PhD in Psychology (Auckland University, New Zealand). She has held executive board positions for the Hearing Voices Network and also for the International Society for Psychological and Social Approaches to Psychosis, in both New Zealand and Australia, and has published journal articles and book chapters in the area of psychosis, with a specific focus on hearing voices, trauma, and recovery.

Paul Brown, MD, is a scholar in Pierre Janet studies. He was trained in London, in medicine (1972), and in psychiatry (1978). He moved to Jerusalem in the 1980s, where his focus was on psychotherapy, notably brief therapy. He went back to Melbourne just before 1990, where his professional interest involved diagnosis, centreing on posttraumatic stress disorder, and, since 2000, stress, suicide, and violence. Inspired by Janet in his clinical practice, he has written several studies on his work.

Karl-Ernst Bühler, Dr. med. habil. Dr. med., is a Professor of Psychosomatics and Psychotherapy at Julius-Maximilians-University in Würzburg, Germany, with a Diplom-Psychologe, and is a consultant for psychosomatics, psychotherapy, and psychiatry. He has made many contributions to international and national journals for psychotherapy, psychosomatics, clinical psychology and psychiatry. His main interests are in philosophical psychology and philosophical psychotherapy as well as in empirical research of psychological causes of depression and existential crises as well as coping with them.

Gabriele Cassullo, PhD, is a clinical psychologist and psychotherapist working in Turin, Italy. Doctor in research in human sciences and non-tenured professor in psychology at the Department of Psychology, Turin University, he is the author of many books and articles on the history, theory, and technique of psychoanalysis. He recently edited *Ferenczi's Influence on Contemporary Psychoanalytic Traditions* with Aleksandar Dimitrijevic and Jay Frankel.

Giuseppe Craparo, PhD, is a psychologist, psychoanalyst, Associate Professor of Clinical Psychology and Deputy Director, MSc Course in Clinical Psychology (Kore University of Enna, Italy). He also is Director of the Psychoanalytic Institute (IPP, Palermo), and a member of the following associations: American Psychological Association, Italian Psychological Association, Italian Society of Psychological Assessment, Association of Psychoanalytic Studies, International Federation of Psychoanalytic Societies. He is the author of several works on psychoanalysis, psychopathology, trauma, and dissociation. Among his books: *Trauma e psicopatologia. Un approccio evolutivo-relazionale* (co-edited with Vincenzo Caretti; Astrolabio, 2008); *Memorie traumatiche e mentalizzazione* (co-edited with Vincenzo Caretti and Adriano Schimmenti; Astrolabio, 2013); *Il disturbo post-traumatico da stress* (Carocci, 2013); *Inconsci, coscienza e desiderio. L'incertezza in psicoanalisi* (Carocci, 2015); *Elogio dell'incertezza. Saggi psicoanalitici* (Mimesis, 2016); *Pierre Janet. Trauma, coscienza, personalità* (co-edited with Francesca Ortu; Raffaello Cortina, 2016); *Unrepressed Unconscious, Implicit Memory, and Clinical Work* (co-edited with Clara Mucci; Karnac, 2017); *L'enactment nella relazione terapeutica. Caratteristiche e funzioni* (Raffaello Cortina, 2017); and *Inconscio non rimosso. Riflessioni per una nuova prassi clinica* (FrancoAngeli, 2018).

Barbara Friedman, MA, LMFT, is a researcher and psychotherapist in private practice in Los Angeles, California, USA, and specializes in the treatment of chronic traumatization and dissociaton. Inspired by the work of Pierre Janet, she co-authored *A Reader's Guide to Pierre Janet* with Onno van der Hart in 1989. In 2007, after two decades of work with challenging cases, she began incorporating principles of neuroplasticity and Comprehensive Energy Psychology with the classic and evolving techniques in trauma treatment.

Gerhard Heim, Dr. rer. soc., Dipl.-Psych., is a psychotherapist (cognitive behavioral therapy) in Berlin, Germany, and has been practicing since 1992. Born in München, he studied psychology and philosophy at the University of Konstanz, wrote his psychological dissertation on attention, laterality, and psychopathology in schizophrenics, and was a clinical psychologist at psychiatric departments in Weinsberg and Berlin. His research interests include psychopathology, history of psychotherapy, and clinical psychology. He has been the president of the Pierre Janet Gesellschaft (founded 2001; www.pierre-janet.de). He has publications on psychopathology, history of psychology, and on topics concerning Pierre Janet's contributions to psychiatry, psychotherapy, and clinical psychology. He is the editor of collected German translated texts by Pierre Janet, such as *Die Psychologie des Glaubens und die Mystik nebst anderen Schriften* (*Psychology of Belief and Mysticism and Other Writings*, 2013) and of volumes with the contributions of the German Pierre Janet Symposias (*Trauma, Dissociation, Personality*, 2006; *Psychotherapy: From Automatism to Self Control*, 2010; *Dissociation and Culture*, 2013; *Key Issues of Psychotherapy*, 2017).

Vittorio Lingiardi, MD, is a psychiatrist and psychoanalyst. He is Full Professor of Dynamic Psychology and past Director (2006–2013) of the Clinical Psychology Specialization Program in the Department of Dynamic and Clinical Psychology of the Faculty of Medicine and Psychology, Sapienza University of Rome, Italy. His research interests include diagnostic assessment and treatment of personality disorders, process-outcome research in psychoanalysis and psychotherapy, and gender identity and sexual orientation. He has published widely on these topics, as the author of several books in Italian and of many international articles including papers in the *American Journal of Psychiatry*, *Archives of Sexual Behavior*, *Contemporary Psychoanalysis*, *Journal of Personality Assessment*, *Journal of Personality Disorders*, *International Journal of Psychoanalysis*, *Psychoanalytic Dialogues*, *Psychoanalytic Inquiry*, *Psychoanalytic Psychology*, *Psychotherapy*, and *World Psychiatry*. He won the Ralph Roughton Paper Award from the American Psychoanalytic Association. He and Nancy McWilliams comprised the Steering Committee of the new edition of the *Psychodynamic Diagnostic Manual* (*PDM-2, 2017*).

Giovanni Liotti, MD, was a psychiatrist and psychotherapist, founder member and past president of the Italian Association for Behavioral and Cognitive Therapies (SITCC), and founder and past president of the Roman Association for Research on the Psychopathology of the Attachment System. He taught at a number of postgraduate schools of psychotherapy in Italy.

His interest in the clinical applications of attachment theory, first expressed in a book co-authored with V. F. Guidano (*Cognitive Processes and Emotional Disorders*, Guilford Press, 1983), focused, in the last thirty years, on the links between trauma, dissociation, and attachment disorganization, a theme explored in a number of journal papers, books, and books chapters. He received the Pierre Janet Writing Award (The International Society for the Study of Trauma and Dissociation, 2005) and the International Mind and Brain Award (University of Turin, Italy, 2006).

Marianna Liotti, MS, is currently serving an internship at the Operative Unit for Eating Disorders of Santa Maria della Pietà, Rome, Italy. She received a master's degree in developmental psychopathology at Sapienza University of Rome, with a dissertation about the role of attachment disorganization, complex trauma, and dissociation on autonomic functions, more specifically on cardiovascular activity. She translated two volumes into Italian, for Raffaello Cortina Editore, *The Neuropsychology of the Unconscious* by E. Ginot and *Healing the Fragmented Selves of Trauma Survivors* by J. Fisher, and she is now working on the translation of the volume *Cognitive Processes and Emotional Disorders* by V. F. Guidano and G. Liotti.

Russell Meares, MD, is Emeritus Professor of Psychiatry at Sydney University, Australia. He trained at the Maudsley and Bethlem Royal Hospitals where he formed an enduring friendship with his mentor Robert Hobson. Together they developed a style of therapy Hobson called the Conversational Model. The basis of their attempt to create a scientifically founded therapeutic approach derives from observations in the clinical sphere, studies of mother–child interaction, neurophysiology, and, more recently, linguistics. These observations included Meares's own, published in a series of papers. Several of these studies tested the effectiveness of the Model in borderline personality.

The Model was initially designed to treat intractable patients for whom Hobson had started a unit at the Bethlem Royal. It has, however, a more general application. Its nature has been described in a series of books, beginning with a preliminary work, *The Pursuit of Intimacy* (1977), and developed in *The Metaphor of Play* (1992, 1993, and 2005), *Intimacy and Alienation* (2000), *A Dissociation Model of Borderline Personality Disorder* (2012), and *A Poet's Voice in the Making of Mind* (2016). These books were complemented by Hobson's *Forms of Feeling* (1985) and a publication with colleagues, *Borderline Personality Disorder and the Conversational Model* (2012).

Andrew Moskowitz, PhD, is a Professor of Psychology at Touro College Berlin, Germany and President of the European Society for Trauma and Dissociation. He has taught for 20 years at various universities in New Zealand, the United Kingdom, and Denmark, and has published extensively on the relation between trauma and dissociation, and psychosis and schizophrenia, from historical, theoretical, empirical, and clinical perspectives. Professor Moskowitz has also researched and published on the relation between dissociation and violence. He is the lead editor of the influential book *Psychosis, Trauma and Dissociation* (Wiley, 2008; 2nd edition, 2019), and has lectured and presented workshops in many European countries and in North

America, on ways of understanding psychosis and schizophrenia from trauma or dissociation perspectives. Professor Moskowitz is also an associate editor of the new journal, the *European Journal of Trauma and Dissociation*.

Clara Mucci, PhD, is a Full Professor of Clinical Psychology at the University of Chieti, Italy, where she was Full Professor of English Literature for several years. A psychoanalyst, member of SIPP (Italian Society for Psychoanalytic Psychotherapy), and training and supervisor analyst for the SIPeP-SF (Italian Society for Psychoanalysis and Psychotherapy-Sandor Ferenczi), she is the author of several books on Shakespeare, psychoanalytic theory and literature, trauma, and personality disorders. Among her publications: *Liminal Personae* (Napoli, 1995); *Tempeste. Narrazioni di esilio in Shakespeare e Karen Blixen* (Napoli 1998); *Il teatro delle streghe. Il femminile come costruzione culturale al tempo di Shakespeare* (Napoli, 2001); *A memoria di donna. Psicoanalisi e Narrazione da Freud a Karen Blixen* (Roma, 2004); *Il dolore estremo. Il trauma da Freud alla Shoah* (Roma, 2008); *I corpi di Elisabetta. Sessualità, potere e poetica della cultura al tempo di Shakespeare* (Pisa, 2009); *Beyond Individual and Collective Trauma: Intergenerational Transmission, Psychoanalytic Treatment and the Dynamics of Forgiveness* (London, 2013); *Trauma e perdono. Una prospettiva psicoanalitica intergenerazionale* (Milano, 2014); and *Borderline Bodies: Affect Regulation Therapy for Personality Disorders* (New York, 2018). She co-edited *Unrepressed Unconscious, Implicit Memory and Clinical Work* (London, 2016) with Giuseppe Craparo. She is certified in the scoring of the AAI (under the guidance of Mary Main and Erik Hesse, and teachers Dino Dazzi and Deborah Jacobvitz) and in the scoring of the Reflective Functioning (under the guidance of Howard Steele). She lectures internationally and is presently visiting scholar at the New School for Social Research, New York.

Ellert R. S. Nijenhuis, PhD, is a psychologist, psychotherapist, and researcher. He engaged in the diagnosis and treatment of severely traumatized patients for more than three decades, and teaches and writes extensively on the themes of trauma-related dissociation and dissociative disorders. He initiated and continues to be engaged in the biopsychological study of complex dissociative disorders. Nijenhuis is a consultant at Clienia Littenheid, Switzerland, and collaborates with several European universities. His theoretical, scientific, and clinical publications include the book *Somatoform Dissociation* (Norton). With Onno van der Hart and Kathy Steele he co-authored the book *The Haunted Self: Structural Dissociation and the Treatment of Chronic Traumatization* (Norton). The first two volumes of Nijenhuis' recent trilogy *The Trinity of Trauma: Ignorance, Fragility, and Control* (Vandenhoeck & Ruprecht) appeared in 2015. The third volume, *Enactive Trauma Treatment*, was released in April 2017. The International Society for the Study of Trauma and Dissociation granted him several awards, including the Lifetime Achievement Award.

Pat Ogden, PhD, is a pioneer in somatic psychology, is the Founder and Education Director of the Sensorimotor Psychotherapy Institute, Colorado, USA, an internationally recognized school specializing in somatic–cognitive approaches for the treatment of posttraumatic stress and attachment disturbances. Her Institute has 19 certified trainers who conduct Sensorimotor Psychotherapy trainings of over 400 hours for mental health professionals throughout the USA, Canada, Europe, and Australia. The Institute has certified hundreds of psychotherapists throughout the world in this method. She is co-founder of the Hakomi Institute, past faculty of Naropa University (1985–2005), a clinician, consultant, and sought-after international lecturer. Dr. Ogden is the first author of two groundbreaking books in somatic psychology, *Trauma and the Body: A Sensorimotor Approach to Psychotherapy* and *Sensorimotor Psychotherapy: Interventions for Trauma and Attachment* (2015), both published in the Norton Series on Interpersonal Neurobiology. She is currently working on a third book, *Sensorimotor Psychotherapy for Children, Adolescents and Families*, with colleagues. Her current interests include developing training programmes in Sensorimotor Psychotherapy for children adolescents and families with colleagues, Embedded Relational Mindfulness, culture and diversity, couple therapy, challenging clients, the relational nature of shame, presence, consciousness, and the philosophical/spiritual principles that guide Sensorimotor Psychotherapy.

Francesca Ortu, PhD, is a Full Professor of Dynamic Psychology at the Department of Psychology, Sapienza University of Rome, Italy. Her research activity is focused in particular on the evaluation of psychodynamic psychotherapies and the study of early relationships in the framework of attachment theory. She has investigated issues concerning the origin of psychoanalysis, devoting particular space to the study of hypnosis and early Freudian theories on hysteria, emphasizing the points of contact with, and distance from, the theories that the French school, and particularly Pierre Janet, were elaborating. She then devoted a series of studies to the analysis of Janetian theory and its clinical importance. She edited the Italian translation of *La médicine psychologique* (Il Pensiero Scientifico, Rome, 1994) and *L'Automatisme Psychologique* (Cortina, Milano, 2013). She co-edited *Pierre Janet. Trauma, coscienza, personalità* (Raffaello Cortina, 2016) with Giuseppe Craparo.

Isabelle Saillot, PhD, is the editor-in-chief of *Janetian Studies* and co-editor-in-chief of the journal *Dogma*. After a Masters in Physics (Université Paris-7), she completed a Masters and a PhD in psycho-anthropology at the Natural History Museum of Paris. In 2004 she founded the Institut Pierre Janet, was its president for eight years, and then became the coordinator of the Réseau Janet (Paris). She divides her time between being a teacher and writer on physics, and doing research on Pierre Janet's work and its relevance for current psychology. Dr. Saillot collaborates with the ESTD (European Society for Trauma and Dissociation), of which she is a founding member and a former French representative. She also works with most of the organizations, in France and elswhere, that are involved in Pierre Janet studies, such as the Centre Pierre Janet, Université de Lorraine, Metz (France), and the Pierre Janet Geselschaft, in Berlin. Since 2009 she has been a board member of the Société Française de Psychologie (founded by Janet in 1901). She gives conferences on the topic of Janet, writes chapters in books, and has several publications in peer-reviewed journals such as *Psychologie Française* and the *European Journal of Trauma and Dissociation.*

Kathy Steele, MN, CS, is a psychotherapy consultation and has been in private practice in Atlanta, Georgia, USA, for over three decades, specializing in the treatment of complex trauma, dissociation, attachment difficulties, and the challenges of complicated therapies. She is an adjunct faculty at Emory University, and a Fellow and past President of the International Society for the Study of Trauma and Dissociation (ISSTD). Ms. Steele teaches internationally and consults with individuals, groups, and trauma programs. She has received a number of awards for her clinical and published works, including the Lifetime Achievement Award from ISSTD. She has published many journal articles and book chapters, and has co-authored three books, including *The Haunted Self* (2006), *Coping with Trauma-related Dissociation* (2011), and most recently *Treating Trauma-Related Dissociation: A Practical, Integrative Approach* (2017).

Caterina Vezzoli, PhD, is a psychologist, psychotherapist, Jungian analyst in private practice, training analyst at the C.G. Jung Institute in Zurich, Switzerland and at CIPA (Centro Italiano Psicologia Analitica), Italy. She is a member of both the IAAP (International Association Analytical Psychology) and the APG (Associazione di Psicoterapia Psicoanalitica di Gruppo), is Vice President of Philemon Foundation, is an active member of Art and Psyche International Group and works as an analyst in Italy and abroad, visiting supervisor in Tunisia, and liaison person for the Malta developing group. Research and training activities in the field of association experiment, analytical psychology, dreams, neuroscience, synchronicity. She has published. in Italian and international journals, has made contributions to collective books, and is editor of *Jung Today* (2009 Nova Science). In her interest in gender studies and women's mysticism she has published on the position of women in history, on the flowering of female mysticism in the first centuries of the first millennium, and the revolution this implied. The interest in synchronicity has been developed with attention to clinical practice and transference and countertransference. Since an early training in psychiatry she has maintained a vivid interest in the field and has recently contributed to the textbook *Manuale di Psichiatria e Psicologia Clinica* (2017).

Onno van der Hart, PhD, is a psychologist and adult psychotherapist in private practice (retired); he is Emeritus Professor of Psychopathology of Chronic Traumatization at the Department of Clinical and Health Psychology at Utrecht University, the Netherlands. He is a scholar in Pierre Janet studies. Both nationally and internationally, he frequently lectures on trauma-generated dissociation, dissociative disorders, phase-oriented treatment of chronic traumatization. He is a past President of the International Society for Traumatic Stress Studies, and is the recipient of a number of awards for his work. With Ellert Nijenhuis and Kathy Steele, he wrote *The Haunted Self: Structural Dissociation and the Treatment of Chronic*

Traumatization (2006). With Suzette Boon and Kathy Steele, he co-authored *Coping with Trauma-Related Dissociation: Skills Training for Patients and Therapists* (2011), and with Kathy Steele and Suzette Boon, *Treating Trauma-Related Dissociation: A Practical, Integrative Approach* (2017).

Bessel A. van der Kolk, MD, is a clinician, researcher, and teacher in the area of posttraumatic stress. His work integrates developmental, neurobiological, psychodynamic, and interpersonal aspects of the impact of trauma and its treatment. He and his various collaborators have published extensively on the impact of trauma on development, such as dissociative problems, borderline personality and self-mutilation, cognitive development, memory, and the psychobiology of trauma. He has published over 150 peer-reviewed scientific articles on such diverse topics as neuroimaging, self-injury, memory, neurofeedback, developmental trauma, yoga, theatre, and EMDR. He is founder and Medical Director of the Trauma Center in Brookline, Massachusetts, USA; past President of the International Society for Traumatic Stress Studies, and Professor of Psychiatry at Boston University Medical School. He is the author of the New York Times Science best seller, *The Body Keeps the Score: Brain, Mind, and Body in the Treatment of Trauma*.

INTRODUCTION

Giuseppe Craparo, Francesca Ortu, and Onno van der Hart

The 1970 debut of Henri Ellenberger's magnus opus, *The Discovery of the Unconscious: The History and Evolution of Modern Psychiatry*, with its beautiful and enlightening chapter on Pierre Janet, has inspired contemporary generations of clinicians to rediscover his ground-breaking studies. Janet's insights and therapeutic approaches remain extremely instructive and relevant to contemporary theory and practice, especially in the area of psychotraumatology. The current book, *Rediscovering Pierre Janet: Trauma, Dissociation, and a New Context for Psychoanalysis*, published almost half a century after Ellenberger's volume, is a testimony to how Janet's legacy can transform present-day understanding and clinical practice. The authors, students of Janet's works who come from different professional and geographical backgrounds, offer a rich variety of integrative perspectives on Janet's original studies that enrich our contemporary understanding of psychotraumatology and its treatment. This book is also an invitation to interested readers to follow up on the many still uncharted aspects of Janet's work that remain to be discovered and understood through a present-day lens.

Following two introductory chapters, this book consists of three parts: Janet's influence on psychoanalysis; Janet's influence on contemporary psychotraumatology; and Janet's influence on current psychotherapy, and ends with an Epilogue. In Chapter 1, "A reader's guide to Pierre Janet: A neglected intellectual heritage," Onno van der Hart and Barbara Friedman provide a summary of Janet's central concepts related to hysteria and neuroses (e.g. dissociation, fixed ideas, violent emotions, psychological misery, the reality function), as presented in his major works on the subject. In Chapter 2, "From consciousness to subconsciousness: A Janetian perspective," Francesca Ortu and Giuseppe Craparo emphasize Janet's conception of subconscious linked to his theory on dissociation. Unlike the Freudian concept of the unconscious, Janet hypothesizes a dissociative rather than a repressed subconscious that is caused by fixed ideas related to a division of the personality in response to traumatic experiences.

Part I, "Janet's influence on psychoanalysis," consists of three chapters. In Chapter 3, "Janet and Freud: Long-time rivals," Gabriele Cassullo analyzes the role of Janet's theory of mind for Freudian metapsychology. The relationship between these two giants of psychology cannot be reduced to a diatribe about plagiarism. According to Cassullo:

> It would be of great value to continue, in the future, the uncovering of Janet's legacy within the Freudian corpus. Due to the conflict between the two, looking for Janet's name in Freud's oeuvre would be of little use; one should look for the concepts instead: not a mechanical task. This inquiry should surely include Freud's gradual elaboration of the concept of *Verleugnung*, disavowal, which is strictly connected to the loss of the *fonction du réel* and culminates with *Splitting of the ego in the process of defence*.

In Chapter 4, "Janet and Jung: A stimulating relationship," Caterina Vezzoli maintains that "Jung developed his own psychology, which from its outset and throughout its development acknowledged the validity of the work of Janet and the French school." According to Vezzoli, Jungian theories on psychological dissociation, the self, psychological complexes, psychological types, individuation, dreams, and synchronicity were also influenced by Janet's works. From her point of view, along with other Jungian authors (for example, Sonu Shamdasani), Jung's theory of the mind is closer to Janet's rather than Freud's. In Chapter 5, "On not taking just one part of it: Janet's influence on object relations theory," Gabriele Cassullo describes Sándor Ferenczi's attempt to synthesize the theories of Janet and Freud. This integration gives birth to some psychoanalytic constructs related to both Fairbairn's developmental theory focused on dissociative mechanisms (Cassullo recalls that Fairbairn used the term *splitting* instead of *dissociation*), and Melanie Klein's theory of the "paranoid-schizoid position." According to Clara Mucci, Giuseppe Craparo, and Vittorio Lingiardi, in Chapter 6, "From Janet to Bromberg, via Ferenczi: Standing in the spaces of the literature on dissociation," recent psychoanalytic developments in the theory and the clinical practice of trauma indicate a movement towards a relational, intersubjective approach, in which real traumatic experiences and dissociation (in accordance with Janet's dissociation theory) have become prominent, as Bromberg's theoretical and clinical studies exemplify.

Part II, "Janet's influence on contemporary psychotraumatology," begins with Chapter 7, "Reflections on some contributions to contemporary psychotraumatology in the light of Janet's critique of Freud's theories," written by Giovanni and Marianna Liotti. They present a Janetian interpretation of the pathological response to a psychological trauma as a passive effect of vehement emotions on higher mental functions. In Chapters 8 and 9, "The holistic project of Pierre

Janet. Part one: Disintegration or *désagrégation*" and "Part two: Oscillations and becomings: From Disintegration to integration," Russell Meares and Cécile Barral emphasize the importance of distinguishing *désagrégation* (a psychologically abnormal condition causing a division of the personality) from *dissociation*. For Andrew Moskowitz, Gerhard Heim, Isabelle Saillot, and Vanessa Beavan, in Chapter 10, "Pierre Janet on hallucinations, paranoia, and schizophrenia," psychopathology is linked to a reduction of psychological force, "which would make the person more susceptible to certain psychological conditions." Therefore, hallucinations, paranoia, and schizophrenia are thought to be interrelated with an insufficient psychological force, which can lead to the expression of actions that are inappropriate to a given situation.

Part III, "Janet's influence on current psychotherapy," contains four chapters. In Chapter 11, "The hypnotherapeutic relationship with traumatized patients: Pierre Janet's contributions to current treatment," Kathy Steele and Onno van der Hart summarize Janet's clinical studies on the therapeutic relationship (*rapport*) with traumatized patients, highlighting his approaches to *somnambulistic influence* and *somnambulistic passion*. These studies inform clinicians on the important role of (auto)hypnosis in therapy. In Chapter 12, "Pierre Janet's treatment of posttraumatic stress," Onno van der Hart, Paul Brown, and Bessel A. van der Kolk show that Janet's phase-oriented treatment for patients with trauma-related disorders preceded modern approaches, and still has much value for current clinical practice. In Chapter 13, "Pierre Janet's views on the etiology, pathogenesis, and therapy of dissociative disorders," Gerhard Heim and Karl-Ernst Bühler present an in-depth study of these important clinical phenomena. They contrast the dissociative nature of hysteria with psychasthenia, the other major category of mental disorders that Janet distinguished. The latter is highly relevant for our clinical understanding and practice. Pat Ogden, in Chapter 14, "Acts of triumph: An interpretation of Pierre Janet and the role of the body in trauma treatment," shows that Janet, more than anyone else, emphasized the importance of completing well-performed actions with a sense of joy; in Janet's words, with an act of triumph. Sensorimotor Psychotherapy places a strong emphasis on this principle.

Finally, in the Epilogue, Ellert R. S. Nijenhuis personifies Pierre Janet with irony in his contribution, "Dissociation in the DSM-5: Your view, *s'il vous plaît, Docteur Janet?*". The result is a critique of the contradictory ways in which DSM-5 conceptualizes and defines "dissociation," "negative" and "positive dissociative symptoms," "dissociative disorders," as well as "conversion" and "conversion disorders." The discourse also includes a well-argued proposal to reconsider Janet's idea that there is a group of trauma-related disorders whose core feature is a more or less profound and elaborate dissociation of the personality. The closing chapter illustrates that studying Pierre Janet's texts does not concern a romantic flight into history. The effort rather is a journey towards conceptual clarity and clinical wisdom.

1

A READER'S GUIDE TO PIERRE JANET

A neglected intellectual heritage[1]

Onno van der Hart and Barbara Friedman

A century ago, Pierre Janet (1859–1947) became France's most important student of dissociation and hysteria. At that time, hysteria included a broad range of disorders now categorized in the *DSM-5* (American Psychiatric Association, 2013) as dissociative, somatization, conversion, borderline personality, and posttraumatic stress disorders. The ICD-10 (World Health Organization, 1992), moreover, correctly regards conversion disorders as dissociative disorders of movement and sensation. Through extensive study, observation, and experiments using hypnosis in the treatment of hysteria, Janet discovered that dissociation was the underlying characteristic process present in each of these disorders.

Unfortunately, his view of the importance of dissociation in hysteria and its treatment was abandoned when hypnosis fell into disrepute. This retreat from hypnosis at the end of the nineteenth century coincided with the publication and popularity of Freud's early psychoanalytic studies. Historically, Janet's considerable body of work was neglected in favour of the rising popularity and acceptance of Freud's psychoanalytic conceptualizations and theories.

Today, renewed clinical and scientific interest in dissociation and the dissociative disorders calls for reexamining the experimental, clinical, and theoretical observations made in psychiatry during the past century. While many psychoanalytically oriented clinicians restrict their historical interest to the study of Breuer and Freud (1895), others have searched for the original sources in French psychiatry, especially those of Janet. Their efforts have been hampered by the difficulty of obtaining the original publications in French, and by the scarcity of these works translated into English.

In the 1970s a change began to occur with regard to Janet. The Société Pierre Janet in France has been reprinting his books since 1973, and subsequently the French publisher L'Harmattan has reissued most of them. In 1973, Claude Prévost published an important book on Janet's psycho-philosophy (Prévost, 1973b).

Numerous articles in French followed. In the English-speaking world a small group of devotees has long recognized the value of Janet's contribution to psychopathology and psychology. With the reprint of Janet's *Major Symptoms of Hysteria* in 1965, the publication of Ellenberger's *The Discovery of the Unconscious* in 1970, and Hilgard's *Divided Consciousness* in 1977, the importance of Janet's contribution to the study of dissociation and related phenomena became better known to the English-speaking world (cf. Decker, 1986; Haule, 1986; Nemiah, 1979, 1980; Perry, 1984; Perry & Laurence, 1984). However, Janet's contributions to the field are not limited to hysteria and dissociation, but encompass a wide range of subjects, as indicated by Ellenberger (1970) and a handful of other English-language publications (cf. Horton, 1924; Bailey, 1928; Mayo, 1948; Havens, 1966; Ey, 1968; Hart, 1983; Haule, 1984b; Pitman, 1984, 1987; Pope, Hudson, & Mialet, 1985). In December 1989, John C. Nemiah, the editor of the *American Journal of Psychiatry*, dedicated his editorial to the centenary of Janet's most important book, *L'Automatisme Psychologique: Essai de Psychologie Experimentale sur les Formes Inférieures de L'Activité Humaine*. Under the title, "Janet redivivus: The centenary of *L'Automatisme Psychologique*," he wrote:

> The recent festivities celebrating the bicentennial of the French Revolution have overshadowed the remembrance of another occurrence in French history that, from a scientific point of view at least, is perhaps of equal magnitude – the publication in 1889 of Pierre Janet's *L'automatisme psychologique*.
> *(1989, p. 1527)*

Nemiah ended his homage as follows:

> [W]e have much to learn from what Janet has to teach us. He was first and foremost a psychologist, and his attention was focused on the experimental side of human life, with a particular concern with its vicissitudes in those suffering from mental illness. 'It is in no way wrong,' he wrote in the introductory chapter of *L'automatisme psychologique*, 'for psychology to probe the varied details of mental aberrations instead of remaining stuck in vague generalizations that are too abstract to be of any practical value. However one looks at it, experimental psychology must be a pathological psychology. ... The method that I have attempted to employ here, without in any to have been successful, is that of the natural sciences. Without bringing any preconceived notion to the problem, I have merely accumulated facts, and, whenever possible, have verified the consequences of these hypotheses by experimentation.'
> The advances in psychiatric knowledge during the 100 years since that was written have not improved on Janet's scientific method and vision.
> *(p. 1529)*

In the same year, a celebration of this centenary took place in Paris, organized by the Société Médico-Psychologique and the Société Pierre Janet. Furthermore, several international journal articles, including the current paper, highlighting Janet's work were published. Since then, interest in Janet's work has steadily grown.

The purpose of this chapter is to review Janet's books on hysteria and dissociation and to provide a summary of the central concepts in each of them. A brief description of Janet's career enables the reader to place these studies in their historical perspective. For a more complete biography, the reader is referred to Ellenberger's encyclopaedic opus, *The Discovery of the Unconscious* (1970).

Pierre Janet

Pierre Janet was born in Paris on 30 May 1859, to an upper-middle-class family. He maintained a distinguished academic standing in the finest French schools, dividing his interests between science and philosophy. At 22, when he embarked upon his professional career as professor of philosophy in Le Havre, two events had had a profound effect upon him. The first, in 1881, was the International Electrical Exposition in Paris, where it became clear that the future would be dominated by science, technology, and electricity. The second, in 1882, was the presentation at the Académie des Sciences and subsequent publication of Charcot's paper, "Sur les divers état nerveux déterminés par l'hypnotisation chez les hystériques" ["On the various nervous states determined by the hypnotization of hysterics"] (Charcot, 1882), which reestablished the scientific status of hypnosis (Ellenberger, 1970, p. 335).

At Le Havre Janet devoted his spare time to voluntary work with patients at the hospital and to psychiatric research. In search of a subject for his doctoral dissertation, he was introduced to Léonie, a 45-year old woman who he proved could be hypnotized directly and from a distance. His experiments were reported in a paper read at the Société de Psychologie Physiologique in Paris in 1885, under the chairmanship of Charcot. Although these experiments (Janet, 1885, 1886a) gave Janet instant fame, he soon realized that many reports of his work were inaccurate. He became suspicious of parapsychological research, preferring instead to pursue systematic investigation of the phenomena of hysteria, hypnosis, and suggestion. Influenced by the work of Ribot and Charcot, Janet dedicated himself to the study of modification of states of consciousness in Léonie and hysterical patients in Le Havre's psychiatric hospital (Janet, 1886b, 1887, 1888). He jokingly named his little ward "*Salle Saint-Charcot*" in the popular fashion of naming French hospitals wards after saints (Ellenberger, 1970). Janet read everything he could on hypnosis, finding a wealth of important clinical descriptions in Alexandre Jacques François Bertrand, Joseph Philippe François Deleuze, and Antoine Despine, the old masters of magnetism. He discovered that important theoretical notions had been developed by early researchers such as Main de Biran, Moreau de Tours, and Taine.

Janet found that the concept of dissociation is a concept first presented in the work of Moreau de Tours in 1845. Its somehow equivalent term, psychological dissolution (*désagrégation psychologique*), also introduced by Moreau de Tours in 1845, was equally well received. Janet's extraordinarily exact and lucid descriptions of experimental and clinical observations (cf. Binet, 1890) of these concepts and his theoretical system continue to receive praise in modern reviews of his works (cf. Pope, Hudson, & Mialet, 1985; Pitman, 1987; Van der Kolk & van der Hart, 1989).

In 1889, Charcot invited Janet to the Salpêtrière, the famous psychiatric teaching hospital in Paris, where he became head of a psychological laboratory. While continuing his vocation as professor of philosophy and publishing a textbook in that field (Janet, 1894a), Janet began to study medicine, completing his studies in 1893 with his doctoral thesis (Janet, 1893a). During this period, he published a number of papers describing his innovative therapeutic approaches to hysteria. As Ellenberger (1970, pp. 764–765) remarked, had Janet published the case histories of Lucie, Marie, Marcelle, Madame D., and the others he had successfully treated at that time, no one would ever have questioned his priority in discovering what was later called cathartic therapy. However, van der Hart and Van der Velden (1987) showed that the Dutch physician Andries Hoek (1868) provided the first case study of cathartic hypnotherapy.

Janet's clinical research at the Salpêtrière became the basis of his dissociation theory of hysteria. These findings formed the thesis for his medical degree and were applauded both within France and internationally. Janet seemed to have a brilliant career ahead when, three weeks after his promotion to Doctor of Medicine in 1893, Charcot suddenly died and a new era in psychiatry began. Many of Charcot's ideas about the presumably physical nature of hypnosis were discarded in favour of the views of the Nancy School of Hypnosis (under Hippolyte Bernheim); namely, that hypnosis was a psychological phenomenon based purely on suggestion. Precisely because of its established psychological nature, hypnosis itself became discredited.

Janet was soon the only one in the Salpêtrière using hypnosis in his research and clinical work. He published many studies on hysteria (cf. Janet, 1898a & b; Raymond & Janet, 1898), then turned his attention to another broad category of neuroses: psychasthenia, with its inherent obsessions, phobias, tics, etc. This resulted in the two volumes on *Obsessions and Psychasthenia* (*Les Obsessions et la Psychasthénie*) published in 1903 (cf. Pitman, 1984, 1987).

Meanwhile, the climate at the Salpêtrière worsened for Janet. Babinski, formerly loyal to Charcot, but invested exclusively in the neurological portion of Charcot's teaching, began to regard hysteria as essentially the result of suggestion, and even as a form of malingering, a disorder able to disappear entirely by the influence of persuasion (Babinski, 1901, 1909). Déjerine regarded hypnosis as morally reprehensible (cf. Janet, 1919; Ellenberger, 1970). In 1910, when Déjerine became director of the Salpêtrière, Janet, the champion of both hysteria and hypnosis, had to leave. Janet was very well received in North and South America where he visited and lectured regularly, beginning in 1904. He received an honorary doctorate at Harvard's tricentenary celebration in 1936. His Harvard lectures in 1906 were published as *The Major Symptoms of Hysteria* (1907b) and are currently garnering much attention.

A decade earlier, in 1896, Janet had become Professor of Psychology at the Collège de France, a famous institute of advanced learning in Paris. First as Ribot's substitute, then as his successor, Janet held this chair until 1934. Many of his courses have been published, complete or in summary (cf. Janet, 1919, 1920, 1926b, 1927a, 1929a, 1929b, 1932a, 1932b, 1925, 1936a; Horton, 1924; Bailey, 1928). Obliged to present a new subject every year, Janet used his classes as a means of combining his psychopathological findings and normal psychology into a unified system. This endeavour began appearing in *L'Automatisme Psychologique* (*Psychological Automatism*), where he remarked that for those who know mental illness well, it is not difficult to study normal psychology (1889).

Janet possessed a remarkable talent for integrating very different materials into a harmonious whole (Delay, 1960). One of these results was the formulation of his psychology of conduct (*psychologie de la conduite*), a major effort to synthesize a multitude of behavioural observations with an evolutionary philosophical approach. In his book, *Les Stades de l'Évolution Psychologique*, he presented a hierarchically ordered classification of human activity from simplest to most complex (1926b). Although Janet's dissociation theory has been rediscovered, there is still little awareness of what treasures are hidden in his later work on the psychology of conduct and in his psychopathological studies, such as those on paranoid schizophrenia (1932c, 1932d, 1932e, 1936a, 1937, 1945, 1947a). Janet's last unfinished work concerning the psychology of religious belief remains unpublished (Janet, 1947b). It is estimated that the published work of this great man, who according to his daughter, did not know the act of rest (Pichot-Janet, 1950), amounted to at least 17,000 printed pages (Prévost, 1973b, p. 10).

Since Janet's primary purpose was to inspire his pupils' independent thinking on the basis of empirical facts, he did not leave a school or ideological movement behind. Instead, time and again, open-minded researchers and clinicians discover that Janet made the same observations as they, and that his theoretical explanations of this information remain viable sources of inspiration. This discovery extends well beyond the field of dissociation.

The following is a chronological review of books that Janet published over a 30-year period. It begins with *L'Automatisme Psychologique* (1889), which first appeared approximately 130 years ago and ends with *Les Médications Psychologiques* (1919). (However, Janet subsequently published a number of other books, a discussion of which is outside the scope of this chapter.) In reading his books, it becomes apparent that one series of works shows Janet's remarkable abilities of classification (abilities that are also reflected in his being an ardent botanist). In these studies, he mapped the various manifestations of hysteria, which then became the foundation of his hypotheses about their origins, nature, and relationship. These hypotheses and observations form Janet's dissociation theory. In another series of studies, the emphasis is on the psychological analysis of one or a few case descriptions in depth. The last book reviewed reflects Janet's attempt to delineate the various forms of psychotherapy he encountered in the literature and the dynamic psychotherapy that he himself practiced as an eclectic psychotherapist.

L'Automatisme Psychologique

Psychological Automatism, Janet's first book in psychology, existed only in French until recently. In 2013 the first translation, in Italian, was published. It introduces his dissociation theory and his model of the functional and structural elements of the mind. It describes psychological phenomena observed in hysteria, hypnosis, suggestion, possession states, and spiritism, though it clearly goes beyond those topics (Janet, 1889). As the book's subtitle, *Experimental-Psychological Essay on the Inferior Forms of Human Activity*, suggests, Janet began with the study of human activity in its simplest and most rudimentary forms. His goal was to demonstrate that this elementary activity forms the psychological automatism: automatic because it is regular and predetermined, and psychological because it is accompanied by sensibility and consciousness (cf. van der Hart & Horst, 1989).

In presenting his model of the mind, Janet distinguished between two different ways that mind functions: activities that preserve and reproduce the past and activities that are directed towards synthesis and creation (i.e. integration). Normal thought is produced by a combination of the two acts that are interdependent and regulate each other. Integrative activity

> reunites more or less numerous given phenomena into a new phenomenon different from its elements. At every moment of life, this activity effectuates new combinations which are necessary to maintain the organism in equilibrium with the changes of the surroundings.
>
> *(Janet, 1889, p. 483)*

In short, this function organizes the present. Reproductive, that is, automatic activities only manifest integrations that were created in the past.

Janet felt psychological automatism was best studied in individuals who exhibit it in extreme degrees, that is, psychiatric patients suffering from hysteria. In them, the integrative activity is significantly diminished, causing the development of symptoms that appear as magnifications of the activity designed to preserve and reproduce the past. Janet discovered that most of them suffered from unresolved (therefore, dissociated) traumatic memories. In this population he studied catalepsy, paralysis, anesthesia, contractures, monoideic and polyideic somnambulisms, and successive existences or multiple personalities. His analysis represented a departure from classical psychology, which made a sharp distinction among intellect, affect, and will. Janet concluded that even at the very lowest level of psychic life, where feeling or sensation exists, movement also exists. Thus, there is no consciousness without activity; even an idea has the natural tendency to develop into an act.

In his structural view of the mind, Janet aligned with earlier French authors such as Maine de Brian, Moreau de Tours, Ribot, and Taine, believing that all human activity had a conscious component. He put this on a par with the inner regulating activities of the mind, the proprioceptive functions as Sherrington (1906) called them. His predecessors and contemporaries generally believed that psychological automatism consisted of acts performed unconsciously and, therefore, mechanically (cf. Despine, 1880). Janet believed that the behaviour patterns he observed were determined by conscious factors, even though they were maladaptive departures from the habitual response patterns of the personality. Using the term "automatic" did not exclude the notion of self-awareness, as the Greek terms *autos* (self) and *maiomai* (striving for, to exert oneself for) are paired in this concept (van der Hart & Horst, 1989). Janet stated that in psychological automatism, consciousness did not belong to the personal consciousness, was not connected to the personal perception, and lacked the personality's sense of self (*idée du moi*). This consciousness existed rather at a subconscious level. As Ellenberger points out, few people realize that it was Janet who first coined the term subconscious (1970, p. 406; cf. Chapter 2). Janet thus differentiated among levels of consciousness. Since the study of elementary forms of activity was a study of basic forms of sensibility and consciousness, he therewith emphasized the unity of body and mind.

Psychological automatism could be manifested in total as well as in partial automatism. The former implies that the mind is completely dominated by a reproduction of past experience, as in the case of somnambulistic states and hysterical crises. The latter occurs when the automatism occupies only a part of the mind – for instance, in cases of systematic anesthesia, where the touch of an object is not registered by the personal consciousness, but is to be found in a second consciousness, a hidden observer, as Hilgard (1977) would say almost a century later.

In both total and partial automatism there exist subconscious psychological phenomena: systems of fixed ideas and functions that have escaped personal control and perception. These dissociated systems are isolated from the personal consciousness. Some of them continue to exist in rudimentary form with a very rudimentary sense of self, as is the case with catalepsy, in which only a single thought and single automatic action appears to occupy the mind. Less primitive is the hysterical crisis, a dissociative episode, complete with amnesia, in which the patient may reenact a traumatizing event. Janet presented this in the case of Marie, reported *in toto* by Ellenberger (1970, pp. 361–364). She suffered from crises in which she continuously reexperienced the trauma of her first menstruation as well as permanent blindness in one eye from an earlier childhood trauma. Janet's treatment demonstrated how correcting Marie's cognitive distortions from the menstrual event at age 13 and modifying the content of the dissociated states in which her trauma at age 6 was reexperienced led to the disappearance of these states and their related symptoms.

Many dissociated elements and systems tend to combine themselves with other such phenomena to form more complex existences. Certain dreams, certain fixed ideas, more or less subconscious, become centres around which a large number of psychological phenomena arrange themselves to become a distinct existence or personality, complete with its own sense of self and life history. These successive existences, or alternating personalities, may interact with external reality, and develop further by absorbing and retaining new impressions. Although he was not so clear in this respect, Janet's examples showed that these existences could also develop higher psychological functions, such as autonomous will and critical judgment.

Binet (1890) pointed out this particular vagueness in Janet's work, which, in our opinion, was related to a paradox Janet encountered. He had intended to study ways in which human activity in its simplest form manifested in hysterics. He found, however, that certain of these dissociated elementary forms of activity were highly developed, including the ability to reason, to make judgments, sustain memories, etc. Contrary to what he expected, integrative and creative activities were present at the level of personality (complete with sense of self), but remained outside of personal awareness in the normal waking state. It was this incongruity, that while studying the most simple he discovered the most complex, that gave the initial presentation of findings in this work its aura of apparent confusion.

Thus, Janet's observations led from the hypothesis of the absence of the function of creative synthesis in the personality to the recognition of the presence of this function in an existence that was dissociated from conscious awareness. Because this very function (often used to connote personality) was unavailable in the waking state but accessible in the hypnotic state, Janet was led first to the discovery of the dissociated existence and then to the necessity of formulating a theory of dissociation.

Janet related the origin of subconscious phenomena in hysterical patients to the narrowing of their field of consciousness. This concept refers to the reduction of the number of psychological phenomena that can be simultaneously united or integrated in one and the same personal consciousness. Some phenomena register in conscious awareness, others are relegated to a subconscious area in much the same way that central and peripheral items in a visual field are noticed. In Janet's view, narrowing the field of consciousness is one of the two basic characteristics of hysteria. The other is dissociation.

Dissociation and mental dissolution (*désagrégation*), terms originally introduced by Moreau de Tours (1845), denote the manner in which this narrowing of the field of consciousness occurs in hysterical patients. Dissociation can be regarded as the form in which this dissolution manifests itself. However, throughout his works, Janet has also used both terms interchangeably. Dissociation occurs when different factors disturb the integrative capacity. This disturbance leads to the division or doubling (*dédoublement*), separation, and isolation of certain psychological regulating activities. These dissociated systems of activities vary in complexity from a simple image, thought, or statement and its attendant feelings or bodily manifestations to the "personality states" of patients with dissociative identity disorder (DID; APA, 2013). These personality states have their own identities, life histories, and enduring patterns of perceiving, thinking about, and relating to the environment (van der Hart & Horst, 1989) – in short, their own first-person perspective (Nijenhuis & van der Hart, 2011).

The dissociative activity clusters or existences either alternate with the personal consciousness in controlling the body or coexist with it. Indeed, in later work, Janet (1909a, 1910b) stated that in certain patients a dissociative personality, which could be evoked in hypnosis, was in fact a healthier state of consciousness than the so-called waking state.

While clinicians such as Bernheim and Babinski regarded hyper-suggestibility as the basic characteristic of hysterical patients, Janet stated that hyper-suggestibility depended on the narrowing of the field of consciousness and the predisposition to dissociation. The patient is suggestible because dissociative parts of his mind lack the higher mental functions of critical judgment. By distracting the patient, the hypnotist is able to communicate directly with these parts. Ironically, Janet also encountered dissociative existences that were not at all suggestible, but showed strong will and judgement of their own.

Janet introduced the concept of psychological misery to denote the mental status of patients in whom the field of consciousness was narrowed and whose integrative powers were strongly diminished, thus allowing dissociative phenomena to occur. In later writings, he placed this mental misery in the broader framework of the oscillations of the mental level that take place in all human beings (1905, 1919, 1920, 1921, 1925, 1934; cf. Sjövall, 1967).

Physical illness, exhaustion, and vehement emotion such as extreme fear and anger inherent in traumatic experiences are primary causes of psychological misery. This state is marked by a serious decline of the integrative power of the mind and, in hysterical patients, an increase in dissociative phenomena. In *L'Automatisme Psychologique* (1889) as well as in an earlier paper (1886a), Janet showed that such intense emotional experiences may become dissociated (complete with amnesia) and then reappear in hysterical crises. They may become subconscious centres around which other psychological phenomena arrange themselves, as in the cases of Marie and Lucie.

A short summary cannot do justice to the wealth of psychological observations and ideas contained in *L'Automatisme Psychologique*. There are many findings in this book that could stimulate future research. One intriguing example concerns the variations in sensory perception in different somnambulistic states. Janet noted that a patient may be predominantly visual in the waking state, auditory in one somnambulistic state, kinaesthetic in another, and even have a state of "perfect somnambulism" in which the balanced integration of all senses exists. It is unfortunate indeed that this book has never been translated. One hundred and twenty years after its original publication in French, and following the Italian edition, an English version would be timelier than ever.

L'État Mental des Hystériques

This book originally consisted of two parts published separately under the same title (*L'État Mental des Hystériques*) with different subtitles. The first part was subtitled *Les Stigmates Mentaux* (*The Mental Stigmata*) (1893a). The second, subtitled *Les Accidents Mentaux* (*The Mental Accidents*) (1894b), was the commercial edition of his medical dissertation, *Contribution à l'Étude des Accidents Mentaux chez les Hystériques* (Janet, 1893b). Both works, translated into English in 1901, are careful descriptive studies based on clinical observations of 120 of Janet's own patients and 20 of his colleagues', one of whom was Despine's patient Estelle (Despine, 1840). Recently Fine and colleagues reported on this case (Fine, 1988; McKeown & Fine, 2008).

On the subject of his own observations, Janet remarked that he was in the habit of writing down everything his subjects and patients said and did, a habit that earned him the nickname Doctor Pencil (1930a). To his analyses of these systematized observations, Janet added his tentative theoretical interpretations, which can be reduced to the same elements as his dissociation theory. These interpretations were experimentally tested in a small number of patients.

Mental stigmata and mental accidents were the terms given to the symptoms of hysteria. In distinguishing between them, Janet employed a well-established classification system that had its roots in the medical tradition of his time. The "stigmata" of hysteria are the essential constitutive symptoms of the illness, as enduring, persistent, and permanent as the illness itself. The patient who may feel himself weakened in some way, but who is unable to specify correctly the symptoms from which he suffers, presents with a relative indifference to his symptomatology. Janet suggests that clinicians should take the initiative in identifying these chronic stigmata, since patients do not usually report them. "Accidents" are the acute transient, paroxystic symptoms that occur intermittently and are experienced by the patients as painful. These accidents can be understood as representations of psychological trauma (cf. Meares, Hamshire, Gordon, & Kraiuhin, 1985). Thus, hysterical anesthesia is a stigma, and an attack (acute episode) of hysteria is an accident. In later work, Janet detached himself from this medically based position, and the concept of personality became dominant in his explanatory view (Janet, 1929a): "The personality is a human construct, generated by human beings with whatever means they have at their disposal … the personality is a work of art build by people, for better or worse, incomplete and imperfect" (pp. 502–503).

In Part One of *L'État Mental des Hystériques*, *The Mental Stigmata*, Janet dealt with anaesthesias, amnesias, abulias, negative symptoms of disorders of movements, and modifications of the character, all of which he regarded as mental stigmata. For each of these negative symptoms (stigmata) he carefully described its different forms and manifestations. With regard to the anaesthesias, he denoted systematic, localized, and general. He regarded hysterical anaesthesia as a strong and continuous distraction rendering the patients unable to attach certain sensations to their personalities because of the narrowing of the field of consciousness. These sensations thus existed in a subconscious manner. The same kind of analysis was made with regard to the amnesias. Using many examples, Janet showed that hysterical amnesia often developed in the wake of vehement emotions aroused and dissociated during traumatic experiences.

Abulia, a concept that receives little attention in current psychiatry and psychology, concerns a degeneration of the will that manifests in tendencies towards indolence, hesitancy, indecision, impotence to act, and inability to focus attention on ideas. Abulia is not limited to hysteria, but in this category of disorders it characteristically presents in the preservation of subconscious acts and the loss of personal perception of acts in current reality. As an essential component of many disorders, this stigma increases in dominance as the patient's state of mind deteriorates. There is a noticeable increase in the tendency to daydream, in apathy or anhedonia, in the patient's proneness to emotional outbursts. This exhaustion of one's vitality and intensification of abulia that Janet observed in his hysterical patients is commonly seen by clinicians today, especially those treating chronic posttraumatic stress disorder (PTSD) (cf. van der Hart, Nijenhuis, & Steele, 2006; Van der Kolk, Brown, & van der Hart, 1989). Titchener (1986) speaks of a posttraumatic decline, of which apathy, a tendency to withdraw from normal interaction with the environment, and a hypochondriacal preoccupation with one's own body are characteristic.

As Janet described the manner in which hysteria modified the character of his patients, we recognize additional observations currently made under the rubric of posttraumatic decline: recurrent dreaming of the traumatizing event, including day-dreaming; constricted affect or alexithymia; and simultaneously, extreme excitability with a tendency to emotional outbursts. It is important that we not limit abulia to being a specific stigma of hysteria. This pattern of (1) weakening of a patient's personal will, decisiveness, and ability to initiate activity; (2) an increase in day-dreaming and apathy; and (3) exaggerated emotional responses underlies a number of currently identified disorders.

Janet concluded Part One with the statement that hysteria is a defect of the unity of the mind, manifesting itself, on the one hand, in a diminishing of the personal synthesis, and on the other, in the preserving of past phenomena, which reappear in an amplified manner.

In Part Two, Janet first tried to unite the infinitely varied spectrum of hysterical accidents by referring to their shared mental aspects: suggestion, subconscious acts, and fixed ideas. He considered that the complete and automatic development of ideas occurred outside of the will and personal perception of the subject: "Suggestions, with their automatic and independent development, are the real parasites of the mind" (1901, p. 267). The performance of acts that result from suggestions is isolated, separated from the personality: that is why they should be called subconscious acts.

Patients suffering from hysteria in a Janetian sense are, as a rule, highly suggestible. Research with patients suffering from dissociative disorders and posttraumatic stress disorder confirms this (Bliss, 1986; Spiegel, Hunt, & Dondershine, 1988). Janet analyzed conditions in which patients are less suggestible. Two of the main conditions of lowered suggestibility were found in subjects who were preoccupied with a certain fixed idea of their own, and being cured. A cure implied a strongly diminished tendency towards dissociating and an increasingly integrated personality. Since no complexly developed dissociative parts (selves) exist in an integrated personality, by definition, there are none to evoke. Artificial somnambulism, in the restricted sense of deep hypnosis, can barely be evoked, whereas a lighter trance state in which continuity of the sense of self is maintained continues to be possible. Although Janet did encounter some exceptions to his rule, he did not give up his position (which is not universally accepted today). Thus, near the end of the treatment, one of his patients, Marcelle, while under hypnosis reported via automatic writing that she was cured forever. As she still showed the dissociative phenomena of deep hypnosis and automatic writing, Janet was pessimistic about her prognosis (1891, 1898a).

While suggestions are generally given by others, fixed ideas usually develop as the result of accidental causes, such as traumatic experiences and hysterical episodes. They tend to dominate the mind completely in dreams and somnambulistic states. They also disturb normal consciousness during the waking state by intruding into it. For example, Janet wrote of a woman walking on the street. She had short dissociative episodes in which she made a curious jumping motion. In hypnosis Janet discovered that she was reenacting her suicide attempt: a jump into the Seine. In an example of a contraction, a sailor continuously walked in a forward bent position, reenacting the trauma of having had a beam fall and press against his chest. Many case examples were cited to show how mental accidents such as dysaesthesias, hyperaesthesias, tics and choric movements, paralyses and contractures are based on fixed ideas. In most cases, patients are amnestic to these fixed ideas, which also affect the stigmata (basic symptomatology) by diminishing the patients' powers of personal perception.

Hysterical attacks are violent, momentary, and periodically recurring events during which the patient's normal consciousness usually disappears. Janet categorized several types of emotional attacks: attacks of tics and clownism, attacks of fixed ideas and ecstasies, and complete attacks. During attacks the underlying fixed ideas are usually transformed into vivid hallucinations and bodily movements. Janet regarded anorexia nervosa in most cases as hysterical in nature. An example of the attack of a fixed idea would be the inner commands an anorexic hears when trying to eat – "Don't eat. You do not have the need to eat."

Janet described the various forms of somnambulism as abnormal states of consciousness, distinct from normal life, which often have their own memories, and for which the subject develops amnesia upon returning to his normal state. This amnesia is due to the fact that the organization of psychological phenomena of the somnambulistic state is united around certain sensations or fixed ideas that are not perceived by the habitual personality. When the patient is cured, these states disappear, that is, they have fused into one state, as Janet quoted from Despine (1840).

Finally, he distinguished the hysterical psychosis that is due to the dominance of abulia (decrease in the level of mental functioning) and an increase in mental confusion. Patients with this disorder tend to confound their waking dreams with normal perceptions and with memories, both normal and traumatic. Their hallucinations are particularly vivid and often involve all the senses (cf. van der Hart, Witztum, & Friedman, 1993).

Janet concluded his psychological analysis of hysteria with the tentative definition that it is a form of mental dissolution characterized by the tendency to a permanent and complete dissociation (*dédoublement*) of the personality.

Although the distinction between mental stigmata and mental accidents is not always clear, it is still the best work to date for instructing clinicians in recognizing the many manifestations of those symptoms that are best explained by Janet's own dissociation theory. It is also an excellent source of reference, demonstrating how much was known about dissociation in the psychiatric world over a century ago. The English edition was reprinted in 1977.

Névroses et Idées Fixes

During and after his preparation of *The Mental State of Hystericals*, Janet published numerous articles in which he presented more detailed descriptions, narratives, and analyses of patients. These papers were collected in the first volume of *Neuroses and Fixed Ideas* (*Névroses et Idées Fixes: Études Expérimentales sur les Troubles de la Volonté, de l'Attention, de la Mémoire; sur les Émotions, les Idées Obsédantes et leur Traitement*) (1898a). Ellenberger (1970) mentions several of these extremely interesting cases in detail.

Fixed ideas (*idées fixes*) are thoughts or mental images that take on exaggerated proportions, have a high emotional charge, and, in patients suffering from hysteria, become isolated from the habitual personality, or personal consciousness (Janet, 1894a, 1898a). When dominating consciousness, they serve as the basis for behaviour. These ideas also manifest themselves in what we now term flashbacks or intrusive thoughts. Janet considered them dissociative phenomena that were parts of subconscious fixed ideas.

Fixed ideas can remain isolated or become linked with new impressions or other fixed ideas. They are perceived during dreams, dissociative episodes such as hysterical attacks, and in many of the communicating devices employed during hypnosis (which is the medium of choice for uncovering and exploring fixed ideas).

Janet made an important distinction between primary and secondary fixed ideas. A primary fixed idea is the total system or complex of images (visual, auditory, kinaesthetic, etc.) of a particular traumatizing event plus the corresponding emotions and behaviours – and, we would like to add, its own sense of self. Secondary fixed ideas have the same characteristics as primary fixed ideas and present after the disappearance (through treatment) of the main fixed idea. Janet classified them into three groups: (1) Derivative fixed ideas result from association with the main fixed idea. For example, if death is the primary fixed idea, a morbid fear of cemeteries or funeral flowers could result. (2) Stratified fixed ideas result from traumata in the patient's life history that were sustained prior to the one that caused the full-blown hysterical or dissociative disorder. We experience this in treatment when the removal of a primary fixed idea is replaced by another fixed idea rather than by the complete elimination of the patient's problem. Stratified fixed ideas correspond to the present-day notion of layers of traumata. Janet advocated a procedure of treating each principal fixed idea until all are addressed, usually beginning with the most recent and proceeding to the earliest. (3) Accidental fixed ideas are absolutely new and produced by an incident in one's present daily life. If treated immediately, they are easy to eradicate. Their existence proves the nature of the patient's mental state of hypersensitivity. Today we would call an accidental fixed idea the conditioned or stress-activated response to a trigger. We recognize this in patients' overreactions or distorted responses to seemingly neutral stimuli in the current environment. In dissociative disorders, accidental fixed ideas would produce a variety of dissociative responses, depending on the nature of the dissociative disorder. In dissociative identity disorder it is often seen as the switch to another dissociative part of the personality (Friedman, 1988).

In treatment, if one discovers the primary fixed idea, one can treat the core of the traumatic problem. This may not, however, resolve the secondary set of problems and symptomatology that require their own treatment. Secondary fixed ideas can produce behaviours in response to previous traumata or in response to the primary fixed idea. If these behaviours alone are eliminated or corrected in treatment, the heart of the problem still exists. Obviously, both need to be considered in conscientious treatment to avoid relapse or partial cure.

The case of Justine provides a rich example of treatment on both levels (1894b). Janet dedicated a 55-page report to Justine, a 40-year-old outpatient at the Salpêtrière. Following a serious contagious disease at age six and a subsequent bout of typhoid fever, she exhibited severe dissociative phenomena, changing from a sweet and gentle girl to an obstinate brat. She became phobic about snails and worms. To cure her of this at age nine, the family physician placed a large snail on her throat. Justine fell over backwards, losing consciousness and breaking several bones. Upon regaining consciousness, she was obsessed by the memory of the snail on her throat.

When her cat was badly injured and put to sleep, Justine reacted with an hysterical attack accompanied by a rash. More seizures and rashes occurred over time; in addition, Justine grew extremely fat. Her mother was a nurse who had to watch dying patients, and Justine sometimes helped her. After this she developed a morbid fear of disease and death. Finally, at age 17, Justine saw the naked corpses of 2 patients who had died of cholera, resulting in her violent fear of cholera. More than ten years later, this image would haunt her during hysterical attacks. Several times a day she would become pale and sweat and shout repeatedly, "Cholera … it's taking me!" She had an ever-present, severe phobia for the word cholera.

In this case Janet observed the fixed ideas in detail, finding that there were primary and secondary fixed ideas. One of his techniques was to evoke and modify the image of this primary fixed idea during hypnosis. In treatment, Janet induced artificial somnambulism and discovered what occupied Justine's mind during an hysterical crisis. She saw the image of the two naked corpses, smelled the revolting stench of decay, heard the tolling of a bell and the cries of those with cholera, and perceived screaming, vomiting, diarrhoea, and cramps of the victims. This traumatizing event involved all her sensory perceptions, forming one fixed idea, one psychological system that completely dominated her consciousness when it arose, leaving no room for other thoughts or actions. Janet found the only way to reach Justine was to enter her private drama as a participant. As she relived the scene in hypnosis, Janet applied his substitution technique, dialoguing with her within this context to modify the contents (cf. Chapters 11, 12, and 13). Over a period of time he was able to suggest gradual transformations of the images: the corpses were provided with clothes, and one was given the identity of a Chinese general whom Justine had seen at a Universal Exposition. When she could see the general stand up and march comically, the images of the traumatizing event ceased in hysterical attacks and persisted only in dreams. Janet addressed this by suggesting innocuous dreams. The trauma no longer occurred in dreams. This success resulted after one year of treatment.

In spite of the transformation of the proprioceptive primary fixed idea, Justine remained phobic to the word cholera. This fixed idea persisted on both the conscious and subconscious levels. While engaging in another activity, Justine could be observed whispering the word cholera. Janet directed his attention to the word itself, suggesting that it was the family name of the Chinese general, and dividing it into three parts: Cho–le–ra. He then had Justine associate the first syllable with different endings in automatic writing, such as chocolate. Next, he used the sound of the first syllable, co- and paired it with different endings: comme, colon, cororiko, etc., until it was no longer associated with the word cholera. In the end, Justine could no longer remember the word that had tortured her, nor did a new cholera epidemic have any effect on her. This phase of treatment lasted ten months.

Janet was planning to rid Justine of her other hallucinations when they disappeared spontaneously. And still the patient was not cured. After the disappearance of the primary fixed idea, secondary fixed ideas began to develop. Instead of the fear of death and disease, Justine exhibited a morbid fear of coffins and cemeteries: derivative fixed ideas. She refused to eat fruit or vegetables: a derivative fixed idea in response to fears of cholera. She also suffered from a multitude of accidental fixed ideas. We can assume that Janet treated them immediately by disconnecting the stimulus (trigger) from Justine's automatic association of it to a trauma. His general approach of educating her mind, and stimulating her integrative capacities, helped Justine to stop the development of these accidental fixed ideas herself.

Janet focused in Justine's case almost exclusively on her traumatic memories regarding the cholera deaths, and on related secondary fixed ideas. He believed that stratified fixed ideas did not play an important role in this case. However, he knew that Justine had suffered, as a child, several frights and emotional shocks (traumatic experiences) without reporting their contents. Today, we would probably pay more attention to the exploration of childhood traumata. For example, we would want to discover if Justine's childhood phobias of worms and snails were related to experiences of sexual abuse.

A final contribution introduced in this work is the phenomenon of the patient's deep involvement with the therapist, known as *rapport magnétique* by the magnetizers (1897; cf. Chapter 11). Janet recognized this intense involvement as a very complex phenomenon. Although erotic elements were present in the rapport, they were not the main therapeutic concern. He viewed the relationship more in terms of an attachment theory in which the need for guidance played the significant role. In treatment, the therapist first assumes the responsibility of directing the patient's mind, then gradually reduces that direction to a minimum. This treatment approach corresponds to modern procedures in which the therapist takes the initiative in building up patients' ego strengths and resources and guides their decision-making processes. As patients acquire the missing skills and employ them in a functional manner, the therapist gradually disengages from the process. Janet believed that therapists should educate their patients to accept their authority and guidance and then systematically reduce their domination of the patients, ultimately teaching patients to do without the therapist. If therapists neglected this point, only temporary cures resulted.

This process could be complicated by *la passion somnambulique*, the patient's overpowering need to be hypnotized by his or her own therapist. This passion can become an addiction and be just as dangerous (cf. Haule, 1986, Chapter 11). Janet concluded that high suggestibility is the mark of a great weakness of mind, which can lead patients to become cathected to both the therapist and the hypnotic state. "Such patients not only crave to be hypnotized, but have a permanent need to confess to the psychiatrist whose picture they keep constantly in their subconscious mind, and to be scolded and directed by him" (Ellenberger, 1970, p. 369). Janet realized that this craving to be hypnotized and guided by the therapist created a problem. At the same time, he deemed the somnambulistic influence indispensable to the cure. In this dilemma, Janet recognized the value of the initial bonding with the therapist, and how the boundary issues in the therapeutic alliance can be confused by the patient's desire for a symbiotic relationship.

Janet's solution was to maintain a delicate balance in both areas. Therapists should utilize the high hypnotizability of the patient without permitting the somnambulistic passion to develop to a dangerous point that makes treatment impractical. In the same way that therapists gradually withdraw from the guidance process and turn it over to the patient, they can use the hypnotic state as a treatment technique without allowing themselves or the altered state itself to become the dominant focus of the patient's attention. Today we know that there is often a point in treatment when it is appropriate to explain this addiction to dissociation to patients with dissociative disorders. We can then teach patients to recognize the onset of the desire to dissociate and teach them the coping skills that would reduce the need to dissociate, or to substitute another activity for the trance state.

Janet discussed this in the case of Justine (1894c). As her treatment progressed, Janet spaced her sessions from several times a week at the beginning to once a month in the third year. By then Justine had frequent visions of Janet in which she heard his voice offering her good advice. This counsel was not a repetition of what Janet had said in sessions, but originated from Justine and was of a novel and wise nature. Although it developed as a result of her association with Janet, it appeared more in the form of introjection than a dependency state.

Janet was quick to point out that reduction of sessions alone did not cure the dependency factor nor the somnambulistic addiction. He told the story of Morel's inpatient who was cured and discharged from the mental hospital. Afterwards, she came to see him at infrequent but regular intervals. When Morel died, she had a relapse and had to be committed permanently. "Let us hope that this accident will not happen too soon to our patients," Janet concluded (Janet, 1894c, 1898a, p. 212).

This book, with its wealth of relevant material, has not been translated into English, nor has the French edition been reprinted before 1989, when this article was first published. Fortunately, a reprint was published in 2007.

The second volume of *Névroses et Idées Fixes (Fragments des leçons cliniques de mardi sur les névroses, les maladies produites par les émotions, les idées obsédantes et leur traitement)* was written in collaboration with Raymond, Charcot's successor at the Salpêtrière (Raymond & Janet, 1898). It contains 152 case presentations shown at the famous Tuesday clinical lessons at the hospital. The first half of the book focuses on mental disturbances such as abulias, mental confusions, deliriums (hysterical psychoses), sleep attacks, somnambulisms, fugues, obsessions, and impulses. Obsessions and related phenomena became the main subject of Janet's studies during these years, resulting in the publication of *Les Obsessions et la Psychasthénie* (Janet, 1903). The second half concentrates on psychosomatic disorders such as disturbances of the sensibility, tics, paralyses, disturbances of language, and visceral spasms. In many concisely described cases the authors show how a disorder developed after patients had been exposed to some kind of traumatizing event to which they responded very emotionally. This volume is a resource of the early, and sometimes very first, documentations of treatment approaches that are so like those found in current literature that one would believe they had been developed only recently (cf. van der Hart, 1988, p. vii).

The Major Symptoms of Hysteria

This book (1907b), published in English in 1907, contains the 15 lectures Janet delivered at Harvard Medical School in 1906. It demonstrates his fine didactic teaching qualities quite clearly. It is both a highly readable introduction to the phenomenology of hysteria and a succinct summary of his extensive studies in the field. In teaching about somnambulism, Janet showed his penchant for paradox:

> Things happen as if an idea, a partial system of thoughts, emancipated itself, became independent and developed itself on its own account. The result is, on the one hand, that it develops far too much, and on the other hand, that consciousness appears no longer to control it.
>
> *(p. 42)*

He advised his students not to be concerned with the obscurity of this remark: "After you have repeated it exactly in the same way with regard to a thousand different phenomena, it will not be long before you find yourself understanding it clearly" (p. 43). By focusing most lessons on various accidents of hysteria rather than on the stigmata, Janet greatly facilitated this understanding in his students.

The lectures contain descriptions and comparisons of the different types of somnambulism. In the generic sense, somnambulism refers to that state of mind in which people are so absorbed in their inner experience that congruent contact with external reality is lost. When they do respond to something in the outer environment, it is perceived as playing a role within the domain of the inner experience. The simplest form of somnambulism is monoideic. This refers to that state of mind in which a single fixed idea (often a traumatic memory) dominates the abnormal state.

In complex somnambulisms like fugues and dissociative identity disorder, reality is not distorted to that degree. The patient in a fugue usually has numerous recollections and exhibits adequate social behavior in order to make the journey that characterizes fugues. Patients with DID can function adequately in society while simultaneously sustaining an hallucination (which Janet [1894b] called *hémisomnambulisme*). For example, they might perceive themselves as wearing a dress when actually wearing jumper and trousers, or hold the self-perception that they are of a different gender than their biological body, yet they enter the appropriate public bathrooms.

As he had done previously (Janet, 1894a), Janet classified the dissociative parts of the personality according to their intellectual and memory capacities. He noted the obvious differences in intellectual capacities of adult alter personalities maintaining jobs and those of traumatized child parts. Regarding memory, he spoke of certain alters having access only to their own past experiences, while other dissociative parts can access the memories of additional parts. All sorts of combinations of intellectual functioning and memory among dissociative parts are possible, Janet noted, predating our discoveries in this area by almost 100 years.

As mentioned earlier, the essence of Janet's concept of hysteria lay in the distinguishing of two layers of symptoms: accidental or contingent symptoms (accidents) and basic, permanent symptoms (stigmata). There are two types of mental stigmata: (1) proper, which appear exclusively in hysteria; and (2) common, which are shared by hysteria and other mental disorders, notably psychasthenic neuroses. Proper stigmata include narrowing of the field of consciousness, the existence of subconscious phenomena, suggestibility, anaesthesia, and amnesia. Common stigmata encompass feelings of incompleteness, lowering of the mental level of functioning, emotional disturbances, troubles of the will, and an inability to begin and end activities.

The lowering of the mental level, which Janet introduced in *Obsessions and Psychasthenia* (1903), is a key concept in his work. In *L'Automatisme Psychologique* (1889), when he spoke of psychological misery, Janet established the important role of the breakdown of higher mental functions in the development of mental disorders. In the last chapter of *The Major Symptoms of Hysteria* Janet gave this notion its place in his theory of hysteria by defining hysteria as a form of mental depression (lowered mental level of functioning) characterized by the narrowing and emancipation of the field of consciousness and an increased tendency towards the dissociation of the systems of ideas and functions that constitute the personality. Lastly, in this book, Janet considered briefly the factors that may cause this lowering of the mental level. Among them were emotional disturbances, for instance, as a response to trauma, and severe physical illness.

So significant were Janet's observations of the presence of physical illness in contributing to the causation of hysteria that, at Janet's centennial, Henri Baruk (1960), a leading French psychiatrist, hailed Janet as having given the clinical basis to the development of modern psychophysiology and expected future discoveries in neurophysiology to derive from Janet's work as well. Because of this emphasis on the presence of severe physical illness in the formation of psychopathology, clinicians now working with dissociative disorders might inquire about this when taking patient histories.

In his Foreword to the 1920 edition of this book, Janet related the development of hysteria to his more recent studies of "the oscillations of the mental level." He dealt with the role of "driving back" or the mechanism of repression, which he addressed in more detail in *Les Médications Psychologiques* (1919, 1925). Janet considered this "incapable of giving a complete explanation of the hysterical neurosis." If there is something like repression, it occurs more in psychasthenia than in hysteria. Janet considered repression to be a result of exhaustion and a severe lowering of the mental level of functioning – not the cause, but the consequence of the psychasthenic depression.

The 1920 edition of *The Major Symptoms of Hysteria* was reissued in 1965 and is still available. We consider it an indispensable introductory work, not only for students of psychotrauma and the dissociative disorders, but for all students of psychiatry, clinical psychology, and neurology.

Les Névroses

Aligned with the previous work is the delightful little book, *Les Névroses* (1909a). It is considered Janet's most concentrated and synthesized work to date (Ey, 1968). Recently a reprint was published (2008), but no translations are available.

In this book Janet systematically compared and contrasted the symptoms of hysteria and psychasthenia, the latter being another fundamental condition of a variety of mental disorders, such as obsessive-compulsive disorder and the phobias (cf. Janet, 1903; Pitman, 1984, 1987). He contrasted the hysterical fixed ideas (as in somnambulism) with the psychasthenic obsessions; the hysterical amnesias with the psychasthenic doubts; the paralyses with the phobias, and so on. While the subconscious fixed idea of an hysteric develops itself completely outside of the individual's personal perception and memory, the obsession of a psychasthenic takes place in collaboration with one's whole personality. Furthermore, it does so without developing itself as completely as a fixed idea. Instead, the psychasthenic is continuously doubting his idea. Janet defined psychasthenia as a form of mental depression characterized by the reduction of psychological tension (see next section), by the diminution of the individual's ability to act on and perceive reality, by the substitution of inferior and exaggerated operations in the form of doubts, agitations, anxieties, and by the obsessional ideas that express these disturbances (1909a, p. 367).

The often-misunderstood notions of psychological force and tension played instrumental roles in many of Janet's psychopathological studies (cf. Janet, 1919, 1921, 1925, 1932; cf. Chapters 9, 11, 12, 13). We return to his *Les Obsessions et la Psychasthénie* (1903) for an elaboration of these concepts. Psychological force is the quantity of basic psychic energy available to an individual. It exists in two forms: latent and manifest. Mobilizing one's energy means transforming one's force from latent to manifest. We can observe a person's psychological force through the number, duration, and speed of his actions. The concept refers to one's basic capacity for psychological functioning. Psychological tension refers to the capacity to use one's psychic energy. The higher one's mental level, that is, the more operations one can synthesize, the higher one's psychological tension. (Obviously, Janet's "tension" has no similarity of meaning to our everyday use of this term.) The fact that patients differ in regard to their available sources of psychological force and psychological tension has important treatment implications (cf. Janet, 1919, 1925; Ellenberger, 1970; Sjövall, 1967; Chapters 8, 9, 11, 12, 13).

Janet's original theoretical model of the mind put forth in his first book, *L'Automatisme Psychologique*, denoted only two levels of mental functions for which one's psychic energy was used: those of synthesis and automatic function. As his work progressed, his experience led him to expand his conceptual model. He developed the ideas of psychological force and tension, and expanded the hierarchy of mental functions to five levels, each of which had a coefficient of reality (1903). The highest level of mental activity was the reality function (*fonction du réel*). This is the function of reality in which one grasps the maximal reality of a situation. It involves the focusing of one's attention on, and simultaneously perceiving fully, the data of external reality of one's own ideas and thoughts. The familiar corollary today is "being completely in the moment." This act requires a synthesis (*présentification*): the formation of the present moment in the mind. "The natural tendency of the mind is to roam through the past and the future; it requires a certain effort to keep one's attention in the present, and still more to concentrate it on present action," as Ellenberger (1970, p. 378) remarked. Janet said:

> The real present for us is an act of a certain complexity which we grasp as one single state of consciousness in spite of this complexity, and in spite of its real duration, which can be of greater or lesser extent ... Presentification consists of making present a state of mind and a group of phenomena.
>
> *(1903, p. 491)*

The five levels of Janet's hierarchy of mental functions that may be used to examine mental health, in descending order, are: (1) the reality function; (2) disinterested activity (habitual, indifferent and automatic actions); (3) functions of imagination (abstract reasoning, fantasy, daydreaming, and representative memory); (4) emotional reactions; and (5) useless muscular movements. The first three levels were considered the superior functions, the last two levels inferior; each set requires a lesser degree of involvement with reality in order to be performed.

A "reduction in psychological tension" (or lowering of the mental level) refers to the lessening of one's ability to use one's psychic energy at a high level of perceptive and integrative functioning. Specifically, it refers to the diminished twofold ability of the individual to (1) perceive fully the details of current reality, coupled with the self-awareness of one's feelings and ideas in that moment, and (2) to act on this reality with intentional imminent behaviour. Instead of engaging with reality in a maximally integrative way, people with psychasthenic depression substitute inferior mental operations in the forms of doubts, agitations, anxieties, and obsessional ideas. The dominance of each type of lowered operational function in response to reality characterizes a different type of disorder, or in Shapiro's terminology, neurotic style (Shapiro, 1965). As noted previously, in hysteria the reduction of psychological tension is characterized by the narrowing of the field of consciousness and an increased tendency to dissociation, and by the emancipation of systems of ideas and functions that, when integrated, constitute the personality (Janet, 1909a, p. 345).

In the final chapter of *Les Névroses*, Janet attempted to give a general definition of the neuroses. He saw them as illnesses affecting the various functions of the organism, mainly by an impairment of the superior parts of these functions. The higher functions are arrested in their evolution, in their adaptation to the present moment, to the present state of the outside world and present intrapsychic state of the individual. At the same time there is no deterioration of the inferior parts of these functions. In short, neuroses are disorders of the various functions of the organism marked by arrested development of the function without a deterioration of the function itself (p. 392).

L'État Mental des Hystériques (Second enlarged edition)

In 1911 an enlarged edition of *L'État Mental des Hystériques* was published. "The mental stigmata" and "The mental accidents" comprised the first part, the second consisted of various articles that were published between 1898 and 1910. One interesting paper dealt with the analysis and treatment of his patient Marcelline, whom Janet saw as a prototype of double personality (Janet, 1910b). A most important paper was "Amnesia and dissociation of memories by emotion" ("L'Amnésie et la dissociation des souvenirs par l'émotion"), presenting the case of Irène (1904), to which Janet referred often in his later work (1919, 1928a, 1925; cf., Van der Kolk & van der Hart, 1991).

Irène was a 20-year-old woman who took care of her terminally ill mother, whose death she experienced as very traumatic. Soon afterwards she became amnestic for the event of her mother's demise as well as for the three months preceding it. She was unable to work, developed severe abulia, and lost all interest in those around her. She was frequently affected by delirious crises in which she very dramatically reexperienced the critical scenes of her mother's last hours and death. Irène was "attached" to the traumatizing event in a way that she could not get beyond. She was unable to adapt to a life without her mother; her behavior resulted from "nonrealization," as Janet (1935b) called it.

Janet's difficult but successful treatment approach consisted of helping Irène restore her memories, first in hypnosis and then in the waking state. She had to transform her traumatic memories into a narrative, a personal account of the event and how it affected her personality. When, after much hard work, she succeeded in this and showed that she actually realized her mother's death and could relate her personal account of this event, Janet noted that her other symptoms, like profound abulia, disappeared. Her mental level of functioning increased, and she became capable of adaptive actions again.

The third part of this book consisted of "the most beautiful and the most original systematic study written on the treatment of hysteria at the end of the last century" (Faure, 1983). In this section, "Le traitement psychologique de l'hystérie" ("Psychological treatment of hysteria") (1898b), Janet emphasized the use of five hypnotic techniques: (1) extended hypnosis; (2) utilizing the temporary absence of symptoms during hypnosis (e.g. letting anorectic patients eat and drink); (3) giving symptom-oriented suggestions; (4) identifying fixed ideas; and (5) treating fixed ideas. The latter two are Janet's most significant and original techniques (cf. Chapter 11).

Janet discovered that, for certain patients, the act of telling their fixed ideas (both in the hypnotic and waking states) functioned as a successful "confession," permitting them to terminate their attachment to the fixed idea. He further observed that this was often insufficient for more severely disturbed patients to detach from their fixed ideas. With them, he tried to break down the fixed idea's entire system of images, feelings, and actions gradually, systematically substituting emotionally neutral or positive content for the traumatic phenomena.

Janet considered the dissolution of fixed ideas indispensable to the cure but, by itself, often insufficient. In his first writings he indicated that special attention was needed to aid patients in attaining higher levels of personality organizations, that is, increased psychological tension. If they remained at a low level, new emotions could be overwhelming, easily giving rise to new fixed ideas and dissociation. Janet described many hypnotic and non-hypnotic techniques aimed at raising a patient's mental level. He also concluded that hysterical patients usually needed long-term treatment to address the complexity of returning them to an adequate level of functioning.

His treatment sessions often entailed having the patient perform everyday life tasks that required graduated amounts of the activity of synthesis – always fostering experiences of success, in Janet's terms, acts of triumph (cf. Chapter 13). This might range from painting or listening to music to translating poetry and sculpting – in essence, art and occupational therapy. At the same time, Janet often advocated a simplification of the patient's home life and interpersonal functioning – stress reduction. His formulae, concrete suggestions and rationale for adding energy and decreasing the patient's energy expenditure, further developed in *Les Médications Psychologiques*, are the bedrock of a comprehensive treatment approach to the massively traumatized or severely dissociative patient (cf. Chapters 11, 12).

Les Médications Psychologiques

The final work in this review is *Les Médications Psychologiques* (1919). *Psychological Healing*, as the English version (Janet, 1925) is entitled, had a special place in Janet's work. The 2-volume, 1,265-page, English edition presents an extraordinarily interesting history of psychotherapy, emphasizing the role of hypnosis and presenting a marvellous survey of Janet's multidimensional treatment approaches. It is here that we find the practical relevance of his concepts of psychological force and tension in designing individualized treatment strategies.

With regard to dissociation, Janet proffers a very valuable chapter on the study and treatment of traumatic memories (in which he is rather critical of Freudian notions). Janet summarizes his approach to this matter thus:

> Strictly speaking, then, one who retains a fixed idea of a happening cannot be said to have a 'memory' of the happening. It is only for convenience that we speak of it as a 'traumatic memory.' The subject is often incapable of making with regard to the event, the recital which we speak of as memory; and yet he remains confronted by a difficult situation in which he has not been able to play a satisfactory part, one to which his adaptation had been imperfect, so that he continues to make efforts at adaptation. The repetition of this situation, these continual efforts, give rise to fatigue, produce an exhaustion which is considerable factor in his emotions.
>
> *(1925, p. 663)*

Psychological Healing is an important source of inspiration and information for the study and treatment of a wide variety of mental disturbances, especially the dissociative and posttraumatic stress disorders (see also Chapters 13 and 14).

Conclusion

It has been Janet's great, though much-neglected, contribution to psychiatry that he formulated the dynamic principles constituting a theory of dissociation: (1) the nature of the structural elements and functions that comprise personality; (2) the nature of the perception of reality and its disturbance in hysteria by the narrowing of the field of consciousness; (3) the nature of conscious activity, especially partial automatism in which a part of one's personality is split off from self-awareness and follows an autonomous subconscious development; (4) the hierarchical classification of the capacity to use psychic energy; and (5) the clear and detailed cases that demonstrate so comprehensively his concepts and treatment strategies for dissociative phenomena in a broad range of disorders.

Modern clinicians have greatly furthered our understanding of the role of dissociation in the development of severe dissociative disorders as defined in the *DSM-5* (American Psychiatric Association, 2013) such as dissociative identity disorder (DID) (e.g., Bliss, 1986; Braun, 1986a, 1986b; Dell & O'Neil, 2009; Kluft, 1985; Kluft & Fine, 1993; Nijenhuis, 2015; Putnam, 1989a, 1997; Ross, 1989, 1997; Steele, Boon, & van der Hart, 2017; van der Hart, Nijenhuis, & Steele, 2006). This understanding has led to important advances in the treatment of patients with these pathologies. It remains apparent, however, that dissociation is also characteristic of a substantial group of mental disorders in which it is still largely unrecognized or confused with other psychological phenomena.

It is the legacy of Pierre Janet that he has left us only the body of his work. He had no disciples, founded no school or group, did no proselytizing. And yet,

> Janet's work can be compared to a vast city buried beneath ashes, like Pompeii. ... It may remain buried forever. It may remain concealed while being plundered by marauders. But it may also perhaps be unearthed some day and brought back to life.
>
> *(Ellenberger, 1970, p. 409)*

For those whose special interests lie in dissociation, the rewards may be well worth the dig.

Note

1 Slightly modified version of van der Hart, O. and Friedman, B. (1989). "A reader's guide to Pierre Janet on dissociation: A neglected intellectual heritage," *Dissociation*, *2(1)*: 3–16, by kind permission of the publisher. The authors wish to acknowledge the helpful comments of Drs. Paul Brown, Rutger Horst, and Richard Kluft.

2

FROM CONSCIOUSNESS TO SUBCONSCIOUSNESS

A Janetian perspective

Francesca Ortu and Giuseppe Craparo

From his earliest attempts at formulating his theories, while repeatedly citing Charles Richet, Theodore Ribot, and Maine de Biran (considered a precursor of experimental psychology), Janet emphasized that mind and body must not be considered as separate entities and that methods of natural science should be used in the study of "human activity in its most rudimentary forms" (1889, p. 19). Defining *L'Automatisme Psychologique* as an essay on objective psychology, Janet (1889) had already adopted the perspective that would eventually lead him to understand the relationship between mental processes and conducts. Janet believed that in studying psychopathology, one must keep in mind at all times that "the patient by definition is different from us and so we can only comprehend his thoughts through his visible actions and not through our own thoughts," and that

> any movement of the limbs, … no matter how simple, is accompanied by a phenomenon of consciousness. Whether it is a position of the limbs, an inclination, convulsions, when the subject seems unaware, reduced to the state of an automaton or whether it is an involuntary movement … we can always assume *and sometimes manage to demonstrate* the presence of phenomena of consciousness … that last as long as the movement itself … in the mind a modification always takes place and it corresponds to the modification that the movement itself seems to undergo. … In short, within any area, from whatever perspective you observe, there are never two separate faculties, one of thought and the other of action; at all times, there is only ever one identical phenomenon, which simply manifests itself in two different ways.
>
> *(pp. 481–482, emphasis added)*

This point of view considers the external, visible action as the fundamental phenomenon, while the internal thought is nothing more than the reproduction of that external action in a reduced and particular form (1889). For Janet, this implies proceeding in a similar manner to that which allowed for the scientific study of an animal psychology, without, however, giving up the consideration of an "interior life." It entails creating a method capable of considering the complexity of human psychological functioning: "It does not involve annulling consciousness but talking about it as if it were a particular conduct, as a complication that overlaps with basic conduct" (Janet, 1926a, p. 204). It is this orientation that Janet termed the psychology of conduct. Is it possible, he asks, to apply a similar type of psychology to man? "This is what I have been trying to do in my teaching for over thirty years" (p. 204).

In Janet's construction of his complex psychological and psychopathological theory, two phases can be distinguished: (I) 1886–1916: the psychology of dissociation; and (II) 1916–1947: the psychology of conduct.

Phase I: 1886–1916: The psychology of dissociation

In three essays published between 1886 and 1888 in the *Revue Philosophique* and later incorporated almost entirely into *L'Automatisme Psychologique*, Janet's studies on "automatic phenomena" (alterations of awareness, memory, and consciousness that appear with the same frequency in hysteria and catalepsy) were focused on two fundamental concepts: personality and consciousness. Janet maintained that the "automatic movements" observable in cataleptics, whether induced or spontaneous as in hysteria,

> are not known by the person since they are determined by sensations not perceptions ... these disaggregated sensations, reduced to the state of a sort of mental dust, are not synthesized into any personality and can therefore be defined as *conscious but not personal sensations.*
>
> *(1889, p. 315, emphasis added)*

That is, while the manifestations of automatism seem to the external observer to be indistinguishable from any other perfectly intelligible act, to the patient who has performed them they appear as manifestations that are totally extraneous to his personality. These phenomena do not integrate into the personality; they show all of the characteristics of a conscious act, except that of being known by the patient who performs them (1889).

Working with somnambulists, Janet observed that the subject's memory of in-trance suggestions depended on the method used to wake him; even though the subject declared that he "knew nothing" about the suggestion, as was clearly demonstrated by his execution of a posthypnotic order, the memory of the suggestion "persisted outside of consciousness" (1886a, p. 586). Janet wondered whether it made any sense to classify manifestations of automatism as unconscious acts and thoughts; perhaps they could be explained more correctly by hypothesizing a "division of consciousness" (*dédoublement de la conscience*) (1886a, p. 588). Indeed, somnambulists were able

> to count the days and the hours separating them from the execution of an in-trance suggestion without having any memory of that suggestion later. How was it possible? We do not know how but outside of consciousness there exists a persistent memory, an ever-vigilant attention and a power of judgment that is able to perform complex operations.
>
> *(1889, p. 263)*

But what sense does it make to speak of "unconscious judgement," Janet asked himself, when one is confronted with a case like that of his patient Lucie? Although this patient declared that she knew nothing about what had happened to her when she was sleepwalking, upon waking she was nonetheless able to write automatically a series of calculations that she had been ordered to do while in the somnambulistic state. "If words are a sign for us of the consciousness of others," Janet asked, "why shouldn't writing also be a characteristic [of that consciousness]?" (1886a, p. 588). Rather than an absence of consciousness, we should speak here of a division of consciousness: "All of the suggestions are necessarily accompanied by a certain degree of unconsciousness or better, a dissociation of the consciousness" (p. 592). In *L'Automatisme Psychologique* (1889), Janet attributed the automatic actions performed by Lucie to the activity of a particular form of consciousness located below the normal consciousness of the individual and described them as "subconscious facts endowed with a consciousness, which is below normal consciousness" (p. 265).

For Janet (1889), automatic phenomena, which can be explained by referring to some simple laws of psychology, are placed within a larger framework, in which it is already possible to glimpse the fundamental principles of the hierarchical theory he subsequently developed (1926a; see Chapter 1). He traced these automatic phenomena back to a rupture in the balance between the two basic activities of the mind that characterize normal functioning: creative activities, which continuously gather phenomena into new syntheses and give life to the personal consciousness of the individual; and repetitive activities, which reactivate old syntheses that in the past had their reason for being. For Janet, psychological synthesis is the main characteristic of consciousness. According to this interpretation, automatic activity is linked to an impairment of psychological synthesis as the consequence of a "narrowing of the field of consciousness." Janet, in fact, considered hysteria as a personality disorder involving a difficulty in reconnecting one's personality with some psychological phenomena (e.g. sensations, ideas, feelings, motor images, and images of memories). At the core of the many and varied disturbances manifested by hysterical and cataleptic patients lies their lack of the capacity to integrate into their personalities those "facts" that are perfectly intelligible to outside observers but which to these patients seem to be totally extraneous to their personality. For Janet, these psychopathologies are characterized by disturbances of the "reflective consciousness" due to dissociative mental states. More precisely, the fundamental disturbance of the "hysterical patient" consists, then, in the interruption of the tendency towards synthesis and towards personality maturation that constitutes the general character of "psychological phenomena," and in the loss of equilibrium between the two fundamental activities – automatic activities and the activities of synthesis – which guarantee "the health of the body and the harmony of the mind." Janet saw "synthesis activity" as an authentically creative activity that reunites the more or less numerous given phenomena with the "new phenomena that are different from their single elements" (1889, p. 483). It is the decrease in the activity of synthesis that leads to an exaggerated development of automatism, that is, to an activity of conservation that tends to bring to light old syntheses that "in a normal individual" have already been replaced by other complex phenomena. Instead, the patient remains stuck in old syntheses. In the emergence of this automatic activity, emotions play a fundamental role; they exert an "action of dissolution" on the mind, decreasing its activity of synthesis and making it momentarily miserable by sowing the seed of a fixed idea within it, which, after a period of incubation will develop and persist. In *L'Automatisme Psychologique*, Janet proposed a model of psychic activity that postulates the existence of different levels of consciousness continuously alternating among each other; he considered the emergence of subconscious activity as the expression of fragmentation, a disturbance characterized by a lack of coherence in human personality, or rather, in the personal consciousness, which does not allow the subject to become aware of psychological phenomena and to recognize them as his or her own.

"By unconscious act (acte *inconscient*), we mean," Janet wrote, "an action which has all the characteristics of a psychological fact, except for one, which is that the person who performs the act is unaware that he is performing it at the time of its performance" (1889, p. 225). This action, still referred to as "unconscious" or "subconscious," has the paradoxical characteristic of appearing to be perfectly intelligible to the external observer, but conversely, completely extraneous (or at least unknown) to the person who has performed it.

In his writings during the last years of the nineteenth century, Janet increasingly focused on the concept of subconscious in conjunction with division of the personality. In these works, Janet clearly aimed at demonstrating the existence of separate elements of consciousness (fixed ideas) in the minds of hysterical subjects – a disaggregation (*désagrégation*) of the personality. These subconscious ideas are the result of traumatic experiences. For this reason, the construct of the subconscious should not to be confused with the Cartesian *cogito* or with an ego in the Freudian sense, although it does clearly belong to the mental sphere. Janet was able to show the close links between automatic actions and personality:

> We believe that it is possible simultaneously to accept both automatism and consciousness, thereby satisfying both those who find in man a form of

elementary activity which is completely automatic like that of an automa-. ton, and those who wish instead to preserve in man, even in his most simple actions, consciousness and awareness. In other words, we do not believe that the activity of a living being that manifests itself externally through movement can be separated from a certain form of intelligence and consciousness which accompanies it internally; *our scope is to demonstrate not only that there is a human activity that deserves to be called automatic but that it is also legitimate to refer to it as psychological automatism.*

(*1889, pp. 2–3, emphasis in original*)

"Automatic actions," Janet wrote in *Névroses et Idées Fixes* (1898a),

are completely connected to our personality, and although they are not completely unconscious, since they often manifest a certain sensitivity and intelligence, they lack that personal consciousness which allows us to be aware of psychological phenomena and to connect them to ourselves. In other words, they are more or less unconscious.

(*p. 391*)

In a number of studies that explored the notions of subconscious fixed ideas and mental contents, Janet's research is focused on the structure and modes of thought. In *L'Automatisme Psychologique,* his explanation of some psychological forms (e.g. somnambulism, automatic writing, catalexis, etc.) was based on a model of psychic activity that postulated the presence, below conscious human life, of a subconscious life made of basic emotions and instincts. The abrupt alternation between these two levels of consciousness was considered responsible for the manifestations of psychological automatism, which shed light on the fragmentation of consciousness, a disturbance that disrupts the coherence of the human personality.

It is in the *narrowing of the field of consciousness* that the roots of hysteria must be sought: "The hysterical personality is unable to perceive all phenomena, it definitely sacrifices some of them. There is a sort of autonomy and the abandoned phenomena continue to develop without the subject being aware of their development" (1889, p. 314). The narrowing of the field of consciousness fostered by the lack of psychological force (see Chapters 10, 12, and 13) brought about by a degeneration of the nervous system thus represents the fundamental phenomenon of hysteria; it allows the multiplicity of symptoms of hysteria to be united into one morbid entity. In this way, it is possible to trace all of the phenomena of automatism back to their essential condition, that is, back to the appearance of a state of anaesthesia and distraction. "This state is linked to the narrowing of the field of consciousness and this narrowing is due to a weakness in synthesis and to the disaggregation of mental compound into several smaller groups than there should normally be" (1911, p. 16).

Dissociation of the personality, then, is the immediate consequence of this weakness in psychological synthesis. According to Janet, we can describe the phenomena in sleepwalking and other subconscious acts as secondary groups, subsidiary systematizations of these neglected psychological phenomena (1911, pp. 278–279).

Unlike hysteria, weakening of consciousness is responsible for the symptoms involved in psychasthenia that are indicative of the specific difficulties these patients have in linking certain phenomena to their personalities. While other people have no difficulty in treating these phenomena as part of their personality, the psychasthenic patient behaves as if she or he did not have access to them:

> The language of these psychasthenic patients seems bizarre or even contradictory: the fact is that their personality disorder is not at all total. It clearly manifests itself in some operations that we could call 'superior': in their capacity for recognition, which normally would make it possible to link new content with older mental content, in their reflective language and in their voluntary acts. However, their mental operations seem to be intact; consciousness, this act whereby various states are brought together to form a oneness, still seems to be present. It is true that the subject maintains that it is not he who performs certain acts, who sees a specific tree, but he definitely has the memory of it, he definitely continues to see the tree. Or, at least, it is evident to us that he continues to see the tree because he describes how it changes; he says: 'the tree is green, its leaves are moving, but I am not the one who is seeing all of this.'
>
> (Janet, 1910a, p. 67)

Thus, the *weakening of consciousness* sheds light on the characteristics of the various symptoms of these two neuroses, introducing several reflections on the subject's *psychological force*. These reflections take into consideration not only the quantity of psychic energy but also the *psychological tension* of the individual, that is, his capacity to elevate energy to a certain level in the hierarchy of functions.[1] *Psychological force*, defined as the amount of elementary energy or, in other words, the capacity to perform a range of both prolonged and rapid psychological acts, exists in two forms: latent and manifest, and it can be mobilized. *Psychological tension* is constituted by the act of concentrating and unifying psychological phenomena into a new mental synthesis, and it varies according to the number of psychological phenomena it synthesizes. Janet also asserts that in understanding neurotic phenomena, it is essential to consider the function of reality. This requires attention, that is, the act of perceiving both external reality as well as thoughts and ideas. The most obvious characteristic of attention is its ability to act on external objects and change reality. The combination of voluntary attention and will makes *presentification* possible, that is, the formation in the mind of the present moment.[2] According to Janet, by considering the capacity for presentification and the force required by this operation, it is possible to construct a sort of coefficient of reality that constitutes a key to understanding psychasthenic phenomena. By considering the psychological force and the psychological tension, and how the two interrelate, it is possible to identify the most suitable treatment for each of the various neurotic conditions.

In *Les Obsessions et la Psychasthénie* (1903), Janet had already abandoned his initial dualistic system (the synthetic–creative activity of thought and the automatic–repetitive activity of doing) for a hierarchical conception of mental levels. The synthetic–creative function of thought was extended to cover the more general role of productive integration, responsible for the progressive disappearance of the various stages of mental evolution. Adopting a genetic perspective, Janet ended up favouring the evaluation of the level of articulation and capacity for thought rather than the complexity of contents.

This fundamental movement from one perspective to another also meant a change in methodology that would have significant implications for Janet's theories. In fact, his abandonment of the static, hierarchical model of his early research in favour of a dynamic conception of the psyche coincided with a greater openness towards historical–evolutionary thought. Studies in psychopathology shed light on the evolutionary history of the species and were, in turn, clarified by that history that amounted to an account of mankind more than to a history of the development of functions.

To avoid running the risk of losing the sense of automatic phenomena by reducing them to reflexes and seeking to explain them merely in the realm of the physiology, it is necessary, according to Janet, to look for an intermediary between consciousness and "unconscious," to study normal distraction – "the long chain of internal words and thoughts that take place and develop almost without our knowledge" (1903, p. 510). These same theories are reiterated in a paper entitled "Les oscillations du niveau mental," which Janet presented at the Fifth International Conference of Psychology held in Rome in 1905. In this paper, Janet reaffirmed the foundations of his theory of psychopathology, locating them now within an evolutionary and developmental framework; he linked the symptoms observed in hysterics and in psychasthenics to oscillations in "force, size, and perfection"; these oscillations "are visible" in the "various mental diseases," particularly in hysteria and psychasthenia. They are also present in normal conditions, for example, in states of fatigue or in intense emotional states:

> It is easy to demonstrate that in hysteria … the symptoms depend on a profound weakening of the psychic life and … they develop through a mechanism that is similar to suggestion … they are psychological symptoms that develop in complete isolation from the will and often from the *personal consciousness* of the patient.
>
> *(1905, p. 111, emphasis added)*

The symptoms of hysteria, Janet continues, demonstrate

> a narrowing of the mind that we can consider a narrowing of the field of consciousness: the mind no longer seems able to operate a unification, a

simultaneous fusion of all of the impressions coming from the periphery which ... in a normal mind are simultaneously grouped together. ... It seems that mental and nervous activity that is too restricted is able to recuperate some activity on the condition that it loses other activity. ... The patient is more or less aware of this impotence and experiences a number of abnormal feelings (for example, feelings of depersonalization) in relation to the depression from these abnormal forces.

(1905, p. 111)

According to Janet, in these two neuroses (but also in depressive states) isolated psychological or physiological phenomena are conserved and exaggerated; these phenomena are often barely conscious or *subconscious*, poorly connected to that mental synthesis that constitutes our personality. They are old phenomena that have been conserved, reproductions of psychological systems that were organized in the past, and it is evident that they are not organized for the present situation. No trace remains, instead, of the complex phenomena that derive from a harmonious functioning of the whole system; there is a reduction of mental synthesis, a narrowing of the field of consciousness; a reduction in consciousness and in personality is ascertainable, particularly in the functions of the present and in the capacity to take into account the present situation and "that which is new in it" and to adapt accordingly.

In "A symposium on the subconscious," published in the *Journal of Abnormal Psychology* in 1907, he reiterated the exclusively clinical meaning attributed to the term subconscious. It refers to specific disturbances of the personality that are observed in patients with hysteria or psychasthenia. These disturbances affect the subject's capacity to integrate his own perceptions into his personality and to recognize himself as the agent of his own actions. Avoiding speculation that would risk letting the discussion slide onto a metaphysical plane, Janet clearly stated that these are psychological phenomena that concern the external world or are grouped around a subject's idea of him- or herself. In both psychasthenia and hysteria, it is possible to demonstrate the presence of serious disturbances of personal perception and of the personality. Despite their apparent differences, it is possible to maintain that "accidents are fashioned on the same model. They are analogous to the depersonalizations of psychasthenics. ... I tried to sum them up under the word 'subconscious,' which, from my point of view, simply designates this new form of the disease of the personality" (1907a, p. 62). In concluding his discussion, Janet maintains that the word "subconscious" is the name given to particular psychological conditions characterized by a dissociation of consciousness caused by fixed ideas. Janet uses the term subconscious due to its connection with psychological dissociation.

The influence of these ideas exactly depends on their isolation. Normally, the ideas of human beings are numerous and mutually oppose each other because they are part of the same consciousness; however, with hysterics this is not the case 'because of the easy dissociability of their psychological unity', as Charcot said, "different individual centres of personal unity may become effective without other areas of the psychological organ being informed by that and participating in the process." These ideas become stronger and stronger, take hold of the mind like a parasite, and cannot be stopped in their development by the efforts of the person because they are unconscious and because they are disconnected from the system of ideas in a second consciousness.

(Janet, 1888, cit. in Bühler and Heim, 2009, p. 195)

Moreover, the paper Janet presented at the Sixth International Congress on Psychology in Geneva in 1909 also addressed the issues of the subconscious and specifically aimed at proposing a clear definition of the concept that would clearly distance it from the idea of the unconscious, which from this moment on was used to refer to speculations of a metaphysical type:

It seems useful here to recall the original meaning in order to avoid becoming engaged in the sterile research that has been grafted on to the first studies and to understand the real problems of the subconscious, an examination of which would prove advantageous. I will only say in this regard that some patients have difficulty linking certain phenomena to their personality while other people have no hesitation in considering [these phenomena] as absolutely personal.

(1909a, pp. 3–4)

The idea of the subconscious, Janet wrote, notwithstanding its philosophical origins, took shape in psychiatric clinics and that is where it should stay. An almost identical theorization and argumentation reappear in an article published in 1910 in the journal *Scientia* that begins with an explication of the different meanings that were by that time being attributed to the terms *unconscious* and *subconscious*:

The studies on the unconscious are very old: they are metaphysical studies that regard the possibility of an intelligence different from human intelligence, that is independent from consciousness and its conduct as we see it in ourselves. The researches on the subconscious are instead much more recent: they consist of clinical and psychological studies undertaken in response to difficulties that arose in the interpretation of some very particular mental disturbances.

(1910a, p. 64)

Fundamentally, the interpretations under discussion are those involving disturbances of the personality. In psychasthenics, this disorder is partial and the disturbance of personal perception does not seem profound; the mental operations of the personality seem to be preserved; the consciousness, this act whereby a multitude of different states are held together in a oneness, appears to be still present. In hysterics, the disturbance of the personality manifests itself in a different way and

> the subject acts as if he is completely unaware of what has just happened; he does not doubt his own memories, he does not say they are extraneous to himself. He simply does not talk about them at all, he ignores them. ... If instead of examining the memories, we examine the movements of these same subjects, we see that hysterics very often perform complex movements which seem intelligent to us – movements that in a normal person would seem to be related to a clear thought – but which these patients claim have for them no relation to a thought, no idea that would account for the movement.
>
> *(1910a, pp. 69–70)*

> On the one hand, these patients affirm that they do not remember, but on the other, they report that they have the capacity "to remember and to move and to hear very well.' ... It is the singular nature of these phenomena presented by hysterical patients, it is the behavior of these patients – whether or not it is comprehensible – which I have tried to sum up in the past with the term 'subconscious,' the 'narrowing of the field of consciousness," the "dissociation of the personality.'
>
> *(1910a, p. 78)*

This same position is also evident in the paper presented by Janet in London in 1913. It contains forceful methodological criticisms of the Freudian theory in general and particularly of its concept of the unconscious and of the mechanism of repression. In a highly polemical tone, not sparing any sarcasm, Janet reiterates here the need to remain on the level of clinical observation, to avoid undue generalizations, and to dodge the organicist threats hanging over the concept of the unconscious. Specifically, the fixed idea (at the origin of hysterical symptoms) is under the threshold of consciousness but its nature is identical to that of the ideas belonging to consciousness (Janet, 1910a).

Phase II: 1917–1947: The psychology of conduct

Janet's adoption of an evolutionary perspective would partially modify his theoretical framework, although he continued to assert the validity of his interpretation of hysteria and psychasthenia as being centred on the concept of the subconscious and his hypothesis regarding the weakening of consciousness. The existence of the subconscious is explained by considerations of a functional nature. The idea that the consciousness could contain all of the psychological operations at the same time seemed absurd to Janet. The consciousness is, in fact, considered a relative phenomenon, a specific effect of *bringing into awareness (mise en conscience)*, which overlaps with other tendencies and conducts.

In this phase, Janet described his theory about the relationship between subconscious and conscious conducts, which led, however, to a partial modification of the meaning of the term subconscious that now came to designate acts that are in an inferior position:

> Psychological acts are connected to one another. There is a first level which I have termed simply reflex, a second level which we have called suspensive, a third level which is that of the totalizing reflex involving sociopersonal acts in which all of the psychic activities come into play. An action may travel across all three levels. Generally speaking, we would say: a phenomenon is subconscious when it remains at a lower psychological level than the other phenomena of the same organism.
>
> *(1926b, p. 96)*

Still in *Les Stades de l'Évolution Psychologique*, Janet (1926b) wrote that

> the acts which remain inferior can be called subconscious acts … in the contemporary world, there are facts written in books and we could say that all of our current evolution consists in transforming the phenomena that exist in the world into books. Clearly there are phenomena that have not yet been written about in books, on every level there are phenomena that do not transform themselves; this means that inferior acts subsist in superior acts. They exist under two forms, as elements of inferior acts and as evolved phenomena that have not yet been transformed.
>
> *(p. 130)*

In *De l'Angoisse à l'Extase* (1928a), Janet emphasized the continuity of this new theoretical framework – in which action had acquired a central position – and of what he referred to as psychological automatism. Janet reaffirmed his belief that the Cartesian perspective that starts with thought and makes action a consequence or a secondary expression of thought must be abandoned in favour of a perspective in which the visible action is the fundamental phenomenon. Thought would be nothing more than a sort of "interior duplicate" or, more precisely, a combination of actions under a particularly reduced form. It was necessary, Janet believed, to express the most elevated psychological phenomena, those most typical of persons, in terms of actions. While the study of conscious thought leads us to exclude a whole series of phenomena from psychological research, observed Janet, it is also true that "behavioral psychology has shown itself inadequate on its own for the study of man" (1928a, p. 203).

Starting from a psychology of conduct, it will be possible not only to identify the links that connect and classify various observations but also to speak of the phenomena of consciousness as a particular action joined together with the elementary actions.

Consciousness and verbal construction – and for Janet consciousness implies, at the outset, having the capacity for verbal expression – allow the totality of the subconscious, present and past, to subsist within it:

> There are things which exist within us that cannot be described with words. We have called these things vague feelings, intuitions, but they are phenomena that have not been transformed into the superior level ... we have often noted that all of the reactions of the inferior level are transformed into acts on the superior level. A more or less considerable part of these reactions continues to retain the inferior form. It is this that has given rise to the acts which have sparked so much controversy under the name subconscious *acts*. We know that man attempts to transform all of his acts into language, but a certain number of these actions are left without any verbal expression, and in some cases, it is even impossible to verbalize them. A subconscious act is simply an action which has conserved its inferior form in the midst of other actions of a higher level.
>
> *(1935a, p. 40, emphasis added)*

Conclusion

As Janet wrote: "The term 'subconscious' ... merely summarizes the singular character of some of the personality disturbances that manifest themselves in a particular neurosis: hysteria" (1910a, p. 64), and later on:

> Since I began using the term 'subconscious' in this purely clinical sense – which I realize is a bit basic – many other authors have begun using it in a much more complex sense. The term is being used to denote extraordinary activities, which, it seems, exist in us without our even suspecting their existence; the term has been used to explain sudden enthusiasms and divinations of genius. This calls to mind an entertaining remark of Hartmann's: 'We can console ourselves over having practical and basic minds, over being so unpoetic and so unreligious; in the deepest part or each of us there exists a marvelous unconscious that dreams and prays while we work to earn our living.' I am careful to avoid discussions of theories that are so consoling and perhaps even true; I limit myself to remembering that I have occupied myself with things that are completely different. The poor patients whom I have studied had no genius: the phenomena that had become subconscious in them were very simple phenomena, which in other people would be part of their personal consciousness and certainly

would not inspire admiration. They [my patients] had lost their freedom to choose and their personal consciousness; they had a personality disorder. It is as simple as that.

(p. 75)

Notes

1 According to Janet, mental functioning is characterized by different levels of consciousness (from elementary activities to complex activities).
2 For Janet, "presentification consists of making present a state of mind and a group of phenomena" (1903, p. 491).

PART I

Janet's influence on psychoanalysis

3

JANET AND FREUD

Long-time rivals

Gabriele Cassullo

> An intimate friend and a hated enemy have always been indispensable
> requirements for my emotional life; I have always been able to create them
> anew, and not infrequently my childish ideal has been so closely approached
> that friend and enemy coincided in the same person.
>
> *(Freud, 1900, pp. 384–385)*

It was not until 1970 that the mutual influence between Janet and Freud was
amply discussed in Ellenberger's *The Discovery of the Unconscious*. In the following
pages, I will try to give an account of Freud's *subjective* view on Janet, and Janet's
subjective view on Freud. This is important, to my mind, in order to understand
any possible compatibility or incompatibility in their theoretical constructions.
We should always keep in mind, however, the words with which Janet closed his
autobiographical account:

> Without doubt, these systematic constructions are very hypothetical
> and temporary. The most interesting part of my work will always be the
> numerous observations I have gathered on both the normal and ailing
> man. I should never have been able to gather them or classify them if I had
> not been directed by philosophical ideas which were always indispensable.
> As William James said, one sees what one is prepared to see, so too, one
> cannot study the psychology of man without guiding ideas, without philo-
> sophical or even religious interests.
>
> *(1930a, p. 133)*

In 1924, in "An autobiographical study," Freud wrote about Janet:

> According to Janet's view a hysterical woman was a wretched creature
> who, on account of a constitutional weakness, was unable to hold her

mental acts together, and it was for that reason that she fell a victim to a splitting of her mind and to a restriction of the field of her consciousness. The outcome of psychoanalytic investigations, on the other hand, showed that these phenomena were the result of dynamic factors – of mental conflict and of repression. This distinction seems to me to be far-reaching enough to put an end to the glib repetition of the view that whatever is of value in psychoanalysis is merely borrowed from the ideas of Janet. The reader will have learned from my account that historically psychoanalysis is completely independent of Janet's discoveries, just as in its content it diverges from them and goes far beyond them. Janet's works would never have had the implications which have made psychoanalysis of such importance to the mental sciences and have made it attract such universal interest. I always treated Janet himself with respect, since his discoveries coincided to a considerable extent with those of Breuer, which had been made earlier, but published later than his. But when in the course of time psychoanalysis became a subject of discussion in France, Janet behaved ill, showed ignorance of the facts and used ugly arguments. And finally, he revealed himself to my eyes and destroyed the value of his own work by declaring that when he had spoken of "unconscious" mental acts he had meant nothing by the phrase – it had been no more than a '*façon de parler.*'

(1925, pp. 30–31)

The thoughts and feelings of Janet towards Freud had been restated just a year before, in 1923, after having been exposed on some previous occasions:

A foreign physician, Dr. S. Freud from Vienna, came to the Salpêtrière and was interested by these last studies [Janet's experiments with hypnotism]. He ascertained the reality of the facts and published some new observations of the same kind. In those he mainly modified the terms I used: he called psychoanalysis what I had called psychological analysis, he named complex what I had named psychological system … he understood as a repression what I had ascribed to a narrowing of consciousness, and he gave the name of catharsis to what I had indicated as a psychological dissociation, or moral disinfection.

(1923a, p. 41)

At the court of Charcot

It all started at the Salpêtrière, in Paris, where the 29-year-old Freud arrived in October 1885 in order to study with Jean-Martin Charcot. At the time, he had left Ernst Brücke's laboratory at the Physiological Institute on the grounds that it would not have enabled him to earn a living sufficient to support a family. As Freud recalls, "the turning-point came in 1882, when [Brücke], for whom

I felt the highest possible esteem, corrected my father's generous improvidence by strongly advising me, in view of my bad financial position, to abandon my theoretical career" (Freud, 1925, p. 10).

At Brücke's lab, Freud also met again his friend Josef Breuer, a 65-year-old researcher and general practitioner who had "developed into one of the most widely sought after doctors in Vienna, physician to aristocrats and members of Vienna's elite" (Makari, 2008, p. 39). Breuer represented an affectively and concretely support-ing figure, someone who really "gave credit" to Freud (Borgogno, 2010). Charcot was to embody, instead, an open door to an unknown scientific universe, in which Freud's intellectual ambitions and emotional interests overlapped (Breger, 2000).

However, in November 1885, a month after Freud's arrival in Paris, Paul Janet – professor of philosophy at the Sorbonne (Brady Brower, 2010) – presented, under the chairmanship of Charcot, the early experiments with hypnosis of his nephew Pierre – a 26-year-old lycée professor – at the Société de Psychologie Physiologique. We do not know whether Pierre Janet and Freud ever met in Paris, but it is hardly conceivable that Freud did not hear about Janet's work, as he was to declare years later (Freud, 1925, p. 13).

From 1885 to 1889 Janet carried on his researches, which were regularly pub-lished in the *Revue Philosophique*, and in August 1889 – after having graduated in philosophy at the Sorbonne just two months earlier – he lectured at two impor-tant psychological congresses, both attended by Freud, that were held in Paris for the Universal Exposition (Ellenberger, 1970, p. 759). In the same year, Janet published his dissertation thesis under the title *L'automatisme psychologique: Essai de psychologie expérimentale sur les formes inférieures de l'activité humaine*, and in 1890, his medical training having just started, he was appointed by Charcot as Director of the Laboratoire de Psychologie Expérimentale at the Salpêtrière.

It is not difficult to imagine that, if Freud saw Charcot as his "ideal mentor," he soon started to see Janet as his "ideal rival," the rivalry being between an out-sider and an insider with relevant connections in academic circles. For his part, Janet developed an image of Freud as an "illegitimate brother" who had come to Paris to steal the master's and his own work.

Yet back in 1885 Janet was more experienced in the treatment of hysterics, he had "a good mind" (as Freud himself admitted to Jung in 1907) (McGuire, 1974, p. 25), was a perspicacious and sensitive clinician (Ellenberger, 1970, p. 350; Breger, 2009, p. 201; Frust, 2008), and had at his disposal the most famous hospital in Europe for research on hysteria. For many reasons, Freud felt himself to be behind, and indeed he was; still, he could rely on Breuer.

In contrast to the cold reception Freud experienced from his professors once he returned from Paris in 1886, Breuer started supporting him and referring patients to him (Breger, 2000, p. 99). Furthermore, before his travel to Paris, Freud had been intrigued by the strange case of a girl (Bertha Pappenheim, or Anna O.) whom, from 1880 to 1882, Breuer had treated intensively by means of what he had described – at the patient's suggestion – as a "talking cure." Freud and Breuer had often discussed the patient, and in Paris Freud had even tried to interest Charcot in the case, but without success (Makari, 2008, p. 40).

Breuer's groundbreaking treatment of Anna O. in 1880–1882, combined with the insights on the case he and Freud reached during their discussions and the new knowledge Freud brought from Paris (and from Nancy, where he had been visiting Hippolyte Bernheim), laid the foundations on which Freud *later* grounded a method for the analysis of the mind that could compete with Janet's rapidly developing "psychological analysis." At the International Congress of Experimental Psychology of London, in 1892, Janet even presented a new procedure – *automatic talking* – consisting of "letting the patient talk aloud at random" (Ellenberger, 1970, p. 366).

In 1893 Breuer and Freud published, in a journal article (titled "On the psychic mechanism of hysterical phenomena") the theoretical premise of their *Studies on Hysteria* (Breuer & Freud, 1895). Janet welcomed it as one of the most significant works of the period, and agreed with them on the relevance of emotions arising during hysterical crises and hypnoid states (Janet, 1893d, p. 432). But he then observed that the link between hypnoid states and hysterical phenomena had already been established by several authors, himself included (Janet, 1893e, p. 19); that Breuer and Freud's remark that hysterics are reasonable when *awake* and alienated during their *dreamlike* hypnoid states was a welcome confirmation of what he had been describing since 1885 as *désagrégation* and *dédoublement de la personnalité* (pp. 25–26); and finally maintained, on the strength of his clinical experience, that he did not believe "that healing occurs in such an easy way, that one has just to make the patient express his fixed ideas to remove them—cure is a terribly more delicate matter" (Janet, 1893a, p. 352).

In order to answer these reasonable critiques, Freud sought to emancipate his theory from Janet's, and for that reason he abandoned Breuer (Breger, 2009). This is how drive theory originated, along with its emphasis on sexuality and all the subsequent breaks – such as those with Breuer, Bleuler, Adler, Jung, etc. – that came with it. However, the first point of differentiation from Janet was the theory of degeneration (Freud, 1894, pp. 46–48).

The theory of degeneration

Biological degeneration was a popular notion in the neurology and psychiatry of the nineteenth century. As George Makari (2008) has written:

> After 1870, biologic inheritance was widely accepted as the cause of psychic functions and the central precondition that led to a mind breaking during accidental events. ... By borrowing his student Charles Féré's notion of a 'neuropathic family' and studying genealogies, Charcot linked a number of illnesses together, attributing all to the same inherited defect. Charcot mapped out family trees that bloomed with hysteria, alcoholism, suicide, progressive paralysis, apoplexy, rheumatic and arthritic disorders.

When challenged as to the common inheritance of these illnesses, Charcot pointed to the neuropathic constellation that could be found among 'Israelites.'

(pp. 34–35)

Similarly, in his comprehensive book, *Faces of Degeneration* (1989), Daniel Pick argues that degeneration theory "needs to be understood as … a complex process of conceptualizing a felt crisis of history" that started "at just the moment when liberal progressivism was so powerfully in trouble" (p. 54). Diagnoses based on degeneration were

a convenient method of explaining away the widely perceived and criticized failure of psychiatry to 'cure' very many of its patients. Incurability … was now affirmed to be an unavoidable fact of nature. The function of the asylum was redefined not as a 'cure,' but as humane segregation of the degenerate and the dangerous.

(p. 55)

By demonstrating that it was possible to give credit to hysterics and do something about them, Charcot shaped a new culture at the Salpêtrière that would "inflame" the future of psychiatry; nonetheless, he kept on asserting that organic *dégénérescence* was a *sine qua non* for mental illness, with *environmental traumas* acting as "accidental triggering factors" (Goetz, Bonduelle, & Gelfand, 1995, p. 262). Janet lifted the theories of Charcot from the level of the brain to that of the mind by transforming "organic *dégénérescence*" into "psychological *désagrégation*" (1893a, p. 497). Then he went beyond his mentor by adding psychological complexity to the combined action of *predisposition and trauma* (Ellenberger, 1970). Freud did the same, but in a different fashion. He developed the concept of *Nachträglichkeit* – that is, the *deferred action* of infantile sexual trauma – which was meant to replace degenerationism (Freud, 1896, pp. 163–166). Not by chance, *infantile sexuality* is the main point of differentiation between Janet and Freud. As he would write to Jung in 1907, "Janet has a good mind, but he started without sexuality and now he can go no further" (McGuire, 1974, p. 25). He could go no further, of course, in the direction Freud envisaged for psychoanalysis.

Maybe because of his Jewish (Rolnik, 2012, p. 7) and humble origins, Freud was quite sensitive to the problem of degeneration (Spiegel, 1986); and it is possible that Janet's ascription of the genesis of hysteria to *misère, faiblesse*, and *désagrégation psychologique* sounded to his ear as unacceptable for that reason. Additionally, if the idea of degeneration could easily be associated with the image of the "uneducated" people that filled institutions like the Salpêtrière, it clashed with the upper-class and cultured patients who consulted Breuer and Freud.

In 1887 Freud started his private practice, and as early as 1888, though still identified with the hereditarism of Charcot, he already underlined that hysterics retain "complete intellectual clarity and a capacity even for unusual achievements"

(1888, p. 53). The idea was further developed in the treatment of Emmy von N. (Baroness Fanny Moser, one of the wealthiest widows in Europe), which exerted a major impact on the evolution of the Freudian theory (Bromberg, 1996). In commenting on the personality of Emmy, Freud harshly attacked Janet for the first time:

> Emmy von N. gave us an example of how hysteria is compatible with an unblemished character and a well-governed mode of life. The woman we came to know was an admirable one. The moral seriousness with which she viewed her duties, her intelligence and energy, which were no less than a man's, and her high degree of education and love of truth impressed both of us [Freud and Breuer] greatly; while her benevolent care for the welfare of all her dependants, her humility of mind and the refinement of her manners revealed her qualities as a true lady as well. To describe such a woman as a 'degenerate' would be to distort the meaning of that word out of all recognition. We should do well to distinguish between the concepts of 'disposition' and 'degeneracy' as applied to people; otherwise we shall find ourselves forced to admit that humanity owes a large proportion of its great achievements to the efforts of 'degenerates.' I must confess, too, that I can see no sign in Frau von N.'s history of the 'psychical inefficiency' to which Janet attributes the genesis of hysteria. ... During the times of her worst states she was and remained capable of playing her part in the management of a large industrial business, of keeping a constant eye on the education of her children, of carrying on her correspondence with prominent people in the intellectual world – in short, of fulfilling her obligations well enough for the fact of her illness to remain concealed.
>
> *(Breuer & Freud, 1895, pp. 103–104)*

Unfortunately, as Freud would learn years later (Tögel, 1999), the personality of Emmy was "split," "double," so that what Freud had been dealing with was – to borrow Sándor Ferenczi's (1932a) expression – the portion of Emmy's personality that had grown out of *identification with the aggressor*. This made her, on one side of the divide, behave obediently with the doctors who tried to help her, but on the other side it impelled her to reject and abandon them as soon as some "dangerous" affective contact was emerging (Breuer & Freud, 1895, p. 105*n*).

A life-long rivalry

Over the years, Freud returned many times to Janet. In two texts published in 1905 ("Fragment of an analysis of a case of hysteria (Dora)" and "Psychotherapy"), he acknowledged the similarity between the French School and psychoanalysis; but stated that Janet's conception of *fixed ideas* was too schematic compared to his own view of *unconscious fantasies*. Janet was interested in the pathological narrowing of consciousness, while Freud was addressing the infinitude of the unconscious.

Moreover, in 1906 Freud mentioned again the problem of degeneration, and also the name of Janet resurfaced. However, in "Creative writers and day-dreaming" (1907), closely connected to the previous work, without mentioning Janet, Freud refers to some phenomena that can only be explained by the concept of dissociation of the ego: "The essential *ars poetica* lies in the technique of overcoming the feeling of repulsion in us which is undoubtedly connected with the barriers that rise between each single ego and the others" (1907, p. 153). What should these barriers be if not dissociative *clivages*? Not by chance, these pages of Freud on part-egos have been used by Bromberg (2006, pp. 58–59).

In those years particularly, the personal, the political, and the scientific intertwined. In fact, Freud wrote to Jung on 14 April 1907:

> Dear colleague, you see, my view of our relationship is shared by the world at large. Shortly before your visit, I was asked to give that report in Amsterdam. I declined in haste for fear that I might talk it over with you and let you persuade me to accept. Then we found more important things to talk about and the matter was forgotten. Now I am delighted to hear that you have been chosen. But when I was invited, Aschaffenburg was not to be the other speaker; two were mentioned, Janet and a native. Apparently, a duel was planned between Janet and myself, but I detest gladiatorial fights in front of the noble rabble and cannot easily bring myself to put my findings to the vote of an indifferent crowd; but my chief reason is that I am eager to hear nothing of science for a few months and to restore my sorely maltreated organism through all sorts of extra-curricular pleasures. Now you will have to measure yourself with Aschaffenburg. I recommend ruthlessness; our opponents are pachyderms, you must reckon with their thick hides.
>
> *(McGuire, 1974, pp. 32–33)*

Here is Jung's report on the "First International Congress of Psychiatry, Neurology, Psychology and Alienists, which was held in Amsterdam" (Makari, 2008, p. 213):

> Dear Professor Freud, Amsterdam, 4 September 1907, just a couple of words in haste by way of abreaction. I spoke this morning but unfortunately couldn't quite finish my lecture as I would have exceeded the time-limit of half an hour, which wasn't allowed. What a gang of cut-throats we have here! Their resistance really is rooted in affect. Aschaffenburg made two slips of the tongue in his lecture (''acts' instead of 'no facts'), which shows that unconsciously he is already strongly infected. Hence his furious attack. Typical that in conversation he never tries to learn anything but goes all out to prove to me what a frightful mistake we are making. He

won't listen to any of our arguments. I have compiled a pretty dossier of his negative affects. All the rest of them are cowards, each hanging on to the coat-tails of the fatter man in front. The discussion is tomorrow. I shall say as little as possible, for every word sacrificed to this kind of opposition is a waste of time. A ghastly crowd, reeking of vanity, Janet the worst of the lot.

(McGuire, 1974, p. 83)

The next step was Professor Stanley Hall's invitation to Freud to deliver lectures at the twentieth anniversary of Clark University, in Worcester, Massachusetts. Janet had already given a similar course, which had "a profound influence in turning attention of our leading and especially out younger students of abnormal psychology from an exclusively somatic and neurological basis to a more psychological basis," as Hall mentioned in the letter of invitation for Freud (Makari, 2008, p. 234). Freud initially declined, on the grounds that the travel was too much for his pocket, but his rival's shadow hovered over his reply to Jung:

I am not wealthy enough to spend five times that much to give the Americans an impetus. ... Janet, whose example they invoke, is probably richer or more ambitious or has no practice to lose. But I am sorry to have it fall through on this account, because it would have been fun.

(McGuire, 1974, pp. 91–92)

In the end, Freud accepted. It was the first time he was to address an internationally renowned audience, and he was anxious. So, he started fantasizing about the reaction to expect from the floor: would his listeners take his part or that of Janet? He wrote to Ernest Jones about the influential American psychologist Morton Prince:

Prince is an upright sympathetic man, very much leaning to our theories and you seem to get yourself into a sort of attachment towards him. Now I have been told in Salzburg that he proclaims my views are mostly taken from Janet and in fact identical with them, I know from Brill and the same from Abraham, that he declined papers sent him on his demand on the account of their containing too much of sexual matter – you say he is not prudish, but he answered Abraham that he could not accept the term "homosexual" because he has so many lay readers (or ladies may be) – his exposition of my remarks on the Unconscious are only bad misconceptions, which make me surmise he has never read the book but only looked at the special item. Now how can you reconcile the words and the deeds of this man, the judgment I must shape of him and the impression he gave you? It might be better to keep from him and to be prepared to his bad intentions veiled by his friendly speaking.

(Paskauskas, 1993, p. 19)

Freud opened his lecture at Clark by giving the credit for the birth of psychoanalysis to Breuer. Then, in the second lecture, he touched on the complex issue of his debt to Janet:

> Janet's hysterical reminds one of a weak woman who has been shopping, and is now on her way home, laden with packages and bundles of every description. She cannot manage the whole lot with her two arms and her ten fingers, and soon she drops one. When she stoops to pick this up, another breaks loose, and so it goes on. Now it does not agree very well with this assumed mental weakness of hystericals, that there can be observed in hysterical cases, besides the phenomena of lessened functioning, examples of a partial increase of functional capacity, as a sort of compensation. … When, later on, I set about continuing on my own account the investigations that had been begun by Breuer, I soon arrived at another view of the origin of hysterical dissociation (the splitting of consciousness).
>
> *(Freud, 1909, p. 22)*

This vignette depicts the classical view on Janet's dissociation from a Freudian angle, a view which unfortunately survives to the present.

However, I am convinced that Freud held in his mind a more complex view of Janet, while he scarcely admitted that in his writings, continuing an internal dialogue with his rival. For example, in 1911 he built on Janet's conception of the *fonction du réel* (the function of reality) to arrive at his own conception of the psychical apparatus. Since he had taken the notion from Janet's 1909 work *Les névroses*, Freud evidently still read Janet and engaged with his thinking. In the same paper, Freud (1911) divides the ego into a *pleasure-ego* and *reality-ego*. Dealing with narcissism, in 1914, he adds a *self-observing agency of the ego*, and again refers to Janet's *fonction du réel*, while in the *Introductory Lectures* he calls this self-observing agency an *ego-censor* (1916–1917). Finally, in 1922, the superego is born. Nevertheless, where did all those egos, or part-egos, or ego-somatic-precursors stem from? Do they fit into Freud's repression or into Janet's dissociation model? Or do they belong to a hybrid model, whose existence Freud never clearly acknowledged, but just used?

In 1910 Freud plainly stated: "We use the collective concept of the 'ego' – a compound which is made up variously at different times" (1910, p. 213). Is the Freudian ego a collective, compound entity? This could explain the treatment of some personality disturbances, with unstable identity, regressive, or borderline states, which do not fall into the classical drive-defence pattern but have, nevertheless, been addressed by means of psychoanalysis, since it has silently incorporated Janet's dissociation model.

Silently, because of the upsurge in the conflict between Freud and Janet. In 1913, the French psychologist presented to the London International Congress of Medicine an open, detailed critique of Freud, which he titled "La psychanalyse." Freud replied a year later with his potently political "On the history of the psychoanalytic movement," and there was another outbreak of the conflict in 1923–1924.

Conclusion

It would be of great value to continue, in the future, the uncovering of Janet's legacy within the Freudian corpus. Due to the conflict between the two, looking for Janet's name in Freud's oeuvre would be of little use. Instead, one should look for the concepts, not a mechanical task. This inquiry should surely include Freud's gradual elaboration of the concept of *Verleugnung*, disavowal, which is strictly connected to the loss of the *fonction du réel* and culminates in a "splitting of the ego in the process of defence."

It should also include, in my opinion, Freud's elaboration of the death drive, which can be understood as a drive towards dissociation. Again, we would be in a hybrid Janetian–Freudian model, seeing that dissociation, in this sense, would not come from a passive fragmentation of the mind, but from an active, disintegrating force (drive).

4

JANET AND JUNG

A stimulating relationship

Caterina Vezzoli

Working on Jung and Janet requires a journey to the late nineteenth and early twentieth centuries, to the Geneva of 1892 when Théodore Flournoy was appointed by the Swiss Government to the first chair in psychology. The recognition of psychology as a science was the most significant event for the psychologists of the time. The journey then proceeds to the Paris of 1902 where Janet formally succeeded Théodule Ribot at the Collège de France and presented his research on automatism and dreams.

By reflecting on the relationship between Jung and Janet, it becomes evident that from the earliest years of his development as a psychiatrist and psychologist, Jung's attitude was that of a free spirit. At the time of the making and development of modern psychology (Shamdasani, 2003) he was experimenting with different approaches in order to find his own method. The French school, with Binet, Ribot, and Janet, was, no doubt, significant for his research, as was the Geneva connection with Flournoy and the approach to occult phenomena so prominent in Jung's early research. This French heritage remained a constant presence in Jung's psychology, as is clear from a remark he made in 1934: "I in no way exclusively stem from Freud. I had my scientific attitude and the theory of complexes before I met Freud. The teachers that influenced me above all are Bleuler, Pierre Janet, and Théodore Flournoy" (1934, p. 535).

In *Experimental Researches* (Jung, 1973) the references to Janet are numerous. In fact, the research on the association experiments carried out at the Burghölzli under Jung's direction shows the contribution of Janet to the understanding of complexes and dissociation.

Throughout his career, Jung recognized and attributed great value to Janet's theoretical and clinical merits. Over the years, Jung developed his own theories on complexes, dissociation, dreams, archetypes, countertransference, individuation, psychoid, psychological types, the self, and synchronicity, but his admiration for Janet and the French school remained a constant.

Experimental research

In 1902 Jung went to Paris to attend Janet's lectures at the Collège de France. Commenting on Janet's influence on Jung, Ellenberger (1970) observes:

> Jung repeatedly referred to Janet (whose lectures he had attended in Paris during the winter semester (1902–1903). The influence of Psychological Automatism can be seen from Jung's way of considering the human mind as comprising a number of sub-personalities (Janet's 'simultaneous psycho-logical existences'). What Jung called a 'complex' was originally nothing but the equivalent of Janet's 'subconscious fixed idea.
>
> *(p. 406)*

In 1902, when he first met Janet, Jung was a young psychiatrist at the Burghölzli Hospital in Zurich, one of the best psychiatric hospitals in Europe, and he was trying to contribute to and elaborate on the theorization of what at the time was called "modern psychology." His approach was "*scientific*," but not strictly positivistic as he was trying to use the best scientific methodology of the time together with clinical observation. He studied association in the "normal individual" (1973), while in *Experimental Researches* he applied the association experiment to the study of subjectivity. In the experiments, he verified that association is anything but free, as it is determined by affective experiences and drives. "Drives" is not a preferred Jungian word; in fact, Jung debated at length about the psychology of instincts that he later associated with the archetype.

At the dawn of the century Jung was using word association experiments rather differently than Wundt had done, as he had never really subscribed to associationism per se. For Jung, research on association was merely a means of inquiry into the structure of the psyche and into the nature of the traumatic experiences that could determine dissociation.

Knowing that Binet was critical of Wundt's associative method and considering the French school to be representative of the best psychiatry of the time, Jung tried to improve the methodology then in use by introducing an experimental apparatus that could include a psychological reading of the results. In fact, at the beginning Jung was interested in working experimentally on differential diagnosis, but this type of research turned out to be unfruitful (Shamdasani, 2003). From then on, Jung's studies were concentrated on an experimental methodology that focused on reaction times and word associations in individuals. The French psychology of the unconscious was the constant point of reference for this early research. In fact, the association experiments confirmed Janet's notion of subconscious fixed ideas.

Dementia praecox

Jung's integration and further development of Janet's psychological theories can be most clearly detected in *The Psychogenesis of Mental Disease* (1982) where he makes references to Janet's books: *L'Automatisme Psychologique* (1889), *Névroses et Idées Fixes* (1898a), and *Les Obsessions et la Psychasthénie* (1903). Especially in the chapters in *The Psychology of Dementia Praecox* frequent references are made to Janet's ideas. The essays collected in this volume were published between 1906 and 1956, and throughout all of these years numerous references to Janet continue to be made.

Following this thread, it is possible to see how Jung's Janetian beginning was then integrated into his own theory. From the outset and throughout the development of his psychology, Jung acknowledged the validity of the work of Janet and the French school.

In his foreword to the first edition of *The Psychology of Dementia Praecox*, dated 1907, Jung specifies that:

> Fairness to Freud, however, does not imply, as many fear, unqualified submission to a dogma; one can very well maintain an independent judgment. If I, for instance, acknowledge the complex mechanisms of dreams and hysteria, this does not mean that I attribute to the infantile sexual trauma the exclusive importance that Freud apparently does. Still less does it mean that I place sexuality so predominantly in the foreground. ... As for Freud's therapy, it is at best but one of several possible methods, and perhaps does not always offer in practice what one expects from it in theory. ... he who wishes to be fair to Freud should take to heart the words of Erasmus: 'unumquemque move lapidem, omnia experire, nihil intentatum relinque.'[1]
>
> *(p. 4)*

The editorial note to *The Psychology of Dementia Praecox* gives the reader additional illuminating information by stating that besides being the culmination of Jung's early research at the Burghölzli, this was the work that engaged Freud's interest in Jung, while at the same time it also contained the elements of their future theoretical divergences.

In chapter 1, "Critical survey of theoretical views on the psychology of dementia praecox," Jung analyzes the literature available at the time on the subject, including experimental research on association, and finds that Janet's concept of *abaisement du niveau mental* can explain the reduced attention and concentration that many of the authors associate with the emergence of unexpected unconscious associations. In the same chapter, dissociation is considered with reference to Janet.

Jung's "autonomous complexes" are likewise explained with reference to Janet's *L'Automatisme Psychologique* (1889). Starting from the autonomous complexes, Jung elaborated on the potential for dissociation of the psyche in normal and abnormal states. The autonomous aspects of the complex are defined as "splinter psyches" or partial personalities. The autonomy of the feeling-tone complexes is defined as the consequence of dissociation that can create double consciousness or split-off personality (1907, §50).

Also of importance in this work is Jung's reference to a book by Frédéric Paulhan, *L'Activité Mentale et les Élements de l'Esprit* (1889), which Binet considered the definitive answer to the sterile doctrine of associationism (Haule, 1984b). This indebtedness clarifies the position of Jung towards Wundiant associationism.

The approach of the French school to dissociation was that preferred by Jung, based on his own research and clinical work at the Burghölzli. Interestingly, in this same chapter there is a discussion of a case analyzed by Breuer and Freud (1893), and Jung's (1907) remarks on the case give the impression that he sees Freud's approach as being in continuity with Janet and the French school.

The main assumption of Jung's experimental researches was that experiences, ideas, and images tend to aggregate into complexes that constitute the building blocks of individual personality. Dissociation can be detected in the experimental situation by the association of words and by the experimental apparatus that went from galvanometric measurements, in the earliest experiments, to the registration of the time of answers. In the experiment, the traumatic contents can emerge from the unconscious and create dissociation in the "dominant personality" with the creation of partial personalities. This of course occurred in the experimental situation as well as in the clinical treatment.

The scientific world of the time was particularly interested in the manifestation of multiple personalities. The old therapeutic tradition of Mesmer and others had already dealt with the multiple-personality phenomena; however, dissociationism attempted to provide a "scientific" theorization of the pathology of these states (Haule, 1984b).

Still used in analytical psychology for both teaching and clinical purposes, Jung's association experiment was originally employed to find evidence of dissociation and to observe the subsequent regression to archaic forms of personality.

Nowadays it is mainly used in didactic settings to show students how life events aggregate into complexes and/or how they can cause the subject to dissociate. It is also used both therapeutically and diagnostically in clinical settings.

The importance of association experiment in the understanding of dissociation becomes clearer when we consider Jung's observation: "When consciousness 'disintegrates' (abaisement du niveau mental, apperceptive weakness), the unconscious parts of the complexes coexisting with consciousness will emerge and will break through into ego-consciousness" (1907, p. 30).

Abaisement du niveau mental and *apperceptive weakness* are clear references to Janet, and quoted from the original text. In the second chapter of *The Psychology of Dementia Preacox*, "The feeling-toned complex and its general effects on the psyche," Jung returns to dissociation, which he has already defined according to Janet and the French school as a *weakening of consciousness* due to the splitting off of sequences of ideas. Janet's formulation sees dissociation as the result of the *abaisement du niveau mental* causing the formation of automatism, as is emphasized in Jung's text.

The events and facts of our life from early infancy onward are stored and aggregated around feeling-tones, complexes that are the scaffolding of our psychic structure. It is evident that while the potential for dissociation can be considered characteristic of the psyche, childhood traumata can determine extreme dissociation and subsequent split-off personalities that are difficult to integrate.

In Jungian theory complexes are partly conscious and partly unconscious, with their own perceptions, feelings, volition, intention. The ego-complex is one among the complexes; consciousness is therefore subject to the influence of emotion pertaining to other complexes such as the mother complex, father complex, persona, shadow, etc. (Kast, 1992). The emotion, the feeling-tone, aggregates experiences and memories in conscious and unconscious clusters that can dissociate from the mental functioning (Knox, 2003) and the ego-complex. Complexes are not necessarily pathological, and for Jung complexes and dissociation can also exist as normal phenomena.

In more recent studies conducted at the University of Milan (Vezzoli et al., 2007), using a modern version of the association experiment, we verified the occurrence of dissociation in non-psychotic subjects. In the association experiment, a word stimulus can elicit answers that indicate the emergence of feelings or emotions that are particularly charged.

In experiments, when the subject is in the presence of a perturbing "feeling-tone," the association chain is interrupted and he or she cannot give the association. The episode or the feeling-tone constituting the autonomous part of the complex cannot be psychically represented nor symbolized. The feeling remains blocked at a pole of the complex and the episode or the feeling-tone is dissociated. The subject takes a long time to recover and to respond to the stimulus. Following the experiment, the origin of dissociation might be clarified and eventually used for the treatment. Needless to say, the analyst's countertransference feeling remains fundamental for the treatment of dissociation.

It is evident that the treatment of dissociation and the integration of the split-off personalities necessarily led to Jung's definitive parting with Freud and his development of his own vision of the unconscious. It was only after this separation, and the consequent elaboration of the structure of the conscious–unconscious system with their different levels interacting continuously, that the treatment of dissociation would become possible. Dissociation can be a regression to other parts of the self that coexist within the personality, not necessarily only a defensive process. In his early elaboration, Jung relied on his experience at the Burghölzli and on Janet.

Critical issues and developments

The years from 1907 to 1913 were ones of great transition for Jung. In 1907 at the Amsterdam Congress Jung openly acknowledged Janet's contribution to the flourishing field of psychopathology.

In 1913, at the International Conference of Medicine held in London, Janet revisited Jung's methodology of the association experiment and expressed a negative evaluation on it because the subjects under scrutiny were known to Jung or to the experimenter, and therefore the experiment could have no diagnostic value. However, by then Jung was already trying to integrate William James's personal equation into his psychological system. His relation with Freud had ended and he was about to embark on what he defined as his most important experiment, *The Red Book*.

In 1905 Binet and William Stern also criticized Jung's method. These criticisms made Jung revise his protocols of research and he recognized that because the influence of the experimenter on the experiment was "an incalculable factor of variation" (Baynes, 1928, p. 108), the results obtained could not be considered valid. The positivistic science of the time offered no solutions for dealing with the experimenter variable. Jung than resorted to James's notion of the experimenter's personal equation.

The problem of the observer captured Jung's theoretical interests for many years and determined his involvement in quantum physics. Criticism of the association experiment led him to discontinue his research on it for the time being, but he remained open to theories that could include the observer.

Personal equation

Jung adopted James' definition of personal equation as including the psychologist's theoretical preconceptions, his personal acquaintance with the subjects investigated, and his "will to believe."

In 1909 James had given a full report on his involvement in the study of the medium Mrs Piper, including, in the report, his theoretical preconceptions – *the will to believe*. The subjectivity of the psychologist was a critical issue, as Jung had already noted in his experimental research. The effect of Binet's, Janet's, and Stern's critiques made him move towards the inclusion of the personal equation in his research.

James and Jung met personally in 1909 at Clark University, where Jung presented on the association experiment. Théodore Flournoy had facilitated the encounter, as he held Jung in great esteem. These details provide a backdrop to the debate that was at the heart of the early development of the "new psychology," with the many participants who were to become the leading figures of the discipline. In a letter to Flournoy, James described Freud as someone who "made on me personally the impression of a man obsessed with fixed ideas" (James, 1909, p. 326).

Jung's investigation into the inclusion of the experimenter pushed his intuition towards the new physics. The early encounters with Einstein and, many years later, with Pauli, as well as the development in quantum physics of the complementarity principle, inspired the exploration of a new area of the psyche and of matter that only today has come to be considered in greater depth (Atmansprachen & Fuchs, 2014).

Symbols of Transformation and the origin of neurosis

In 1912, Jung was invited for the second time to Fordham University, a Jesuit university in New York City, this time without Freud. Before leaving, he sent Freud his newly published book *Symbols of Transformation* (Jung, 1952), and on the first page he wrote: "laid at the feet of a master from a disobedient but grateful student" (Shamdasani, 2012).

In this text, Jung asserts that neurosis is caused by innate sensitiveness or weakness; we could say, in a certain sense, that Jung is returning to Janet. While *Symbols* could be considered Jung's major work on his theory of neurosis, it also recalls Janet's theory of psychic exhaustion (1975, §519). He clearly states that the sexual paradigm cannot be considered the unique reason for the development of neurosis.

With *Symbols of Transformation* Jung is expressing and giving definitive structure to the opinion he had already outlined in a milder form in the 1906 foreword to *The Psychology of Dementia Preacox*. He definitively refuted Freud's position on the sexual nature of libido, without excluding sexuality. At this point he could freely elaborate on the nature of the unconscious. To him, the unconscious was not a "cauldron" of repressed incestuous desires but rather the source of creativity as well as destructiveness.

Jung presupposes the coexistence of different layers of consciousness and unconsciousness that interact continuously, as he had been asserting since the beginning of his research on complexes more than ten years before. He is also trying to elaborate on how stable consciousness can be.

A delineation of the structure of consciousness–unconsciousness and the different layers of the psyche is a recent acquisition that comes from contemporary neuroscientific research. Jung called psyche what today we call brain–mind system. Hobson, in his research on sleeping and dreaming (Hobson, Pace-Schott, & Stickgold, 2003), specifies that the brain–mind is a unified system whose components interact dynamically to produce continuously changing states. This insight is fundamental in understanding dissociative dynamics.

The structure of consciousness will be the basis of Jung's research on psychological types.

Origin of mental diseases

In the paper "The content of psychoses" (1914, §325/332), Jung questioned the scientific paradigm of his time that saw mental diseases as illnesses of the brain. He gave a statistic on the patients admitted to the Burghölzli in the prior four years and showed that only 9 per cent of this population had brain anomalies that included, using the terminology of the time, imbeciles and the feeble-minded who presented cerebral alterations and malformations of certain parts of the brain. Jung concluded that the anatomical approach missed the point in understanding mental diseases. Future psychiatric understanding, he thought, could only be by way of psychology.

Jung had always been very interested in the study of the brain. At the beginning of his research at the Burghölzli he worked in the anatomy laboratory dissecting brains. His references to the pathology of the brain are therefore accurate. In *Mental disease and the psyche* (1928, §496), Jung cites Janet as the French psychopathologist who settled the question of the organic basis of neurosis.

The Red Book

Between 1913 and 1917 Jung dedicated his attention to what he considered his most important experiment (2009), in which he elaborated on his dreams and unconscious fantasies. He worked on them both verbally and in pictorial form and developed the method of "active imagination." In 1914, at the outbreak of the First World War, Jung began a year-long pause in the writing of *The Red Book* and started a correspondence with Schmid (Jung & Schmid-Guisan, 2013) about introversion and extraversion. Recently published, this correspondence shows that Jung was verifying his hypothesis with somebody he considered extraverted and so the opposite of his own introverted personality type.

In 1917, edited and translated by Constance Long, Jung's book, *Collected Papers on Analytical Psychology* (1917a), was published. Part of this book would later be included in the *Collected Works*. It is very interesting to read the old edition after the publication of *The Red Book*. Jung's journey to the discovery of his personal equation and myth was a transforming experience guided by the creativity of the unconscious that transformed consciousness. From this experience, Jung re-emerged and reformulated his theories. In this first edition of the *Collected Papers* we can see that he is striving to formulate his newly conceived ideas that would reach theoretical maturity in the subsequent years.

"The conception of the unconscious" (1917b), Jung expounds his notions of the *collective mind* representing collective thought, the *collective soul* representing collective feelings, and the *collective psyche* representing the general collective psychological function. To explain these newly coined concepts Jung quotes Janet's *L'Automatisme Psychologique: Essai de Psychologie Expérimentale sur les Formes Inférieures de l'Activité Humaine* (1889), and states:

> To quote P. Janet, the collective psyche contains the "parties inférieurs" of the mental function which being fixed and automatic in its action, inherited and present everywhere, is therefore super-personal or impersonal. The conscious and the personal unconscious contain as personal differentiations the "parties supérieures" of the mental function, therefore the part that has been acquired and developed ontogenetically.
>
> *(1917b, p. 451)*

Consciousness and unconscious

The great theme that captivated the interest of psychologists in the last years of the nineteenth century was ancestral memories. Many had written and elaborated on the ancestral unconscious, and even though these works were often dismissed as unscientific, they nevertheless contributed to the debate on the unconscious.

In his work "The role of the unconscious," published in English in 1918, Jung starts by recognizing the great contributions of Janet and Ribot to the study of the unconscious. One of the main points is the distinction between the personal and supra-personal or collective unconscious.

Ribot had differentiated three levels of the unconscious: the first, called the hereditary or ancestral unconscious; the second, the personal unconscious stemming from coenesthesia; and the third, the personal unconscious containing the residual affective states and events of life. Ribot attributed the effect of transference to unconscious material contained in the third level of the personal unconscious. It was August Forel who introduced Ribot's ideas at the University of Zurich and at the Burghölzli (Shamdasani, 2003).

In "The role of the unconscious" Jung aligns himself with Janet and Ribot in criticizing Freud's unilateral approach to the unconscious. He adds his own observations on the compensatory function of the unconscious and on symbolization. By discussing "when an image is a symbol," Jung places the patient at the centre of the interpretation and not the content, in the tradition of Janet and of many of the psychologists of the French school. His reasoning is that the images coming from the unconscious are not symbolic per se. The analyst's conscious attitude should be open to evaluating the oneiric contents and images, according to the patient's present moment and situation; only after this reflection can the oneiric contents be considered symbolic or non-symbolic. The unconscious symbolic function is, paradoxically, double, as it can reveal or hide its content. This attention to the patients' oneiric productions and symbols comes from Jung's work with psychotic patients whose symbolic function is compromised. In the analytic relationship, the patient's material has to be analyzed in the context of his or her situation.

Jung, of course, elaborated further on the collective unconscious, the archetype, and the psychoid level of the psyche. However, it seems important to mention from where he started.

In *The Master and his Emissary* McGilchrist (2009), in reflecting on the structure of the brain, cites a passage from "The role of the unconscious":

> Just as the human body represents a whole museum of organs, with a long evolutionary history behind them, so we should expect the mind to be organized in a similar way ... We receive along with our body a highly differentiated brain which brings within its entire history, and when it becomes creative it creates out of its history – out of the history of mankind ... that age-old natural history which has been transmitted in living form since the remotest times, namely the history of the brain structure.
>
> *(McGilchrist, 2009, p. 8)*

McGilchrist's aim is to demonstrate, with the support of neuroscientific studies on the structure and interaction of the two hemispheres, that the brain reflects human evolutionary history. He wants to show how the higher functions arose out of the underlying subcortical structure concerned with biological regulation at an unconscious level.

I have cited Jung in this context not to claim any ascendency, but rather to show how these general intuitions were commonly shared in the context of the French School environment, and how Janet and Ribot were profoundly aware of this history.

Jung attributed great importance to the analyst's countertransference feelings. In his praxis, he considered the impact of the personal equation on the analytic relationship as well as the importance of an analytic attitude that can read the oneiric contents as an expression of the patient's needs and pathology.

Dreams

Jung had read Freud's *The Interpretation of Dreams* in 1900; and in January 1901 in a paper entitled "On dreams" he expressed his differences with the Viennese analyst: dreams were not always wish fulfilments; they were frequently undisguised, and the content of dreams was related to the state of consciousness. In 1912, in *Symbols of Transformation* (Jung, 1952), he would return to the differences between himself and Freud and his theorization would remain unaltered.

There are unpublished works where Jung reviewed the literature on dreams with the intention of creating a history of dreams and their interpretation from antiquity to modern times (Shamdasani, 2003). In fact, it was Janet who in 1919 sharply criticized Freud for not considering that the disorders of memory influence the recollection of dreams as well as the narrative on awakening. Janet's evaluation of Freud on dreams was severe and clearly expressed the opinion that Freud had theorized based on partial truths.

Jung's first publication, "On the psychology and pathology of so-called occult phenomena" (1902), was centred on Flournoy's work *From India to the Planet Mars* (1900). In the passages on dreams Jung stated that he did not believe dreams used censorship and he drew attention to Janet's and Binet's emphasis (Shamdasani, 2003) on the relation between dreams and the level of dissociation. He specifically refers to Janet when speaking about hysterical forgetfulness as a significant factor in the genesis of dreams (Jung, 1902).

In *The Psychology of Dementia Praecox*, Jung states: "Dreams are an apperceptive weakness par excellence as it is particularly clear from their predilection for symbols" (1907, p. 26). The reference to Janet is clear. As for the work on occult phenomena, we should not forget that at the time psychology and spiritualism were part of the new interest in understanding the mysterious processes of the mind. In 1898, for example, Janet had already done studies on parapsychological phenomena in dissociation.

Moreover, in "General aspects of dream psychology" (1916/1948), in discussing transference Jung observes:

> Transference is answered by a counter-transference from the analyst when it projects a content of which he is unconscious but which nevertheless exists in him. The counter-transference is then just as useful and meaningful, or as much of a hindrance, as the transference of the patient, according to whether or not it seeks to establish that better rapport which is essential for the realization of certain unconscious contents. Like the transference, the counter-transference is compulsive, a forcible tie, because it creates a 'mystical' or unconscious identity with the object.
>
> *(p. 273)*

In this work first published in 1916 and finally revised in 1948, Jung is well aware of the dangers created by the dynamics played by the unconscious projections activated in the analytic relationship. He ponders at length on the unconscious resistances and on how the analyst has to work to make conscious what is unconscious in him as well as in the other. However, his reference to the compulsiveness and the mystical ties with the object send us back to the conception of the unconscious that he initially elaborated on the model of Janet and Ribot.

The concept of countertransference was elaborated over the course of many years, drawing on the images of the alchemical text *Rosarium Philosophorum* (Jung, 1946), from the formulation of the collective unconscious and from quantum physics, all theories that contained the same initial realization that the experimenter was part of the experiment.

Transference and countertransference are indissoluble aspects of the analytic relationship.

Psychological types and consciousness

Jung first presented his thoughts on types in Munich at the psychoanalytic Congress in 1913. Subsequently, Jung would say that he had been trying to reach for a position that differed from that of Freud and Adler. However, a year later he was analyzing the extreme case of introversion and extraversion in schizophrenia and hysteria and questioning if there really was such a thing as a "normal human type" (Shamdasani, 2003).

In "The content of psychoses," Jung states:

> Introversion and extraversion are dependent on my energetic conception of psychic phenomena. I postulate a hypothetical, fundamental striving which I call libido … libido does not have an exclusively sexual connotation … libido is intended as energetic expression of psychological values.

> The introverted types direct his libido chiefly to his own personality
> ... The extraverted type directs his libido outwards ... The introverted
> sees everything in terms of value of his own personality; the extraverted is
> dependent on the value of the object.
>
> *(1914, p. 190)*

He adds that Freud is decidedly a champion of extraversion and Adler a champion of introversion, which explains why they find it very difficult to understand each other.

Over the years, to the introverted and extraverted psychological types he added the four functions and then further elaborated on the dominant and inferior functions plus the combination of the functions with introversion and extroversion. *Psychological Types* was published in 1921.

In this text, when working on the definition of fantasy as irruption of unconscious contents, Jung refers to Janet and the automatisms that create dissociation. In fact, Jungian typology can be better understood if considered as a self-experience in the process of exploration of different layers of consciousness that also includes the unconscious.

The system of complexes as made of different layers brings with it the idea that images, dreams, and active imagination have to be considered not as ego experiences, that is, the experience of coping with the world, but rather as self-experience. Therefore, typology is an experience of consciousness that includes the unconscious layers.

The psyche is made up of many different layers, and consciousness emerges out of different functions and out of different combinations between functions and the introversion and extraversion typologies. Consciousness, then, emerges out of complexity.

Conclusion

I will conclude with a last citation from Jung himself in which he summarized the evolution of the concept of the complex. In 1957, in his preface to Jolande Jacobi's book, Jung writes:

> This fact, that there are well-characterized and easily recognizable types of complex, suggests that they rest on equally typical foundations, that is, on emotional aptitudes or instincts. In human beings, instincts express themselves in the form of unreflected, involuntary fantasy images, attitudes, and actions, which bear an inner resemblance to one another and yet are identical with the instinctive reactions specific of Homo sapiens. They have a dynamic and a formal aspect. Their formal aspect expresses itself, among other things, in fantasy images that are surprisingly alike and can be found practically everywhere and in all epochs, as might have been expected. Like the instincts, these images have a relatively autonomous character;

that is to say they are 'numinous' and can be found above all in the realm of numinous or religious ideas.

(pp. 532–533)

In more than 50 years the early experimental researches had grown far beyond the initial nucleus. This brief passage summarizes in a nutshell one of the dense concepts in the history of Jungian psychology – the complex and its derivatives. The relatively autonomous character of images and their likeness to the instincts tells us that the early notion of the evolutionary history present in our human body and minds have been developed further. The instincts and the numinosity of religious ideas speak of the psychoid layer of the psyche where matter and psyche meet. This is the new field of synchronistic phenomena that is being explored in parallel with quantum physics.

Note

1 Erasmus, Adagia (move every stone, try everything, leave nothing unattempted).

5

ON NOT TAKING JUST ONE PART OF IT

Janet's influence on object relations theory

Gabriele Cassullo

As far back as 1981, Emanuel Berman – who dedicated his doctoral thesis to multiple personality disorders, and thus anticipated the present renewal of interest in Janet – dealt with the general distrust of psychoanalysts towards Janet's concept of dissociation. Berman showed that, even if Freud's *"anti-Janet* stand" (1981, p. 285) led to an ostracism of theories based on "dissociation," the notion continued to resurface – though often in a covert form – so that in time it has been incorporated into many psychoanalytic theories.

Some few years later, Janet became the "forefather" of a new theoretical trend investigating multiple personality and posttraumatic stress disorder, and reasserting the centrality of dissociative processes of the mind (e.g., see Chapter 1; Nemiah, 1984; Putnam, 1989b; Van der Kolk & van der Hart, 1989). But, this time around, it was Freud's contributions to the field that were dismissed (Gullenstad, 2005).

In the same years, the psychoanalyst Jules Bemporad admitted: "We may have been a bit hasty in burying Janet, and his ghost continues to reappear in very strange guises" (1989, p. 635). And in 1995, Philip Bromberg built on Bemporad's metaphor:

> If one wished to read the contemporary psychoanalytic literature as a serialized Gothic romance, it is not hard to envision the restless ghost of Pierre Janet, banished from the castle by Sigmund Freud a century ago, returning for an overdue haunting of Freud's current descendants. With uncanny commonality, most major schools of analytic thought have become appropriately more responsive to the phenomenon of dissociation, and each in its own way is attempting actively to accommodate it within its model of the mind and its approach to clinical process.
>
> *(1995, p. 189)*

Taking one step back, the reciprocal influence between Janet and Freud had been amply discussed in Ellenberger's *The Discovery of the Unconscious* (1970), which also showed how Janet's shadow hovered over Breuer's conception of *hypnoid states* (Breuer & Freud, 1895, p. 286), Bleuler's and Jung's elaboration of *schizophrenia* and *introversion* (McGuire, 1974, p. 160; Falzeder, 2007, p. 358), and Adler's *inferiority complex*: "an extension" of Janet's *sentiment d'incomplétude* (Adler, 1912, p. vi).

A few years after Ellenberger's study, Claude Prévost (1973a) made one of the most careful analyses of the *querelle* between Janet and Freud. He maintained that the image that Freud and Janet gave of each other was largely based on a "misunderstanding," which "crystallized the reciprocal vision of the two men in a partial or mistaken picture" (p. 65) – a misunderstanding originating in personal rivalry, since both wanted to stand as the heir of Charcot (Pérez-Rincón, 2012), rather than in any theoretical incompatibility.

Sándor Ferenczi

Ferenczi's interest in the work of Janet preceded his encounter with Freud (Cassullo, 2018), and continued all through his life. However, Janet's influence on Ferenczi has hardly been discussed in psychoanalytic journals. One of the reasons is that a number of papers in which Ferenczi credited Janet's work are not available in English. However, they have been included in the Italian edition of Ferenczi's collected works (directly translated from the original Hungarian and German), in which one can count up to 25 entries for Janet, while the English edition does not even list Janet's name in the index, and quotes him fewer than five times.

Be it as it may, even in the years when he was regarded as a "standard bearer" for the Freudian cause, Ferenczi acknowledged Janet's role in "Exploring the unconscious":

> Charcot, Möbius and Janet made it clear that … the human mind is … a most complex structure, of which consciousness shows only the exterior façade, while the true motor forces and mechanisms are to be found in a third dimension, that is, in the depth of the mind behind consciousness. It is true that these scientists … continued to believe that divisibility and disintegration of consciousness is to be found only in a pathological affected mind, which perhaps is congenitally too weak for the necessary synthesis, for integrating the forces of the mind. They did not notice that hysteria only shows in an exaggerated and distorted form what occurs in every human being.
>
> *(1911, p. 309)*

One can recognize the Freudian version of the story. Nevertheless, Ferenczi is among the few Freudians to mention Janet's work as a *sine qua non* for psychoanalysis: "It was only when Charcot and Janet, and later Breuer, ... applied the psychological approach to the study of *hysteria* that those developments brought up by Freud's researches became possible" (1913, p. 2).

In later years, Ferenczi increasingly stressed the relevance of the "exogenous factor" (external trauma) in producing psychopathology, and compared his view to Janet's (1914, p. 134; 1936, p. 133). Particularly, the psychological fragmentation that follows a traumatizing event, with consequent *narrowing of the field of consciousness* (this is a concept of Janet, 1889, 1907b; here mentioned by Ferenczi, 1919, p. 116) and reorganization of the posttraumatic mind in a variable topography in which "dead zones" (e.g. connected to bodily-emotional states) can give way to "overbuilt areas" (e.g. intellectual survival-strategies) (see Ferenczi, 1932a, 1932b).[1] At the same time, Ferenczi continued to follow Freud in assigning a structuring role for the personality to sexual development, as well as to the quality of the early dependency from (today we would say attachment to) caregivers in fostering either a dissociative or a resilient personality, when confronted with stressful and traumatizing events in life (see Dimitrijevic, Cassullo, & Frankel, 2018).

In this regard, we should stress that Janet took the concept of dissociation mainly from the psychiatrist Jacques-Joseph Moreau (nicknamed de Tours) (Janet, 1889, p. 461). The latter observed that "in order to explain madness there must be an *excitation* as a primary fact that generates the phenomena of delusion and *molecular* disaggregation" (p. 461, emphasis in the original). Janet questions the need for this excitation, and prefers to call it "a depression and weakness," a lowering of the individual's mental level or integrative capacity. And at the end of *Psychological Automatism* he returns to this point by asking:

> How a psychologist of Moreau (de Tours)'s standing could ever write such a surprising sentence: 'In becoming an idiot, a subject pass through a psycho-cerebral state which, if it was to continue to develop, would make a man of genius out of him or her'? How could he believe that illnesses of the nervous system and madness itself can strongly promote the development of intelligence? This is probably due to such a term, 'excitation,' which Moreau (de Tours) uses again and again for designating madness. No, no matter what the analogies in external circumstances are, madness and genius are two extreme and opposite terms of the whole psychological development.
>
> *(p. 485)*

Here we come to the great divide between Janet and Freud. Janet put the lower and the higher expressions of the human mind on opposite sides. Conversely, as we also know from his studies on Leonardo and other men of genius, Freud did not. In his model of the mind, psychological misery and genius are not incompatible. Not by chance, Freud started from the very point Moreau (de Tours) underlined (without ever mentioning him), and which Janet refused, that is: *a primary traumatic neural excitation* (occurring in infancy, Freud added). And this is what brought him to his theories on infantile sexuality, drives, the primal scene, and so on, which differentiates his model from Janet's.

Again, Ferenczi combined the two by underlying that there can be a "sudden, surprising rise of new faculties after a trauma," which he named "traumatic progression" (1932a, p. 229), but at the cost of the general integration of the personality and of the capacity of the ego to tolerate or regulate further excitations without falling apart (dissociating). By postulating that dissociation is the result of a *weakness of the ego* (Janet) in regulating *excitations* coming from bodily and/ or environmental sources (Freud), Ferenczi, thus, paved the way for Fairbairn's object relations theory.

Ronald Fairbairn

The Scottish psychoanalyst Ronald Fairbairn is widely known for his reformulation of Freud's libido theory in terms of "a theory of development based ... upon object-relations" (1941, p. 31). His motto was "libido is not primarily pleasure seeking, but object seeking" (1946, p. 137). In doing so, he opened the way for subsequent relational orientations, all based on the assumption that the individual's search for "simple tension-relieving implies some failure of object-relationships" (p. 140). Yet Fairbairn was also one of the first major theoreticians of psychoanalysis to break the ostracism against Janet and to propose a systematic integration of Janet's and Freud's models of the mind (Davies, 1998).

Fairbairn's interest in Janet dates back to his doctoral thesis in Medicine, titled "Dissociation and repression" (Fairbairn, 1929). However, in the following ten years he put Janet aside and dived deep into the Freudian libido theory, so that there is no further record of Janet's name in his essays during this period.

It was only in 1940 that Fairbairn's early interest in Janet's studies of dissociative processes resurfaced. This is because Ferenczi's original mixture of Freud and Janet had landed in Scotland through the work of the psychiatrist Ian Suttie (Cassullo, 2010, 2014). As Clarke (2011) recently demonstrated, Suttie had a *direct* impact on Fairbairn from 1940 onward. Therefore, Suttie's belief (echoing Ferenczi's) that the dissociation of mental states that are – or better, should have been – connected to the traumatic aspects of infantile dependency is to be considered as the *main disposition* to psychopathology and social maladjustment, is at the very root of Fairbairn's (1940) influential study on schizoid phenomena, which launched a subsequent reformulation of Freud's libido theory in terms of "a theory of development based essentially upon object-relations" (Fairbairn, 1941, p. 31).

Unfortunately, a difficulty in recognizing Janet's influence on object relations theory arose from Fairbairn's use of the term *splitting* instead of *dissociation*. Yet, apparently, Fairbairn made no distinction between the two:

> A theory of the personality based upon the conception of splitting of the ego would appear to be more fundamental than one based upon Freud's conception of the repression of impulses by an unsplit ego. The theory

which I now envisage is, of course, obviously adapted to explain such extreme manifestations as are found in cases of multiple personality; but, as Janet has pointed out, these extreme manifestations are only exaggerated examples of the dissociation phenomena characteristic of hysteria.

(1952, p. 159)

The specific concept of splitting of the personality was, of course, one originally introduced by Bleuler to explain the phenomena of schizophrenia; but, in my opinion, there is no fundamental distinction between the process of hysterical dissociation, to which Janet drew attention, and that splitting of the ego which is now recognized as a characteristic feature of schizoid states.

(1953, pp. 14–15)

In fact, Janet's dissociation had *directly* influenced Bleuler in his development of the classical concept of splitting (in German *Spaltung*) in schizophrenia (cf. Chapter 9; Moskowitz & Heim, 2011). The reason why Fairbairn used the word "splitting" instead of dissociation is that he wanted to address the same psychopathological entity that Bleuler identified with his definition of schizophrenia, and which Fairbairn dynamically explained by his concepts of "schizoid mechanisms" and the "schizoid position." Melanie Klein was to rely on the same concepts when she formulated her influential theory of the "paranoid-schizoid position":

[Fairbairn] calls the earliest phase the 'schizoid position' and states that it forms part of normal development and is the basis for adult schizoid and schizophrenic illness. I agree with this contention and consider his description of developmental schizoid phenomena as significant and revealing, and of great value for our understanding of schizoid behavior and of schizophrenia.

(Klein, 1946, p. 100)

When this paper was first published in 1946, I was using my term "paranoid position" synonymously with W.R.D. Fairbairn's "schizoid position". On further deliberation, I decided to combine Fairbairn's term with mine … using the expression "paranoid-schizoid position."

(Klein, 1952, p. 293)

Later on, Klein and Fairbairn developed their own models of the mind: a more drive-oriented one in Klein's description; a more relation-oriented one in Fairbairn's. Nevertheless, the shadow of Janet and of his studies on dissociative processes stands at the roots of both.

Finally, in a remarkable summary of his ideas titled "Observations on the nature of hysterical states" (1953) Fairbairn gave his last word about Janet, Freud, and their influence on object relations theory. He starts by recognizing Janet's achievement, not only in identifying hysteria as a recognizable clinical state, but mainly in trying to provide an explanation of the genesis of the phenomena displayed by his hysterical patients by formulating his classical concept of "dissociation."

From the standpoint of this concept, the hysterical state is essentially due to inability on the part of the ego to hold all the functions of the personality together, with the result that certain of these functions become dissociated from, and lost to, the rest of the personality and, having passed out of the awareness and control of the ego, operate independently. The extent of the dissociated elements was described by Janet as varying within wide limits, so that sometimes what was dissociated was an isolated function such as the use of a limb, and sometimes a large area or large areas of the psyche (as in cases of dual and multiple personality); and the occurrence of such a dissociation was attributed to the presence of a certain weakness of the ego – a weakness partly inherent, and partly induced by circumstances such as illness, trauma, or situations imposing a strain upon the individual's capacity for adaptation (Fairbairn, 1953, p. 13).

Then Fairbairn introduces what has become the classical distinction between dissociation and repression, which he had already discussed in his doctoral thesis (1929). Dissociation is "a passive process," "a process of disintegration due to a failure on the part of the cohesive function normally exercised by the ego" (1953, p. 13). Instead, Freud's repression is an "active process."[2] Why? Because what Freud took from his visit to Charcot, in Paris, was a specific interest in the phenomena of the "hysterical counter-will": that is, a behaviour of the subject that runs against his or her conscious motivations. In other words, on his return from Paris, Freud was already developing a rudimentary theory about resistance, repression, unconscious conflict between drive and defence, and even dream-work. This theory undoubtedly relied on the work of Charcot and Janet (Freud's denial about this appears today quite specious), but went beyond it.

> Can it be a matter of chance that attacks in young people of whose 'good upbringing and manners' Charcot speaks highly take the form of ravings and abusive language? This is no more the case, I think, than the familiar fact that the hysterical deliria of nuns revel in blasphemies and erotic pictures. In this we may suspect a connection that allows us a deep insight into the mechanism of hysterical states. There emerges in hysterical deliria material in the shape of ideas and impulses to action which the subject in his healthy state has rejected and inhibited, often by a great psychical effort. Something similar holds true of a number of dreams, which spin out further associations that have been rejected or broken off during the day. I have based on this fact the theory of 'hysterical counter-will' which embraces a good number of hysterical symptoms.
>
> *(Freud, 1892, p. 138)*

In Freud's view, if counter-will takes "a great psychical effort," it must be "an active force." He would later call this force *resistance*, as it paralleled and opposed the efforts he was making in order to hypnotize and cure his patients. In Fairbairn's view, this is what Freud initially added to Janet's edifice: no matter how traumatized, weakened, depressed the ego of the patient may appear, a part of it fights, and with great energy, against therapy and the therapist itself (Fairbairn, 1953, p. 14).[3] Fairbairn imagined it as a split-off "internal saboteur" (1953), born out of introjection of the traumatizing aspects – way too exciting or too rejecting – of reality. "Be this as it may," as Fairbairn (1953) writes:

> it was to explain the resistance that Freud postulated the process of repression; and, since resistance is an active process, it was as an inherently active process that repression was conceived by Freud. It is largely for this reason that the concept of repression has come to supersede that of dissociation. For ... it lends itself ... to providing the basis for a comprehensive investigation of the dynamics of the personality; and, in actual fact, it is the foundation-stone upon which the whole explanatory system represented by psychoanalytical theory has been built. At the same time, I must record the opinion that the eclipse of the concept of dissociation ... has not been altogether an unmixed gain. According to Janet, as we have seen, the dissociative process characterizing hysteria was a manifestation of ego-weakness; and, although it did not take Freud long to recognize that hysterical symptoms were the product of a defense springing from weakness of the ego, the presence of such a weakness is not inherent in the concept of repression as such.
>
> *(p. 14)*

In other words, the weaker the ego is, the harder it has to fight in order to protect its weakness. And it may do so, according to Fairbairn, by a particular kind of splitting of the personality, which is called repression. It is not true that Freud did not touch on these aspects, as he did so in his theory on narcissism, and later on by developing an ego psychology within the structural model framework (Fairbairn, 1953, p. 15). But such a theory was never fully integrated with the initial drive–defence model and, in my view, this largely happened as a consequence of Freud's refusal to acknowledge Janet's contribution on dissociation, in order to keep his own model sharply distinguished from the latter's. Nevertheless, Freud could not avoid returning again and again to the trauma–dissociation problem, until the very end of his life. In fact, in 1937–1938 he wrote:

> The aetiology of every neurotic disturbance is, after all, a mixed one. It is a question either of the instincts being excessively strong – that is to say, recalcitrant to taming by the ego – or of the effects of early (i.e., premature) traumas which the immature ego was unable to master.
>
> *(1937, p. 220)*

The traumata … concern impressions of a sexual and aggressive nature and also early injuries to the self (injuries to narcissism).

(1938, p. 120)

All these phenomena [of traumatic origin], the symptoms as well as the restrictions of personality and the lasting changes in character, display the characteristic of compulsiveness; that is to say, they possess great psychical intensity, they show a far-reaching independence of psychical processes that are adapted to the demands of the real world and obey the laws of logical thinking. They are not influenced by outer reality or not normally so; they take no notice of real things, or the mental equivalents of these, so that they can easily come into active opposition to either. They are as a state within the state, an inaccessible party, useless for the common weal; yet they can succeed in overcoming the other, the so-called normal, component and in forcing it into their service. If this happens then the sovereignty of an inner psychical reality has been established over the reality of the outer world; the way to insanity is open.

(1938, pp. 123–124)

A "state within a state," an "inaccessible party." Those are all metaphors that clearly display a dissociative personality structure, rather than an inhibited-repressing one. Many psychoanalysts have witnessed in their daily work dissociative phenomena, and some of them, such as Ferenczi and Fairbairn, wanted to acknowledge this by integrating it within psychoanalytic theory. As I have tried to describe, object relations theory was born out of these attempts.

Conclusion

I touched on the *querelle* between Janet and Freud in order to argue that their rivalry fostered clinical and theoretical advances when the ideas of the other were included in one's own frame of reference, whereas it produced "developmental arrests" in the field when they were excluded.

I then argued that, despite Freud's "*anti-Janet* stand" (Berman, 1981, p. 285), Ferenczi started the first attempt at a *theoretical synthesis* of the models of Janet's and Freud's in psychoanalysis. This was developed further by Suttie (1935) and led to the foundation of a more effective theoretical systematization, reached by Fairbairn, which we call now the object relations theory.

Notes

1 As van der Hart (unpublished) underlines, "while Janet (1909b) emphasized that the vehement emotions involved in traumatic experiences produce their disintegrating effects in proportion to their intensity, duration and repetition, Ferenczi … formulated this insight even more clearly in terms of trauma-generated dissociation of the personality." Ferenczi observed that "[i]f the shocks increase in number during the

development of the child, the number and the various kinds of splits in the personality increase too, and soon it becomes extremely difficult to maintain contact without confusion with all the fragments each of which behaves as a separate personality yet does not know of even the existence of the others. Eventually it may arrive at a state which – continuing the picture of fragmentation – one would be justified in calling *atomization*. One must possess a good deal of optimism not to lose courage when facing such a state, though I hope even here to be able to find threads that can link up the various parts" (1932a, p. 229, emphasis in the original). For further comparisons between Janet and Ferenczi, see: van der Hart, Nijenhuis & Steele, 2006; Howell, 2005; Howell & Itzkowitz, 2016.

2   This makes Janet the forefather of "deficit theories," as Freud is for "conflict theories." However, this distinction follows more our need for clear-cut definitions (and for keeping the traditions of Janet's and Freud's separated) than the reality of things. In Fairbairn's theory, in fact, "repression and splitting of the ego represent simply two aspects of the same fundamental process" (1953, p. 15).

3   Ferenczi would call it a part of the personality that *identified with the aggressor* (1932a). His discussion of *introjective mechanisms* – which dates back to his first psychoanalytic contribution (1909) – made him a forerunner of object relations theory and a precursor of Fairbairn's view of the "introjection of the bad object" (Clarke, 2014), that is, of its unsatisfying or even damaging aspects. In his last and decisive paper "Confusion of tongues" (1932a), Ferenczi observed: "Through the identification, or let us say, introjection of the aggressor, … [the traumatizing external element] becomes intra- instead of extra-psychic; the intra-psychic is then subjected, in a dream-like state as is the traumatic trance, to the primary process, i.e. according to the pleasure principle it can be modified or changed by the use of positive or negative hallucinations. In any case the attack as a rigid external reality ceases to exist and in the traumatic trance the [subject] succeeds in maintaining the previous situation" (p. 228).

6

FROM JANET TO BROMBERG, VIA FERENCZI

Standing in the spaces of the literature on dissociation

Clara Mucci, Giuseppe Craparo, and Vittorio Lingiardi

As Henri Ellenberger (1970) wrote, Pierre Janet's work may be compared to a great city buried under the ashes, similar to Pompeii, a place that one day might be rediscovered and brought back to life again. This has been in several respects Janet's destiny: his corpus has signified a vital transplant of ideas and discoveries that have influenced the contemporary discourse on several pathologies, and most especially on dissociation. A similar destiny awaited Sándor Ferenczi, who after decades of obscurity has now influenced and informed contemporary psychoanalytic views of trauma and dissociation, not least with his concept of identification with the aggressor on the part of the victim of violence and his therapeutic approach as it appears in his *Clinical Diary* (1932b).

Between the end of the nineteenth century and the first decades of the twentieth, Janet paved the way for a view of a mental malfunctioning resulting from severe traumatization that we now understand as dissociation. Freud, Janet, and Ferenczi are depositories of views of trauma theory, repression, and dissociation that reciprocally complete each other only recently we have begun to integrate. What still remains to be clarified is why, if dissociation itself had been described as a psychopathological root in *Studies on Hysteria* (Breuer & Freud, 1895), Freud decided to leave aside this finding and to propose repression as the cause of mental illness. As regards the work of Janet and Ferenczi, it is on the terrain of trauma theory and therapeutic practice that their relevance stands out, a realm in which contemporary tragic events linked to wars, genocides, child abuse and neglect, etc. have led to further investigation.

Our contribution situates itself in this trend of reevaluation of two eminent pioneers of psychological and psychoanalytic thought and practice. Janet and Ferenczi have allowed contemporary psychoanalysis to reincorporate the dissociative elements in the functioning of any psychic structure and to stress the importance of working with these parts in therapy in a reciprocal process of regulation, as highlighted by Philip Bromberg (1998, 2006) and further explicated by recent neuroscientific developments (Schore, 2012; Schumpf et al., 2014).

The relevance of Janet's and Ferenczi's contributions is fully acknowledged by the Psychodynamic Diagnostic Manual (PDM-2) (Lingiardi & McWilliams, 2017, 2015), an international resource grounded in psychodynamic clinical models and theories, and explicitly oriented towards case formulation and treatment planning. According to PDM-2, over the last decades "clinicians and researchers have resumed the study of trauma and dissociation that had largely been eclipsed by the Freudian concept of repression" (Lingiardi & McWilliams, 2017, p. 182), "Janet has been 'rediscovered'" (p. 200), and "psychodynamic authors have approached dissociative psychopathology from many different starting points" (p. 200). Contemporary psychoanalysts have in fact

> returned to the teachings of Janet and Ferenczi for the prevalence of trauma-related distress, developmental impact, and psychopathology in a wide variety of traumatized populations, including combat veterans but extending to concentration camp survivors and their offspring, victims of childhood physical, sexual, and emotional abuse and neglect, and victims of terror, torture, displacement, refugee status, and human trafficking.
>
> *(p. 182)*

"Standing in the spaces" of psychoanalysis at the turn of the century, Janet and Ferenczi have clearly contributed to what only now we are starting to appreciate in full. Only recently have Janet's major works been reprinted in French and appeared in English and in Italian for the first time; while Ferenczi's *Clinical Diary*, written in 1932 and containing his most revealing ideas about trauma, "fragmentation" (his word for dissociation), and therapy, was published (both in French and in English) only in the late 1980s, after several detours (Bonomi, 2017).

Janet (1889), with his concept of *désagrégation psychologique* stemming from overwhelmingly stressful events, points to an understanding of severe mental illness, closer to present views of both trauma and dissociation (see Masud Kahn on cumulative trauma, 1963; Van der Kolk, 1996; Van der Kolk & der Hart, 1989; van der Hart, Nijenhuis, & Steele, 2006; Bromberg, 1998, 2006). Emphasizing the importance of the early relationships for the child and of any traumatic factors in the upbringing and the environment created for him or her by family dynamics, Ferenczi (1932b) also hinted at the destructive outcome of traumatization resulting in "fragmentation" of the immature psyche and the possible subsequent identification with the aggressor, resulting in "splits" in personality.

Not by chance, early relational trauma as misattunement between child and caregiver, or even severe neglect and abuse (in a continuum of severity) of children, are currently seen as etiological factors for future mental and organic pathology (see Schore, 1994; 2003; Cozolino, 2002; Fonagy & Target, 2003; Liotti & Farina, 2011; Lyons-Ruth & Jakobvitz, 2008).

Early traumatization and abuse in family relationships protracted over time are likely to leave a vulnerability, not only for possible subsequent development of dissociative disorders, borderline pathologies, posttraumatic stress disorders, somatoform disorders, substance abuse, and alcoholism but also for organic illnesses, such as, among others, coronary, circulatory and heart problems as well as liver and immunological diseases, as the epidemiological research carried out in the US since the 1990s on ACE (Adverse Childhood Experiences) has highlighted (see Felitti & Anda, 1997, 2010).

Repression versus dissociation: Freud and Ferenczi

A century ago Freud (1915) stated:

> We have learned from psychoanalysis that the essence of the process of repression lies, not in putting an end to, in annihilating, the idea that represents an instinct, but in preventing it from becoming conscious. When this happens, we say of the idea that it is in a state of being 'unconscious,' and we can produce good evidence *to show that even when it is unconscious it can produce effects*, even including some which finally reach consciousness … *Everything that is repressed must remain unconscious*; but let us state at the very outset that *the repressed does not cover everything that is unconscious. The unconscious has the wider compass: the repressed is a part of the unconscious.*
>
> *(pp. 166–167, emphasis added)*

In this passage, Freud clearly states that the repressed and the unconscious are not one and the same thing: the repressed is only a part of the unconscious (and is precisely what has undergone repression), and a wider area has to be defined as un-conscious, meaning, non-conscious, the effects of which are felt in behaviour and attitudes in human beings and can retrospectively be reconstructed or, as Freud says, "translated" back to consciousness. While this statement might help us understand that there is a part of the unconscious that is not repressed, for example, "un-repressed" and yet unconscious, as Mauro Mancia highlighted over a decade ago (Mancia, 2006), linking the "unrepressed unconscious" to what contemporary neuroscience includes under the rubric of implicit memory, leaves open the question of what constitutes the part of the unconscious (*Ucs*) that, not being repressed, nonetheless possesses the features of the *Ucs*. Does this part belong to the "dissociated"? Does it consist of that which is not intentionally repressed but which is nonetheless split off from consciousness because it is unbearable?

Repression, on the contrary, for Freud has to do with an active decathexis of material or contents that have undergone a process of repression by a more mature subject, a defence, Freud argued, initiated intentionally and subsequently forgotten: "the essence of repression lies simply in turning something away, and keeping it at a distance, from the conscious" (Freud, 1915, p. 147).

On several occasions in *Studies on Hysteria* (Breuer & Freud, 1895), the existence of dissociation is posited and described. Only in subsequent writings did Freud erase his view of dissociation as the early response of an overwhelmed young subject (a response we now understand as encoded in implicit memory[1]) in favour of a voluntary form of repression, implying an older, more mature subject (what would be, in our contemporary language, encoded and subsequently rejected by explicit memory).

In "Sketches for the 'preliminary communication' of 1893" (1892), written right before *Studies on Hysteria*, Freud argued (in point 3) that the memory creating the content of hysterical attacks is a "second state of consciousness" (p. 151). It is absent from the memory of the patient, but if he or she succeeds in carrying this memory through to consciousness the capacity to evoke an attack ceases. In point 4 he adds that the problem of the origin of the content of the memory in hysterical attacks is closely aligned with the question of what conditions are normally present when an event is admitted into the "second state of consciousness." If the event is deliberately forgotten, this physical activity is transformed into a hysterical attack.

In "On the psychical mechanism of hysterical phenomena: preliminary communication" (Freud, 1893), we read:

> each individual hysterical symptom immediately and permanently disappeared when we had succeeded in bringing clearly to light the memory of the event by which it was provoked and in arousing its accompanying affect, and when the patient had described that event in the greatest possible detail and had put the affect into words.
>
> *(p. 57)*

> Again the "intentional aspect" is explained as follows: "it was a question of things which the patient wished to forget, and *therefore intentionally repressed*, from his conscious thought and inhibited and suppressed" (p. 61, emphasis added). And the author goes on: "The second group of conditions are determined not *by the physical states in which the patient received the experiences in question.*"
>
> *(emphasis added)*

Very clearly Freud talked of a "splitting in consciousness" in the case of Miss Lucy R. in *Studies on Hysteria*, but for him what causes the split in consciousness (originating hysterical symptoms) is an "intentional act":

> The actual traumatic moment, then, is the one at which *the incompatibility forces itself upon the ego and at which the latter decides on the repudiation of the incompatible idea. That idea is not annihilated by a repudiation of this kind, but merely repressed into the unconscious.* When this process occurs for the first time there comes into being a nucleus and centre of crystallization for the

formation of a psychical group divorced from the ego – a group around which everything which would imply an acceptance of the incompatible idea subsequently collects. *The splitting of consciousness in these cases of acquired hysteria is accordingly a deliberate and intentional one. At least one is often introduced by an act of volition; for the actual outcome is something different from what the subject intended.* What he wanted was to do away with an idea, as though it had never appeared, but all he succeeds in doing is to isolate it psychically.

(*Breuer & Freud, 1895, p. 188, emphasis added*)

Here Freud hints at a "splitting in consciousness" as a reaction to trauma but he also posits an intentional desire to erase the disturbing idea that as a consequence has become repressed and has created a symptom in its turn. In place of a memory that is repressed, a symptom is created, something embedded in the body. This seems the point at which "splitting in consciousness" and "repression" as traumatic concepts are conflated in the symptom formation of a hysterical woman. It is evident that the "splitting of consciousness" he described does not arise from the immaturity of the overwhelmed psyche.

It is important to note that the distinction between a state in which the subject intentionally represses an idea or content (and is therefore in a more mature state) and a state in which the subject undergoes the traumatic process that leads to symptoms instead of memories because of immaturity and fragility is already there: the two ways of reacting to a traumatizing event – repression with intentional processes implying the subject's effort, and dissociation, implying (besides the implicit memory encoding we now understand) an overwhelming bodily reaction – are something Freud considered but decided to leave aside and exclude from his future theorization on trauma.

Historically, the path of splitting, or rather dissociation or fragmentation, would have been the pathological reaction described by Janet as a response to the traumatic shock or by Ferenczi when he talks about fragmentation of the personality. Here is his famous entry on "Fragmentation" in his *Clinical Diary* (1932b):

A child is the victim of overwhelming aggression, which results in 'giving up the ghost,' ... with the firm conviction that this self-abandonment (fainting) means death. However, it is precisely this complete relaxation induced by self-abandonment that may create more favorable conditions for him to endure the violence. ... Therefore, someone who has 'given up the ghost' survives this death physically and with a part of his energy begins to live again; he even succeeds in reestablishing unity with the pre-traumatic personality, although this is usually accompanied by memory lapses and retroactive amnesia of varying duration. But this amnesic piece is actually a part of the person, who is still 'dead,' or exists permanently in the agony of anxiety. The task of the analysis is to remove this split.

(*p. 39*)

The extraordinary accuracy of this description of the dissociative traumatic reaction, which might even result in a fainting of the body, a freezing response, has been confirmed by neurophysiological findings, for example the vasovagal response leading to lightheadedness, confusion and unconsciousness (compatible with the "retraction of the field of consciousness," as described by Janet, 1907b; Porges, 2011). More than a defence, and certainly not an intentional or even partially intentional defence, the neurophysiology of trauma describes an integrative failure of mental and psychical resources as a response to the external overwhelming experience, more than an intrapsychic defence at work (Liotti, 2006; van der Hart, Nijenhuis, & Steele, 2006).

In another revealing passage, Ferenczi (1932b) describes how the overwhelming experience leaves a permanent mark and results in a splitting in the personality, and ultimately in a change in the victim's behaviour:

> From the moment when bitter experience teaches us to lose faith in the benevolence of the environment, *a permanent split in the personality occurs.* ... Actual trauma is experienced by children in situations where no immediate remedy is provided and where adaptation, that is, a change in their own behavior, is forced on them – *the first step towards establishing the differentiation between inner and outer world, subject and object. From then on, neither subjective nor objective experience alone will be perceived as an integral emotional unit* ...
>
> *(p. 69, emphasis added)*

As a consequence of trauma, the child adapts his or her behavior to the environment, and in this way a permanent cognitive distortion and a twist in personality are initiated. For Ferenczi, trauma also bears the traces of an external, overwhelming interpersonal experience that has become internalized, intrapsychic, but maintains an interpersonal force in so far as the relationship with the external world is concerned – a sort of IWM ("internal working model") in Bowlby's (1969) terms, or a representation, a system similar to Bucci's (1997) symbolic and sub-symbolic communications. Moreover, what Ferenczi stressed in his trauma theory and its clinical implications is that the child will very likely internalize the aggressiveness and the dissociated sense of guilt of the persecutor (which are also extremely important elements for future pathology).

Anticipating Ferenczi's traumatic and dissociative model, Janet emphasized the idea that at the basis of pathological hysteria lay a *désagrégation psychologique* or dissociation of the personality that was the contrary of that synthetic and integrated superior function in which higher levels of consciousness rested (1889, 1907b).[2] For Janet an environmental trauma, not necessarily a sexual trauma, had arrested the cognitive and affective development of the subject and caused the "retraction of the field of consciousness" so typical of the traumatic effect. Several studies by Janet stressed the relevance of environmental conditions, or primary relations as we would call them today. As Giovanni Liotti has clearly underlined in a recent reconsideration of Janet's critique of Freud's assumptions:

Janet's idea that the pathological response to psychological trauma, once the above-mentioned vulnerability has been posited, is the passive consequence of the overwhelming emotion over the superior forces of consciousness (namely, that it is a functional deficit induced by the traumatic memory), is clearly opposed to Freud's idea that pathology depends on an active defence on behalf of the ego aiming at excluding uncanny emotions and representations from consciousness.

(2014a, p. 32, translated)

In underlining the deliberate and intentional defence of repression of an idea (and a memory), which creates in turn a symptom rooted in the compromise formation between the repressed idea and the pain of the unacceptability of the idea to consciousness, Freud opened the road to a psychoanalysis (as opposed to Janet's "psychological analysis") in which the more mature intrapsychic reaction is emphasized over the collapse of a dissociated and divided body. In Freud's theorization, the libido system and the drive were to prevail over the relational, intersubjective, environmentally determined quality of the mind–body system (all elements that subsequent interdisciplinary studies on how the subject is born have supported, as is evident from studies in infant research, attachment, and interpersonal neurobiology or regulation theory).

In addition, in describing a theoretical system that privileges the way the ego responds with defensive strategies as a way to protect itself, Freud creates a top-down model that modern neuroscience seems to have replaced with a bottom-up model, as in Porges's findings: the response goes from the bottom – from the stem – to the cortex, which is rather dysfunctional in its response (Liotti, 2014a, p. 35; Porges, 2011).

As a consequence of this Freudian attitude, the pathology that Freud studied and treated was more likely to be of a neurotic and less severe type than the severely traumatized patients Janet and Ferenczi were willing to treat. This is also why the dissociative road to pathology is more in line with present-day severe borderline pathologies. As Allan Schore notes:

Freud's idea about trauma must be reassessed (Van der Kolk, Weisaeth, & van der Hart, 1996) and … the concept of dissociation must be reincorporated into theoretical and clinical psychoanalysis. It is now clear that dissociation represents the most primitive defense against traumatic affective states and that it must be addressed in the treatment of severe psychopathologies.

(2003, p. 246)

The contribution of Pierre Janet

In *L'Automatisme Psychologique*, Janet (1889) posited the so-called *désagrégation psychologique* as the basis of hysterical pathology and the phenomenon he calls "automatism," which contrasts with the crucial *synthetic or integrative function* that characterizes mental health. Janet believed that some hysterical symptoms depend on the existence of subsystems of the personality dissociated from personal consciousness, working and living autonomously, with their origin going back to the past and specifically to traumatizing events.

Janet attributed a central role to environmental trauma, especially when it takes place during critical moments of affective and cognitive development. The trauma need not be especially sexual in nature, as in Freud's first writing, but it results in the dissociation and disorganization of the personality of the individual. As a consequence, the encoding of the overwhelming event is impossible and leads to the development of those "fixed ideas," often corresponding to "frozen emotions"; they are due to sudden or terrorizing shocks and are rigidly excluded from personal consciousness. These traumatic memories, if repeated during the developmental phases, or if particularly intense in their nature, may be pushed outside of the flux of personal consciousness to the point of creating secondary dissociated personalities (called "subsequent existences"). These psychological groups generally reemerge suddenly and intensely. Another feature of hysterical symptoms is, in fact, the automatic and intrusive reactivation of traumatic memories that have contributed to the formation of the symptoms themselves (1928a).

"Psychological analysis" (compared to Freudian "psychoanalysis"), for example, the method that Janet theorized for the analysis and treatment of the phenomenon of automatism in hysterical patients, therefore leads to the revelation of the traumatizing event behind his or her subconscious fixed ideas and their symptoms. These subconscious fixed ideas are at the same time causes and effects of a mental weakness or "psychological poverty" and tend to change very slowly; hysterical crises are almost "masked performances" of these subconscious ideas, and these disorders seem to transform subjects into real "living statues." Bringing those subconscious ideas back to consciousness is not a sufficient condition for the resolution of a trauma-generated mental disorder (a similar statement was made by Ferenczi and is nowadays considered more and more relevant in contemporary relational approaches; Ellenberger, 1970). Finally, for Janet, a "narrowing of the field of consciousness" seems to be one of the two fundamental characteristics of these patients, different from psychologically healthy people, in whom the creative activity of consciousness tends to be associated with the active "synthesis" of memories and sensations linked to the experience of selfhood and, therefore, to an integrated construction of identity and personality.

In a subsequent study, *L'État Mental des Hystériques* (1893a, 1894b), Janet argued once again that hysteria can be conceptualized as a mental disorder essentially derived from the lack or perturbations of the function of psychological synthesis, which underlies even more clearly those symptoms now called "dissociative," so that the resultant environmental dysfunction may be traced back to such impairments in the developmental process. Later on, in *L'Évolution Psychologique de la Personnalité* (1929a), Janet discussed the theme in its extreme consequences, suggesting that this lack of synthesis and personal coherence might depend on the primary relationships of the child that basically affect the course and development of his or her sense of individuality. The relevance of the social component is underlined on several occasions in the work. According to Janet, all superior psychological functions, such as thought, will, or memory, evolve as a reflex and as a consequence of social influence on the individual.

In other studies, Janet (1898a, 1903, 1909a) extends his reflections beyond the field of classical hysteria, including the description of outpatients in his clinical exemplifications. In these studies, hysteria is considered as distinct from another category of disorders, *psychasthenia*, which includes a great number of neurotic disorders, such as obsessions and phobias. In contrast to hysteria, in these conditions fixed ideas may also be conscious (Ellenberger, 1970). These works bear witness to the important evolution of Janet's thought in comparison to *L'Automatisme Psychologique*, where the author assumed just two levels of functioning of the consciousness: the function of synthesis and the automatic one. In explaining psychasthenia, however, Janet refers to a wider theoretical system, where consciousness is at the top of the integrative function. In addition to the concept of synthesis, he introduces both the notion of *presentification*, that is, the active capacity of the mind to concentrate on the present moment without confusing itself with past memories (Janet, 1928b), and the so-called *fonction du réel* ("function of the real"), which consists of the capacity of the mind to act on external objects and on reality, modifying them according to the aims of the subject.

Janet's topicality

The primacy that Janet assigned to creative activity and the integrative functions of consciousness has important connections with some contemporary models, in particular, with developments in trauma theory and models of dissociation. The description of the *fonction du réel*, for instance, implies not only a relationship with the social environment but also an awareness and attention to inner states and to one's own beliefs, as well as to those of others; this function additionally expresses an individual's capacity for self-determination and contributes to the development of the personality (van der Hart et al., 2006). We can identify some analogies between this notion and the function conceptualized as *mentalization*, which refers to the ability to understand interpersonal behaviour in terms of mental states, a capacity acquired through primary attachment relations (Fonagy & Target, 2003, p. 339). It implies both a self-reflective and an interpersonal component, which is fundamental in the organization of the self and in affective regulation (see also Liotti & Farina, 2011). If difficulties occur in primary relationships, the individual may undergo a disorganized development, to the point of experiencing some parts as "alien" or as not really belonging to the self (Fonagy & Bateman, 2005). The establishing of an "*alien self*" may provoke a fragmentation in the continuity of the subject if there are subsequent traumatic experiences within the family or during crucial stages of growth, so that a healthy development of the reflective function is weakened. This process becomes the pathological nucleus in some features of the border-line personalities (Bateman & Fonagy, 2015; Fonagy et al., 2014; Liotti, 2014b; Liotti & Gilbert, 2011).

Within the wide corpus of theories and research studies on attachment, our discussion will give a particular relevance to the hypotheses of Giovanni Liotti (2006; Liotti & Farina, 2011) on trauma and on dissociative development. A connection seems to exist between disorganized attachment in the child and the development of a vulnerability to future disorders, if protective or reparatory factors do not occur in one's experience. Disorganized attachment can be described as a breakdown of behavioural strategies due to the unresolved conflict between contradictory views both of the caregiver (as a source of protection and danger at the same time) and of the self (Main & Hesse, 1990). Disorganized attachment has received increased attention, especially thanks to the studies of Lyons-Ruth and colleagues (see Lyons-Ruth et al., 1991; Lyons-Ruth, Bronfman, & Parsons, 1999; Lyons-Ruth & Jacobvitz, 2008). This attachment category seems to be more frequent when the caregiver suffers from unresolved trauma, mourning, depression, substance abuse, or personality disorders (Carlson & Sroufe, 1995; Main, 1995; Main & Morgan, 1996).

According to Liotti (2006), trauma, dissociation, and disorganization in attachment constitute three aspects of a single psychopathological process. It seems inevitable that reference be made here to what Bowlby (1969) defined as internal working models (IWMs), structures of memories and expectations that develop on the basis of different attitudes of the attachment figures in respond-ing to the requests of the child. In other words, by the end of the first year of life, IWMs are modeled through the interaction between child and caregiver, which are first stored in the implicit memory circuits and later organized into semantic, explicit memories that can be narrated. Particularly important is the IWM of disorganized attachment, which can be conceptualized as a pattern strictly related to dissociative responses to traumatizing events (Cassidy & Mohr, 2001; Liotti & Farina, 2011). The development of a disorganized IWM, estab-lishing multiple, incoherent, and non-integrated (dissociated) perceptions of the self and others, seems to be connected to the simultaneous (and incompatible) activation of both the attachment motivational system, on one side, and the defensive system, on the other. This conflict results in the impossibility of mak-ing use of coherent strategies of behaviour, which recalls the breakdown of the integrative functions of consciousness that are typical of dissociative phenom-ena, as Janet had already described.

According to Liotti, therefore, we need to pay special attention to the rela-tional dynamics of the single event, suggesting that both the meaning of trauma and connection with an attachment figure (in conjunction with frequency and intensity) might prevent the integration of the event within the conscious structure, explaining dissociative reactions. In other words, if trauma is connected to attachment figures, the child has to dissociate this reality from his or her consciousness ("this is not happening; it is not happening to me; it's not Mum or Daddy who are doing this to me"). A reaction is thoroughly described in specialized literature as well as in literary fiction, as in the five novels by Edward St. Aubyn that recount the story of Patrick Melrose (even if it is quite an autobiographical narration), who had to come to terms with a devastating childhood, an abusive sadistic father, and a masochistic alcoholic mother. Patrick withdraws into dissociative experiences ("the escape when there is no escape"; Putnam, 1992, p. 104) by "observing from above" the violence he is undergoing or by becoming literally the gecko near the window who can escape by vanishing behind the wall:

> The harder he struggled, the harder he was hit. Longing to move but afraid to move, he was split in half by this incomprehensible violence. Horror closed in on him and crushed his body like the jaws of a dog. After the beating, his father dropped him like a dead thing onto the bed. ... He did not know who this man was, it could not be his father who was crushing him like this. From the curtain pole, if he could get up on the curtain pole, he could have sat looking down on the whole scene, just as his father was looking down on him. For a moment, Patrick felt he was up there watching with detachment the punishment inflicted by a strange man on a small boy. As hard as he could Patrick concentrated on the curtain pole and this time it lasted longer, he was sitting up there, his arms folded, leaning back against the wall. Then he was back down on the bed again feeling a kind of blankness and bearing the weight of not knowing what was happening. He could hear his father wheezing, and the bedhead bumping against the wall. From behind the curtains with the green birds, he saw a gecko emerge and cling motionlessly to the corner of the wall beside the open window. Patrick lanced himself toward it. Tightening his fists and concentrating until his concentration was like a telephone wire stretched between them, Patrick disappeared into the lizard's body.
>
> *(St. Aubyn, 2012, pp. 71–72)*

According to Bromberg (1998, 2011), dissociation serves the paradoxical purpose of maintaining a sense of internal continuity, avoiding the traumatic dissolution of a sense of self and of identity. In his view, dissociation may be regarded as a continuum that goes from a healthy capacity to fluctuate and to keep a sense of unity within the multiple aspects of the self, to dissociation as a rigid defence against intense, cumulative, relational traumatic experiences that impair fluidity and coherence. "Health is the ability to stand in the spaces between realities without losing any of them" (2011, p. 51). Also, "this is what I consider the ... capacity to feel like one self while being many" (1996, p. 10).

In agreement with Russel Meares (2012a, p. 10), Bromberg believes that the main characteristic of personality disorders is a rigid use of dissociation aimed at defending against the overwhelming affects linked to the traumatic experience:

> Defensive dissociation shows its signature through disconnecting the mind from its capacity to perceive that which feels too much for selfhood to bear. It reduces what is in front of someone's eyes to a narrow band of perceptual reality that lacks emotionally personal relevance to the self that is experiencing it ('whatever is going on is not happening to *me*').
>
> *(2011, p. 50)*

Splitting and fragmentation of the personality in interpersonal trauma

Ferenczi's theory of trauma (1932a, 1932b) has greatly contributed to a better understanding of dissociative phenomena. To Freud, Ferenczi replies that

> the obvious objection that we are dealing with sexual fantasies of the child himself, that is, on hysterical lies, unfortunately is weakened by the multitude of confessions of this kind, on the part of patients in analysis, to assaults on children.
>
> *(1932a, p. 95)*

For the Hungarian analyst, the majority of abuses are not acknowledged, or their real meaning is denied in the relationship with the caregiver. The major consequence is what he terms "identification with the aggressor," by which the child internalizes not only the aggressiveness of the persecutor but also his or her own split guilt (Ferenczi, 1932a, 1932b, pp. 189–190).

Dissociation and interpersonal trauma such as abuse, severe deprivation, incest, or violence, in contrast to psychic traumatization stemming from natural catastrophes or events in which human responsibility has not had a role (see the distinction between man-made trauma, in which a relationship is implied, and natural catastrophes like earthquakes or typhoons, Van der Kolk, 2014), are therefore strictly connected, especially if the event takes place within the most significant relationships for the child. The denial of its real meaning (abuse, incest) becomes an attack on the sense of the self, creating a fragmentation and a void, an erasure that, in some cases, may be converted into identification with the aggressor. The child's development is characterized by dissociative processes, in which split personalities or fragments mark out the self. The way for the child to overcome the traumatic pain and to survive is "by loss of consciousness, compensating fantasies of happiness, splitting of the personality" (Ferenczi, 1932b, p. 80).

In a paragraph "on the long-term effect of forcibly imposed, obligatory active and passive genital demands on young children," Ferenczi wrote:

> The girl feels soiled, indecently treated, would like to complain to her mother, but she is prevented by the man (intimidation, denial). The child is helpless and confused, should she struggle to prevail over the will of adult authority, the disbelief of the mother, etc. *Is it the whole world that is bad or am I wrong? – and chooses the latter.*"
>
> *(1932b, p. 80, emphasis added)*

The very distinction between what is intrapsychic and interpersonal is deleted, because of the identification with the aggressor and the adaptation to the requests (and distortions) of the environment, as we have seen in the famous quote (reported on p. 79), about the abused child "giving up the ghost" (1932b, p. 39).

This passage is surprising for its anticipation of what neuroscience has described as the deactivation of the parasympathetic system induced by trauma-induced dissociation, as set forth by Allan Schore (1994, 2001, 2009, 2011, 2012) and by Stephen Porges (2011) in his account of the vagal response to trauma.

Recent studies in neuroscience employing neuroimaging and especially Functional Magnetic Resonance Imaging (fMRI) have shown the link between trauma-induced dissociation and alterations in the right hemisphere (Meares, Schore, & Melkonian, 2011; Schore, 2009). McGilchrist (2009) described dissociation as "a relative hypofunction of the right hemisphere. Dissociation is, furthermore, the fragmentation of what would be experienced as a whole – the mental separation of components of experience that would ordinarily be processed together, again suggesting a right-hemisphere problem" (pp. 235–236). Lanius and colleagues (2005) have observed through fMRI that dissociation in traumatized patients activates the right hemisphere mostly. According to Schore (2011), "neurobiologically, dissociation reflects the inability of the right brain cortical-subcortical implicit self-system to recognize and process the perception of the external stimuli" and integrate them with internal stimuli "on a moment-to-moment basis" (p. xxiii). This failure of integration, continues Schore,

> of the higher right hemisphere with the lower right brain and disconnection of the central nervous system from the autonomic nervous system induces an instant collapse of both subjectivity and intersubjectivity. Stressful affects, especially those associated with emotional pain are thus not experienced in consciousness (Bromberg's 'not-me' self-states).
>
> *(2011, p. xxiii)*

At the same time, we know how highly controversial is this neuroscientific approach. According to Mark Solms and Oliver Turnbull (2002), for example, "all of the attempts to dichotomize the basic mental functions of the left and right hemispheres have proved futile, and it is likely that there is no single fundamental factor that distinguishes the functions of the two hemispheres" (p. 244).

What everyone agrees on is that when the caregiver is not sufficiently attuned to the child or is emotionally unable to regulate the child's affective internal states, the affect regulation in the dyad and the child's capacity to self-regulate are both impaired. These observations help us to understand the paradigm shift in contemporary psychoanalytic models of psychopathogenesis: from oedipal repression to pre-oedipal dissociation (Schore, 2012, p. 126).

One last reference from Ferenczi's *Diary* points to the importance of adaptation to the environment resulting from maltreatment:

> from the moment when bitter experience teaches us to lose faith in the benevolence of the environment, a permanent split in the personality occurs. … Thus, the splitting of the world, which previously gave the impression of homogeneity, into subjective and objective psychic systems; each has its own way of remembering, of which only the objective system is actually completely conscious … Only in sleep do we succeed, by means of certain external rearrangements … in calling off this guard. Actual trauma is experienced by children in situations where no immediate remedy is provided and where adaptation, that is, a change in their own behavior, is forced on them – the first step toward establishing the differentiation between inner and outer world, subject and object. From then on, neither subjective nor objective experience alone will be perceived as an integrated emotional unit.
>
> *(1932b, p. 69)*

Contemporary views of dissociation and traumatic memories

At the end of the 1970s, studies on Vietnam veterans, a deepening knowledge of child abuse issues, and a new understanding of what can be considered traumatic led to the formation of the diagnostic category of posttraumatic stress disorder (PTSD), which was introduced in *DSM-III* in 1980 (APA, 1980). Memory disturbances (both amnesia and intrusive flashbacks) are among the most disquieting symptoms of posttraumatic pathology, and the identification of PTSD opened a dialogue about the possibility of retrieving memories of abuse, even after a considerable period of time (Harvey & Herman, 1994; Herman & Schatzow, 1987; Mucci, 2008; Sandler & Fonagy, 2011; Van der Kolk & van der Hart, 1991). Studies have now shown that traumatic memories due to early maltreatment, abuse, or other early relational trauma are encoded in a different way than nontraumatic memories (Tulving & Thomson, 1973).

They can also be considered as memories registered in what Mancia called "the unrepressed unconscious" (Mancia, 2006; Craparo & Mucci, 2016; Craparo, 2017a, 2018), that is, early memories encoded in the body and in the limbic system, and connected to the preverbal views of the subject and therefore acting as guides for his or her IWMs, the inner representations of self that, although neither conscious nor repressed, nonetheless unconsciously guide behaviour and self-esteem. This is also consonant with Freud's conviction that "not all that is unconscious is repressed" (1923, p. 8).

According to Janet (1919, 1925), only a portion of the interaction between individuals and the environment enters the conscious processes. In normal situations, information is automatically integrated on the basis of that which already exists. Storage and categorization are fundamental mechanisms in the organization of memory. For Janet, the memory system and its integration are at the core of healthy functioning. When frightening experiences cannot be related to pre-existing information, they are split from personal consciousness through dissociation and become pathological fragments, the so-called subconscious fixed ideas mentioned above. These fragments affect behaviour and mental functioning and make memories of the event weak and fragmented. A lack of integration explains the violence of the affects linked to the reactivation of such traumatic memories.

Contemporary studies show that if the hippocampus has not completely matured (which occurs at the age of three or four) a person may only remember the *quality* of the event without context, meaning, or significance. Even afterwards, the functioning of the hippocampus can be damaged so that memories are difficult to situate in a definite time and space, especially in the case of prolonged stressful situations (Van der Kolk & van der Hart, 1989). The consequence is that one has amnesia for a specific event while preserving the feelings or emotions linked to it (Jacobs & Nadel, 1985; Sapolsky, Krey, & McEwen, 1984), together with the inability to reevoke the event using explicit memory.

For Janet (1889, 1909b), retrieving the amnestic experiences can only take place in a mental state similar to that which existed during the original event. Contemporary neurobiologists have found that it is easier to retrieve a memory encoded in implicit memory in states of hyperarousal or fear similar to the moment of inscription (Van der Kolk, 2014). This might explain why the therapeutic context, even if it implies a protected and safe setting, may in some cases reactivate implicit memories of past emotional situations to the point of clarifying certain contents and episodes that could not have been understood or remembered in the past (Boeker et al., 2013; Fonagy, 1999; Lingiardi & De Bei, 2011). This is the paradoxical status of the traumatic "knowing and not knowing," as described by Dori Laub (1992, p. 184), which is the privileged terrain of psychotherapy with early traumatized patients.

In the so-called "unrepressed unconscious," primitive memories are impressed in the body–mind system and encoded before they could be verbally defined and qualified by a specific meaning (Brooks-Brenneis, 1996; Liotti, 2007; Rothschild, 2000; Solomon & Siegel, 2003). In conjunction with either very early relational traumatization or overwhelming experiences for the immature child, a primitive and massive kind of dissociation tends to be established while trauma is happening (peri-traumatic dissociation; see Putnam, 1989b), very often with depersonalization and derealization (Van Buren & Alhanati, 2010; Van der Kolk & van der Hart, 1989).

The different ways in which memories are stored influence their retrieval and elaboration. According to Meares (2009), traumatic experiences are stored not in the episodic memory system but in an earlier and more primitive memory system, at least in individuals who are growing up. The inappropriate reactivation of traumatic experiences in the therapeutic relationship is a consequence of their defective encoding, so that traumata are not remembered as single events but as a form of negative knowledge about oneself (due to their inscription in the implicit memory).

In the therapy with victims of abuse and maltreatment, the internal identification with the aggressiveness of the abuser and the internalization of his or her split-off guilt leads to complex work with both the parts of the self identified with a victim and the parts of the self identified with the persecutor, which also explains why the aggressiveness is directed against oneself and one's body. It is only when both the identifications with the victim and the persecutor are worked through, released, and finally given up that the traumatized person is reborn and healed, really going beyond trauma (Mucci, 2013, 2018).

Trauma and dissociation in the contemporary relational approach: The contribution of Philip Bromberg

Philip Bromberg (1998, 2006, 2011) proposes a clinical theory based on a relational model that posits dissociation at its centre. According to his hypothesis, since the mind does not start as a single entity but develops multiple discontinuous and discrete states, "self-states are what the mind comprises. Dissociation is what the mind does" (2006, p. 2). Moreover, he postulates an ordinary dissociation characterized by flexible relationships among self-states that allows humans to deal with the ever-shifting requirements of life's complexities through the use of creativity and spontaneity.

Pathological dissociation is activated to protect subjects from traumatic dissolution when the illusion of continuity becomes too dangerous to be maintained due to incompatible affects and perceptions that cannot be symbolically understood by the subject and to the discrepancies among experiences that cannot be tolerated.

Like Janet, Bromberg believes that early relational trauma severely damages the integrative functions of the mind. In accordance with studies on traumatic memories, Bromberg postulates that early relational trauma might create retroactive amnesia, in which somatic memories devoid of symbolic form are not representable in conscious-explicit form. Bromberg refers to these as "the shadow of the tsunami" (2011, p. 165).

In Bromberg's clinical theory, dissociated experiences cannot be verbally communicated but can be observed in behavioural patterns within interpersonal relationships, including therapy (Lingiardi, 2008). The clinician should pay particular attention to the emerging states of the dissociated self that can take the shape of an *enactment* (Craparo, 2017b), here conceived of as a dyadic event in which therapist and patient are linked through a dissociated mode of relating in which each is in a not-me state (Bromberg, 2011, p. 151).

In so far as enactments imply an action (see Gabbard, 1995, p. 478), they can make past dynamics and unconscious elements thinkable. The action is first an implicit and affective representation of the event that might subsequently be mediated by the language of both participants as a first step toward representability (Bromberg, 2011; Schore, 2012).

As Bromberg suggests, the therapist has to agree to experience countertransferentially the traumatic states of the patient in order to function as an emotional regulator and integrative co-agent. However, if clinicians show a refusing attitude or fear of or detachment from these dissociated states, they not only miss a fundamental step towards a therapeutically meaningful change but risk retraumatizing patients. These enactments may, for instance, repeat a pathological object relation by intensifying the affective dysregulated states (Levy & Lemma, 2004; Schore, 2012; Van der Kolk, 1989). This is entirely congruent with Ferenczi's therapeutic attitude, which can be synthetized as "mutuality" and reciprocity in his technique. For Ferenczi it is the analyst's attitude as a totally "benevolent and helpful" witness (1932b, p. 24) to the pain of the patient, that is the element that allows the latter to go beyond the simple "abreaction" of the traumatic past, making the reinscription of a new experience possible, thanks to the joint effort of the psychoanalytic couple and the use of their dissociative parts.

As repetitions of the past in the present within the therapeutic relationship, enactments permit the reconnection of emotional and affective aspects of memories, while reinscribing, even at implicit levels, new relational experiences, a sort of "repetition with a difference" (Fineman, 1988). For Ferenczi, in fact, it is the real participation of the analyst, "benevolent and helpful," that enables the reconstruction of the missing links in the story of the subject. It is the emotional participation of the analyst that makes the body a sentient body and restores unity where there was fragmentation:

> The analyst is able, for the first time, to link *emotions* with the above primal events and thus endow that event with the feeling of a real experience. Simultaneously the patient succeeds in gaining insight, far more penetrating than before, into the reality of these events that have been repeated so often on an intellectual level.
>
> *(1932b, p. 14)*

A mere intellectual approach to these phenomena would lead the affective part to go even further out of control and strengthen the dissociation (Bromberg, 2006). During this phase, difficulty may arise in distinguishing between reliving the events as if they were in the present and going along with the patient through the past and arriving at a different perception of it. In addition, this allows an event that has long been intrapsychic (and has formed the particular lenses through which the patient views reality) to become interpersonal. What is created is therefore new implicit relational knowledge between the me (conscious) and not-me (unconscious) (Bromberg, 2011).

Within the nonlinear dynamics of the therapeutic process, language is a unifying and synthetizing element, though it is insufficient. Experience is not only symbolized by words but also given meaning by the varied contexts of the relational exchange that is communication. In other words, language not only conveys meaning but also creates the meaning itself as the result of a relational process (Boston Change Process Study Group, 2007, 2008; Bromberg, 1998; Levine, Reed, & Scarfone, 2013; Stern et al., 1998).

In the wake of Ferenczi's reciprocal analysis – which is centred on recognition rather than interpretation and based on the analytical process as co-creation of history and meaning – and followed by the theorizations of Fairbairn, Sullivan, Winnicott, and Balint, the fundamental element of this method is that the multiple realities contained in the various states of the self have the opportunity to connect (Bromberg, 1998). They can connect, thanks to the presence – witnessing of the therapist's own states of consciousness, which are freely put into play. To put it in the words of Janet (1889), consciousness arises from the constant tension between an organism's natural tendency to synthesize and a reality that continuously disorganizes it and tends to make it dissociated.

A good analytic relationship, Bromberg states, enables the patient to transform his or her dissociative defences into meta-reflective qualities that allow one to include and integrate past, present, and future. Even if no therapy can radically transform one's affective memory, the therapeutic relationship – the special climate of understanding and introspection typical of intersubjectivity – seems to be able to create new emotional memories, stories, and possibilities that will over time inhibit the automatic repetition of dysfunctional behavioral, emotional, and cognitive schemas. The therapeutic relationship also appears to restore the healthy function that dissociation once prevented. There exists a form of memory that is charged with emotion and meaning but lacking in words.

Many of our patients are haunted by implicit traumatic emotional memories that cannot be expressed in words. Not because these words are removed or hidden, but because they have yet to be pronounced. Our task as clinicians is to learn how to pronounce these words "for the first time" together with our patients. If we succeed in doing this it is thanks to the fabric that Janet and Ferenczi first, and later Bromberg, wove using the precious threads offered by the early Freud.

Notes

1 Implicit memory, a concept that has come into use only in the last 30 years, can be considered the psychobiological base of the unconscious in its most comprehensive meaning of "what is not conscious." It influences relevant aspects of our life and is involved in our motivational and affective processes.
2 Both Janet and Ferenczi emphasize the bodily reaction and the absence of personal consciousness, and of subjectivity, in traumatic states, leaving the traumatized subject literally in a place of estrangement.

PART II

Janet's influence on contemporary psychotraumatology

7

REFLECTIONS ON SOME CONTRIBUTIONS TO CONTEMPORARY PSYCHOTRAUMATOLOGY IN THE LIGHT OF JANET'S CRITIQUE OF FREUD'S THEORIES[1]

Giovanni Liotti and Marianna Liotti

This chapter compares Pierre Janet's views on the dissociative responses to psychological trauma with those influenced by the psychoanalytic theory of defence mechanisms, in order to examine their accordance with some findings of contemporary psychotraumatology studies. We agree with Russell Meares's statement that both psychoanalysis and Janet's psychological analysis seem often compatible with clinical observations and with data from contemporary neuroscience (Meares, 2012a, p. 27). Our aim, therefore, is not to argue in favour of one of those theories and against the other. Rather, we mean to highlight the relevance of Janet's ideas for contemporary psychotraumatology without implying that the psychoanalytic ones are less – or more – relevant.

A brief reminder of how Janet summarized the main diverging features between his theory and psychoanalysis will provide the starting point for our reflections on the different interpretations of some contemporary psychotraumatology studies suggested by the two theories.

How Janet stated the main differences between his theory and Freud's

In his contribution to the XVII International Congress of Medicine held in London (Janet, 1913) and in a later book (Janet, 1923a), Janet summarized in three arguments the main differences he detected between his own theory, which he had christened "psychological analysis," and Sigmund Freud's psychoanalysis:

1. The notion of a *narrowed field of consciousness* as a direct and passive effect of the vehement emotions experienced during and after a traumatizing event is different from Freud's idea of an active psychological *defence mechanism* developed to banish from consciousness unacceptable mental contents.

2. Janet's view of the subconscious (*le subconscient*) as an expression of a complex *hierarchy of mental functions* – whose lower level of automatic operations (*automatisme psychologique*) does not involve any type of consciousness, while the higher levels culminate with fully fledged reflective consciousness – markedly diverges from Freud's concept of the dynamic *unconscious* as a product of defence mechanisms.

3. Janet hypothesized that human behaviour is driven by a variety of psychobiological systems (*action tendencies*) stemming from both evolutionary processes and individual development, thus rejecting what he called "Freud's *pansexualism*" as a case of unrestrained generalization.

Three questions emerge from this summary of the differences between Janet's psychological analysis and Freud's psychoanalysis. The first concerns the nature of the response to psychological trauma: a passive narrowing of the field of consciousness or an active defence of the ego against the mental pain of traumatic memories? The second question is which general theory could better account for the defective conscious access to traumatic memories (and related mental contents): a theory of consciousness as a multi-layered process whose higher layers may be hindered by adverse experiences, or the idea of a vast reservoir of unconscious mental contents and processes created by ego defences? The third question regards the basic motives that underpin mental processes and overt behaviour (including those involved in the responses to trauma): are they to be conceived as a multiplicity of motivational systems with different inborn foundations, or as two antithetical instincts or drives (Eros and Thanatos)?

These three questions provide a useful template to reflect on some research findings in contemporary psychotraumatology, with the aim of illustrating the persistent interest of Janet's hypotheses.

Narrowing of the field of consciousness or a defence against mental suffering?

It is unclear if Janet thought that a preexistent inherent deficit of higher mental function was necessary in order to let the vehement emotions associated with traumatic experiences and memories narrow the field of consciousness – i.e. to cause a pathological lowering of mental functions (*abaissement du niveau mental*). This was, according to Janet, the origin of the posttraumatic dissociation characterizing the conditions that about a century ago went under the name of hysteria, and today are described as borderline (Meares, 2012a), somatoform, and dissociative disorders. Janet's work and the reviews of his theory available nowadays (see, for instance, Ellenberger, 1970; Heim & Bühler, 2006; Meares, 2012a; Ortu, 2013; van der Hart & Horst, 1989; van der Hart, Nijenhuis, & Steele, 2006; Van der Kolk & van der Hart, 1989) suggest his belief in a multiplicity of factors predisposing to posttraumatic dissociation. Janet thought that the predisposition to dissociation was due to an amalgam of innate temperamental factors (which are, as we know today, genetically determined) and of early experiences, both crucial for personality development. This view parallels the findings of contemporary research evidencing that dissociation is deeply influenced by infant attachment disorganization (Dutra et al., 2009; Ogawa et al., 1997), while such disorganization is, in turn, influenced by genetic and temperamental factors (Gervai, 2009; Luijk et al., 2011).

It can be argued, therefore, that Janet's theories on the vulnerability to post-traumatic dissociation anticipated the contemporary debate on the interdependence between relational and genetic/temperamental variables in the genesis of early attachment patterns (Gervai, 2009; Luijk et al., 2011), and on the influence of these patterns on the development of the higher mental functions putatively hindered by dissociation, such as the capacity for mentalization (Enskin et al., 2017; Fonagy & Target, 2006). Janet's interest, reported by Ellenberger (1970), in the studies of American scholars (e.g. Cooley, 1902) on the role of social factors in personality development supports this hypothesis. Janet's theory that, given the vulnerability mentioned above, the pathological response to psychological trauma is a disintegration of higher mental functions due to vehement emotions, is clearly different from Freud's understanding of pathology as dependent from an active ego defence, aimed to banish from consciousness overwhelming emotions and representations. On this subject, discussing his first clinical observations, Janet wrote:

> 'the traumatic memory presented itself in a peculiar way: it could not be expressed during waking and it reappeared only in special circumstances, during another psychological state … a particular change of consciousness that I tried to describe … as sub-consciousness by disintegration. This dissociation … seemed related to a state of exhaustion, determined by various causes and specifically by emotion.'
>
> *(1923a, p. 37)*

Janet summarizes the difference between this point of view and Freud's theory in the following words: "Dr. S. Freud regarded as repression what I deemed a narrowing of the field of consciousness. But, above all, he converted clinical observations and a therapeutic method with specific and limited indications in an enormous system of philosophical medicine" (1923a, p. 38).

In other words, Janet regarded the dissociative outcomes of traumatizing events and memories as a passive "mental exhaustion," a pathological narrowing of the field of consciousness (*rétrécissement de la conscience*) that took place in individuals predisposed to it by temperament and by early adverse experiences. This view is clearly different from the idea that posttraumatic dissociation is, instead, an active and motivated mental operation, an "act of will," as Freud stated: "I was repeatedly able to show that the splitting in the content of consciousness is the result of an act of will on the part of the patient; that is to say, it is initiated by an effort of will whose motive can be specified" (1894, p. 46).

The theory according to which posttraumatic dissociation represents a defence against mental suffering, namely a psychological mechanism that is somehow motivated, even if unconscious, was, and indeed still is, an important one in the whole field of psychotraumatology, not only in psychoanalytic literature (see, for example, Dell, 2009). Nonetheless, on this matter even psychoanalytic authors have expressed reservations, based on clinical and research findings, both in an indirect (Lyons-Ruth, 2003) and in a direct way (Howell, 2011, pp. 35–36; Meares, 2012a, pp. 139–147). An increasing number of psychoanalysts regard it as possible that an important facet of the response to traumatizing events could have not an actively defensive nature, but – as Janet thought – an automatic and physiological one. They hypothesize the existence of a different and independent aspect from the defensive one, even if both can be present in dissociative processes (see, for instance, Craparo, 2013, 2017a, 2017b). The renewed appreciation of Janet's theory of dissociation is wittily conveyed by the often-quoted words of Bromberg, himself a psychoanalyst:

> If one wished to read the contemporary psychoanalytic literature as a serialized Gothic romance, it is not hard to envision the restless ghost of Pierre Janet, banished from the castle by Sigmund Freud a century ago, returning for an overdue haunting of Freud's current descendants.
>
> *(1998, p. 189)*

Outside the psychoanalytic field, a growing number of theoretical and clinical perspectives are explicitly based on Janet thesis more than on Freud's (Liotti & Farina, 2011; Ogden, Minton, & Pain, 2006; Ogden & Fisher, 2015; van der Hart, Nijenhuis, & Steele, 2006).

The results of research studies in the domains of psychology and neuroscience can also be used to support the Janetian hypothesis that the narrowing of the field of consciousness in response to psychological trauma is not primarily an ego defence or a consequence of the defensive "act of will" described by Freud. An example is provided by Horowitz and Telch's (2007) research study. Subjects in a dissociative state induced via audiophonic stimulation experienced heightened pain in response to a standard cold pressor test, in comparison to control subjects who were in an unaltered state of consciousness. Altered states of consciousness similar to the narrowing of the field of consciousness observed by Janet, therefore, do not always exert a self-protective function in the presence of painful experiences. If posttraumatic dissociation involves an altered state of consciousness, the latter may not necessarily represent a defence against pain. Other experimental data show, however, an association between altered states of consciousness and analgesia.

The polyvagal theory (Porges, 2007, 2011) can reconcile evidence that altered states of consciousness can reduce the intensity of perceived pain with research findings that point to the opposite. The brain system designed to cope with environmental threats and traumatic experiences operates through shifts between autonomic hyperactivation (mediated by the orthosympathetic system) that can amplify pain and fear, as in the experiment conducted by Horowitz and Telch (2007), and hypoactivation (a hypoaroused state mediated by the vagus nerve), that can instead be associated with numbing and analgesia (Porges, 2011). This psychobiological system, which governs the sequence freezing, fight, flight, faint, is represented in the brain stem (Panksepp & Biven, 2012) and does not require any conscious decision (any "act of will," in Freud's terminology) in order to influence pain perception and consciousness.

Data from neuroimaging studies seem at the very least to be compatible with Janet's idea that, in response to the activation of traumatic memories, what occurs is a direct and passive lowering of the mental level rather than the employment of an active intrapsychic defence (for a review of these neuroimaging studies, see Liotti & Farina, 2013). These studies show *decreased* metabolic activity within the neocortical areas associated with the higher-order conscious functions and therefore putatively involved in any "effort of will" by the ego (Freud, 1894, p. 46). The posttraumatic reduction of metabolic activity in neocortical areas seems to reflect Janet's concept of a narrowing of the field of consciousness (lowering of the mental level) more directly than Freud's idea of a deliberate, however unconscious, act of will (Liotti & Farina, 2013). It seems unlikely, *prima facie*, that an effort of will is associated with a decreased metabolic activity exactly in those cortical areas that should putatively be active during volitional processes.

Intuitive support for Janet's theory may be also found in neuroscientific studies concerning the effect of chronic traumatization on dendritic growth in the prefrontal cortex (PFC). A series of studies in rodents demonstrated that exposure to cumulative trauma induces loss of dendrites in the PFC (Ansell et al., 2012). In contrast to the PFC, chronic stress increases dendritic growth in the amygdala, thus accentuating the imbalance of amygdala over PFC function. The loss of PFC gray matter as a consequence of chronic trauma has also been seen in humans. Structural imaging has shown that the number of adverse events a person has been exposed to correlates with smaller PFC gray matter. Those who have reviewed all these replicated studies (Ansell et al., 2012; Arnsten et al., 2015) draw the conclusion that exposure to cumulative traumatic stress markedly impairs the executive functions of the PFC and simultaneously strengthens the emotional responses of the amygdala, a conclusion favouring Janet's dissociation theory rather than Freud's hypothesis that splitting is the result of an act of will, in so far as choosing and willing are based on efficient executive functions.

Studies of the brain's bioelectrical activity in pathological conditions associated with posttraumatic dissociation also favour Janet's dissociation theory. The analysis of event-related potential (ERP) in subjects suffering from posttraumatic syndromes evidenced a deficit in the synthesis of the two major components of the P300 wave. This synthesis represents an aspect of the attentional functions and could be seen as a manifestation of coordination between brain areas, integrating stimulus, and response (Meares, 2012a, p. 58). Thanks to this synthesis, P300 usually appears as a monophasic waveform. In posttraumatic syndromes, instead, it remains split in its two main components, P3a and P3b (the first originating mainly from prefrontal areas, the latter deriving mostly from parietal activity), which appear as two different peaks. It seems, then, that posttraumatic syndromes are characterized by a reduced coordination between the activities of brain areas that usually function together, an interpretation supporting Janet's idea that the narrowing of the field of consciousness in response to traumatizing events and memories is expressed in the failure of the mental synthesis of personal identity (*synthèse personnelle*: Janet, 1889, 1907b). Another study of brain bioelectrical activity, based on the EEG coherence technique rather than on evoked potentials, showed a deficit of cortical connectivity in complex posttraumatic stress disorder (Farina et al., 2013) that possibly reflects a narrowing of the field of consciousness.

Different hierarchical levels of mental activity or an unconscious created by ego defences?

The second main criticism made by Janet of Freud's theory regards the relationship between conscious and non-conscious mental processes and contents. This criticism could be reformulated, using the contemporary language of neuroscience, in terms of a different focus assigned by the two authors to top-down and bottom-up brain–mind processes. These two kinds of processes comprise the recursive interaction between lower brain–mind functions and higher ones. In his attempts to understand the genesis of posttraumatic dissociation, Janet conceived of a bottom-up mechanism, proceeding from the lower mind–brain levels towards the higher ones (vehement emotions disrupting the functions of consciousness). In contrast, Freud's theory of the origins of the dynamic unconscious focused on mental activities (the ego defences) going in the opposite direction and involving top-down processes (Liotti & Farina, 2013).

According to Freud, a defensive exclusion from self-awareness of disturbing emotions and other mental elements is made possible by higher-level mental functions, linked to ego mechanisms. Janet, instead, believed that the higher levels of human consciousness, characterized by volition and choice (that is, non-automatic functions), compose the apex of a brain–mind hierarchical system whose lower levels are essentially automatic (psychological automatisms; see Janet, 1898). Full consciousness involves a high degree of psychological tension (*tension psychologique*, Janet, 1920) that collapses during a vehement activation of the automatic, lower levels of the mind–brain. When the psychological tension collapses, a mental state deprived of reflective awareness (namely, the subconscious) is left, and it is accompanied by the manifestation of psychological automatisms that characterize both dreams and dissociative states during waking, including posttraumatic dissociative symptoms.

Janet criticized Freud's theory mainly on the basis of the above-summarized ideas. According to Janet, Freud's theory was an unwarranted generalization of the clinical observations about subconscious phenomena that the French author had confined to traumatic memories and to the consequent disaggregation or dissociation of consciousness. Freud's generalization, according to Janet, ended up in "an enormous system of philosophical medicine" (1923a, p. 38) in which almost all mental processes, even those not associated with traumatic memories, were seen as a consequence of defensive ego mechanisms. Freud thus rejected the possibility that such processes could be the manifestation of psychological automatisms that are usually hidden, being embedded in the functions of an unaltered consciousness. Janet (1907b) called such functions *synthèse personnelle* (personal synthesis, corresponding to consciousness of the self), *fonction du réel* (reality function, remarkably similar to the contemporary notion of working memory), and *présentification* (the ability to differentiate past from present, fantasy from reality). At the risk of summarizing his theory too superficially, we could say that Janet suggested that conscious functions are organized in a hierarchical system, in which the highest levels are reality function and *présentification*, the intermediate level is personal synthesis, and the lower level is the domain of subconscious automatisms. A high degree of psychological tension at the lower levels, caused by the vehement emotions of traumatic memories, brings forth a lowering of the psychological tension at the higher levels. The consequence is the manifestation of psychological automatisms in the context of an altered state of consciousness.

This summary illustrates Janet's focus on bottom-up processes in his theory of the genesis of posttraumatic symptoms. Freud, on the contrary, focused on the ego functions (higher-level mental processes) to explain the exclusion from consciousness of drives and emotions, and the creation of the dynamic unconscious as a result of repression. Freud thereby assigned a primary role to top-down processes in the genesis of pathological symptoms, both those associated with traumatic memories and those linked to internal conflicts between id and superego forces.

Above, we discussed the contemporary neuroscientific studies (Ansell et al., 2012; Arnsten et al., 2015) supporting the idea that cumulative trauma increases the activity in the lower-level emotional brain (e.g. the amygdala) and hinders the functions of the higher-level prefrontal cortex. The results of these studies are in keeping with the bottom-up aspects of Janet's theory concerning the genesis of posttraumatic dissociation. Now we shall examine more carefully the explanation of the bottom-up influence of trauma provided by the polyvagal theory (Porges, 2011).

According to polyvagal theory, human reactions to traumatizing events are governed by a survival defence system basically shared by all vertebrate species and located mainly in the brain stem. This system involves in its operations the structures and networks of the autonomic nervous system: the neural network called reticular formation that controls the activation of the sympathetic system and the nucleus of the vagal nerve (parasympathetic system). The nucleus of the vagal nerve comprises three parts (ventral, dorsal, and ambiguous) with notably different functions during the exposure to environmental stressors – hence the term "polyvagal." During the exposure to a traumatizing event, and very likely also during the automatic retrieval of a traumatic memory, the survival defence system exerts a bottom-up influence on the higher brain functions that is much more rapid and powerful than any top-down influence the frontal cortex may exert on the brainstem. The bottom-up influences of the survival defence system on the neocortex could contribute to the explanation of the impaired cortical functions during the retrieval of traumatic memories, the reduced rate of dendritic growth in the prefrontal cortex (PFC) after cumulative trauma, and the deficits in cortical connectivity evidenced by the studies quoted in the preceding paragraph.

In clinical practice, a consideration of the influences exerted by the survival defence system on the higher mental functions could explain the vehement emotional responses related to the surfacing of traumatic memories during dialogues with trauma survivors. These responses may be seen as manifestations of the failed emotional regulation caused by the bottom-up hindrance to the PFC. The activation of the survival defence system may also explain – without any necessary reference to the concept of dissociation as an ego (top-down) defence against mental pain – the dissociative symptoms so typical of the survivors of chronic childhood trauma. Dissociative experiences and symptoms may be the expression of trauma-related dysfunctions of consciousness caused by bottom-up processes, and akin to the *abaissement du niveau mental* (lowering of the mental level) first hypothesized by Janet.

Multiplicity of psychobiological systems or conflict between Eros and Thanatos?

According to Janet (1926b), the motivational dynamics of the human mind should be regarded as the outcome of a multiplicity of action tendencies rather than being reduced to one drive (libido, Eros) or to two antithetical drives (Eros and Thanatos). Each action tendency, it should be noticed, regulates not only overt behaviours but also affects and thoughts (see van der Hart, Nijenhuis, & Steele, 2006, for reflections on Janet's theory of action).

Janet hypothesized, in accordance with Darwin's theory, that evolutionary pressures selected multiple action tendencies in order to cope adaptively with different environmental challenges. Each action tendency is aimed at a specific goal and is expressed in a sequence of phases (latency, preparation, activation, performance, and termination). This orderly sequence of different phases cannot be captured by the energetic concept of drive discharge advanced by Freud. Rather, it should be conceived as an organized system (van der Hart, Nijenhuis, & Steele, 2006).

The concept of action system in Janet's theory is akin to the concept of behavioural control system advanced by Bowlby (1969), in so far as the latter does not implicate any mechanism of drive discharge, but is conceived as a goal-corrected system organized along cybernetic principles. The concept of action system is also compatible with the idea of motivational system advanced by Lichtenberg (1989). In general, the contemporary contributions to the study of motivation (Bowlby, 1969; Cortina & Liotti, 2014; Gilbert, 1989; Lichtenberg, 1989; Liotti, 2016; Panksepp & Biven, 2012) insist on a multi-motivational perspective and are therefore more in accordance with Janet's theory of the multiplicity of action systems than with Freud's theory of two antithetical drives (Eros and Thanatos). The contemporary contributions to the study of motivation agree on the idea that motivational processes are the expression of psychobiological systems, each organizing and controlling mental activities and overt behaviour so as to direct them towards a specific goal endowed with evolutionary value. In other words, these systems are conceived as adaptations selected, in accordance with Darwinian principles, during the ages of the evolution of vertebrates leading to *homo sapiens.*

In the domain of contemporary psychotraumatology, the evolutionary approach to the study of motivational systems has been influential in inquiries on infant attachment disorganization as an antecedent of dissociative processes and a risk factor for posttraumatic dissociation (Liotti 1992, 2004, 2009, 2014b, 2016; Liotti & Farina, 2011; Lyons-Ruth, 2003; Schore, 2009). Longitudinal and pro-spective research studies, together with the converging results of many cross-sectional studies, demonstrated beyond any reasonable doubt the association between infant disorganized attachment and, in later life, dissociative tendencies linked to increased risk of posttraumatic dissociation (Cassidy & Mohr, 2001; Dozier, Stovall-McClough, & Albus, 2008; Dutra et al., 2009; Lyons-Ruth & Jacobvitz, 2008; Ogawa et al., 1997). The antecedents of infant attachment dis-organization have also been the object of many controlled research studies (for a review, see Lyons-Ruth & Jacobvitz, 2008), whose converging results point to two major risk factors: (1) the frequent interruption of the attachment figure's caregiving behaviour by expressed fear and/or aggression, and (2) the disorgani-zation of the caregiving system in the attachment figure expressed as caregiv-ing helplessness (Solomon & George, 2011). Genetic and temperamental factors play a modulatory rather than a causal role in the disorganization of the infant's attachment system (Gervai, 2009).

In the multi-motivational evolutionary perspective, infant attachment disor-ganization can be described as the outcome of the simultaneous and conflicting activation of two inborn motivational systems: the attachment system and the survival defence system (fight–flight). The first one motivates the infant to search for protective proximity to the caregiver, asking for help and comfort, while the second motivates it to flee from the attachment figure and/or to try to fight against her or him (Liotti, 2014b, 2016; Liotti & Farina, 2011). Such a simultane-ous and conflicting activation of the two systems explains the paradoxical behav-iour of the disorganized infant (e.g. the infant may freeze – a behaviour typical of the survival defence system – interrupting the approach to the attachment figure motivated by the attachment system), and is reflected in the experience called fear without solution (Cassidy & Mohr, 2001).

The conflicting simultaneous activation of two motivational systems that characterizes attachment disorganization could be expressed, according to the classic psychoanalytic theory, as a conflict between life (Eros) and death (Thanatos) drives – the first manifested in the search for proximity to the mother and the second in the destructive aggression against her. This psychoanalytic interpretation of early attachment disorganization, however, cannot explain the results of controlled research studies concerning the developmental pathways opened up by disorganization of infant attachment as elegantly as the evolutionary multi-motivational theory does. Between the third and the sixth year of life, the vast majority of children whose attachment was disorganized during the first eighteen months of their life develop characteristic controlling strategies in the interaction with the attachment figure (Lyons-Ruth & Jacobvitz, 2008). The first of these strategies is called controlling–caregiving, and is characterized by the inversion of the normal direction of care-seeking and caregiving between children and parents. Children adopting this strategy behave as if they are more often motivated to take care of their parents than to ask for the parents' care. The second relational strategy adopted by children who have been disorganized in their infant attachments is called controlling–punitive and is characterized by behaviours aimed at dominating the parent in situations where one could expect to observe care-seeking (attachment) behaviour.

According to the psychoanalytic theory of two basic instincts, the controlling–caregiving strategy could be interpreted as a solution of the conflict between Eros and Thanatos through the prevailing discharge of the libidinal drive, while the prevailing discharge of the destructive drive in the effort to solve the conflict could explain the controlling–punitive strategy. This classical psychoanalytic interpretation, however, does not explain the reason why the direction of care-seeking and caregiving is inverted in the controlling–caregiving strategy; why does the prevailing Eros not simply take the form of increased care-seeking behaviour, and show up as a paradoxical effort of children to take care of the parents? A multi-motivational explanation of the controlling strategies, which is closer to Janet's idea of multiple-action systems, does not incur this difficulty. According to multi-motivational theories, there are good reasons for shifting from a disorganized attachment motivation to another inborn motivational system whenever the interpersonal context allows one to do so. The subjective experience of attachment disorganization, involving fright without solution and fragmentation of the self (dissociation), is very painful, so it is rewarding to avoid it. Thus, in the controlling–caregiving strategy, the care-seeking (attachment) motivation is substituted by the caregiving one, while in the controlling–punitive strategy it is substituted by the competitive one aimed at dominance (for a description of the different systems identified in the evolutionary multi-motivational theory – attachment, caregiving, sexuality, competition for dominance, cooperation – see Cortina and Liotti, 2014). This explanation of the genesis of the controlling–punitive strategy in the activation of the competitive system is closer to the observation of the type of aggressive behaviour one sees in it than it is to an explanation in terms of destructive aggression (Thanatos). The controlling–punitive strategy involves the type of relatively benign ("ritualized," in the language of ethologists) aggression characteristic of the competitive motivational system aimed at achieving dominance, not the destructive aggression characteristic of the fight–flight motivational system, and is more remindful of the death instinct.

Concluding remarks

Besides being compatible with the results of some research studies in contemporary psychotraumatology, Janet's critique of Freud's theory is influencing the development of new clinical strategies in the psychotherapy of trauma survivors. An example of these strategies is provided by the clinical practice known as stabilization, which consists in preparing the field for the exploration of traumatic memories through psychological interventions aimed at coping straightforwardly (i.e. without any previous interpretation of ego defences) with the patient's narrowing of the field of consciousness. The sensorimotor approach to the psychotherapy of trauma-related disorders, for instance, suggests that one should address the narrowing of consciousness from the beginning of psychotherapy, and it considers the roots of this narrowing to lie in the instability of the autonomic system caused directly by traumatic memories, rather than in the side effects of ego defences against mental pain. Sensorimotor interventions focus primarily on the patient's distressing bodily experiences rather than on trauma-related emotions and thoughts; the latter are addressed only after a degree of autonomic stabilization has been achieved. Sensorimotor interventions, therefore, seem to operate via bottom-up brain–mind processes (cf. Chapter 13; Ogden, Minton, & Pain, 2006; Ogden & Fisher, 2015). The usefulness of a preliminary autonomic stabilization for the later therapeutic work on traumatic memories is supported by empirical studies (Cloitre et al., 2012), although it is still debated whether or not such a stabilization is a priority for the majority of chronically and severely traumatized patients (Cloitre, 2016; De Jongh et al., 2016).

To have rescued Janet's theory from almost a century of disregard – even oblivion – is a great merit of those theorists and clinicians (some of them contributors to this book) who value the vitality of theories more than their own persuasions, be those persuasions close to Freud's contributions or otherwise.

Note

1 Giovanni Liotti's (2014a) article "Le critiche di Pierre Janet alla teoria di Sigmund Freud: corrispondenze nella psicotraumatologia contemporanea" (published in *Psichiatria e Psicoterapia*, Vol. XXXIII, 1, pp. 31–40) has been thoroughly revised, expanded, and updated by Marianna Liotti. This chapter is the result of both authors' joint contributions.

8

THE HOLISTIC PROJECT OF PIERRE JANET

Part One: Disintegration or *désagrégation*

Russell Meares and Cécile Barral

At the beginning of the twentieth century, two men emerged as leaders of one aspect of a cultural revolution. They depicted a world of human experience that was alarmingly unlike what was visible on the surface. Although the ideas underlying the work of these two men were, to an extent, complementary, they were also contrasting and opposed. One man was working towards a holistic, or synthetic, view of reality, towards harmony, while the other was analytic, breaking the world of appearance into its component parts. This man's expressions were pervaded by themes of violence and primitive sexuality. For the other, these were secondary phenomena.

The personalities of the two men were, like their approaches to reality, contrasting. The one whose drive was towards coherence projected a reserved, courteous, apparently conventional persona. His detractors called him "bourgeois." The other was a more dominating character. It was he, as the century wore on, who came to be seen as the personification of this new view of mankind. However, nearing the end of the century, his domination waned and the other man's value was recognized anew.

Despite their differences, these men were seen as main figures in the larger movement of those times that reflected, it seemed, a radical shift in Western consciousness. When their work was displayed, with that of their colleagues, in London for the first time, Virginia Woolf, in her characteristic way, announced: "On or about December 1910, human character changed" (Woolf, 1950, p. 91).

These men, of course, were Henri Matisse and Pablo Picasso. Their rivalry mirrored in a remarkable way that between Pierre Janet and Sigmund Freud, whose respective synthesizing and analyzing approaches provided views of psychic life that were both complementary and opposed. Their observations and theories led to changes in the way that human consciousness might be conceived, which paralleled the view of human reality implicit in the new art. They spoke, unknowingly, as voices of the changed zeitgeist of Europe.

The change was seismic in its suddenness and effect. It cannot, of course be dated exactly as Woolf, half-humorously, had done. It was most clearly manifested during the years 1905 to 1913. At the beginning of this period, in 1905, the first form of Einstein's relativity theory was published. Old distinctions between space and time, energy and matter, were thrown into doubt. The implications of science were both exciting and ominous. Kandinsky, who seems to have had a supremely acute sensibility, wrote of his profound shock on hearing of Rutherford's theories, which emerged about this time, that the atom could disintegrate. He was shaken, to a state approaching dread; he felt the whole notion of reality was under threat, that nothing was stable.

The new art expressed and contributed to this mood. In 1905, the imagery of the group, of which Matisse was considered the leader, was exhibited and received with public outrage. A critic called them "Les Fauves," the wild beasts. In 1907, Picasso painted his iconic vision, "Les Demoiselles d'Avignon," which is perhaps the centrepiece of his oeuvre. The eyes and faces of the brothel women in this painting are both frightening and frightened, the visages of trauma, a theme fundamental to both Janet and Freud. It was during this time that Janet and Freud achieved international recognition for their ground-breaking theories. Janet was invited to lecture at Harvard in 1906, and Freud at Clark University, Massachusetts, in 1909. What had caught the world's attention was the idea that we are powerfully influenced by forces of which we are unaware, that are "unconscious."

In speaking of Janet, it is hard not to mention Freud, since they are so often linked together as co-founders of modern psychodynamic theory (e.g. Jung, 1948, p. 477; Ellenberger, 1970). Our subject, however, is Janet. Consequently, we can only touch upon the work of Freud in the briefest way.

We have been asked to write about the relevance of Janet's ideas to the understanding of borderline personality disorder (BPD), and its treatment. We do so from a perspective in which BPD is conceived as having a disintegrative basis, of traumatic origin (Meares, 2012a), and in which treatment is approached by means of the Conversational Model (Hobson, 1985; Meares, 2004; Meares et al., 2012). Our contribution is divided into two halves. The first (RM) focuses on the theme of disintegration, the notion of what Janet called *désagrégation*; the theme of the second concerns that which is disintegrated, the ongoing experience of self that Janet conceived as a dynamic hierarchy, involving oscillations and becomings of personal being (CB).

Janet's project

Janet and Freud reached these pinnacles of recognition from very different directions. Freud arrived via neurology; Janet was a philosopher, who had become a psychiatrist and a psychologist in order to understand better the nature of human consciousness, that sense of ordinary existing, which we are calling "self." We have begun our brief attempt to summarize his pathway to that end with a visual analogy that we hope gives a picture of the sense of what Janet was trying to do, compared with Freud's project, which is clearer than what can be conveyed by paragraphs of prose. The contrast between the two systems resembles that between, say, Matisse's "Harmony in Red (*La Desserte*)," painted in 1908, and Picasso's first cubist images, painted the following year, in which a theory is imposed upon, and organizes, the data of experience. The resemblance, however, between the two pairs of rivals is not identical. The painters developed a wary friendship, and creative conversation, in which their complementarity was recognized (Spurling, 1998, 2005). Janet and Freud did not recognize it, to say the least.

Both Janet and Matisse, who were widely read, were products of an intellectual milieu dominated by the philosophy of Henri Bergson. Janet was a friend and school fellow of Bergson, while "Bergsonian intuition offers an especially striking parallel with Matisse's thoughts on painting" (Flam, 2015, p. 33). By "intuition" Bergson meant what we now call empathy, the capacity to, as it were, transport oneself to the interior of an object in order to sense its essential quality (Bergson, 1913). It was through such means that Matisse would attempt to capture the central features of that which he observed; then he would amplify those features. The outcome of this representation is an image that is not a copy but a larger shaping of that which was given by the immediate sensory process.

Matisse's approach resembles that of the therapist whose work is guided by the Conversational Model (Hobson, 1985; Meares & Hobson, 1977; Meares, 2000, 2004, 2005), who is seeking to potentiate the emergence of self in someone in whom this experience has been denied through repetitive trauma. This approach, we believe, is consistent with, and to some extent anticipated by, Janet in his later writings.

Our two essays have the aim of showing the trajectory of Janet's thought from its beginning, which focused on states of disintegration (*désagrégation*), through to his later works, which reflected an attempt to build a picture of mind necessary to the understanding of mental illness, and to a treatment involving the aim of integration or synthesis. Our path through the vast terrains of Janet's writing is directed to showing its relevance to modern understanding and treatment of trauma, particularly as it has damaged personality development.

The early work: Hysteria

Janet's quest for the nature of self led him to immerse himself in the personal reality of those whose sense of existing was upset; seriously ill people, suffering a condition then called "hysteria." Most of the patients diagnosed would now be said to have "borderline personality disorder (BPD)" (Meares, 2012b). In these subjects, the sense of self is stunted, deformed, or even lost (Meares, 2012a). It was as if Janet sensed that, although the elusive character of self is difficult to grasp, the way towards it might start with what is not self, that "being" might be discovered through its absence.

Before Janet, the condition was vaguely defined. Janet's approach to the puzzle presented by hysteria was truly scientific. He committed himself to scrupulous observation of the phenomena in order to discover "rigorous laws" underpinning the "surface phenomena" (1901, p. 484). He based his findings on hysteria on a study of 120 patients, an extraordinary evidential database. What emerged was a picture of a condition resembling the current BPD diagnosis. It was a syndrome of severe personality disorder associated with multiple bodily ills. Its manifestations were protean. However, as Janet pointed out, against a current orthodoxy, the multiplicity of symptoms did not imply that hysteria was not a specific disorder. He considered that, among the many symptoms of the disorder, one group was pathognomic. He called them the "stigmata," the "marks," which identified the illness. They were essentially those of loss of function, particularly of motor power, sensation, and memory. It is of interest that these same symptoms may be the cardinal features of BPD. The ninth diagnostic criterion of BPD in *DSM-IV* (APA, 1994) – dissociative symptoms and paranoid ideation – has "excellent specificity, that is, rarely occurs in other diagnostic groups" (Skodol et al., 2002, p. 937).

Freud rejected the notion of the stigmata, influencing the manner of diagnosis of "hysteria" in the twentieth century, which led to disastrous outcomes (e.g., Slater, 1965). On the other hand, it was shown that a diagnostic method based on Janet's stigmata isolated a condition that was discrete and had diagnostic stability (Meares & Horvath, 1972).

Désagrégation and dissociation

The great significance of Janet's work is the "law" that he derived from his observations. It underpinned his understanding of the basis of the mental stigmata and the mental accidents.

The central fact of the Janetian opus is the phenomenon of *désagrégation*. Janet found that his patients suffered "a want of mental unity" (1901, p. 222), a failure properly to integrate the various phenomena of mental life into a coherent whole. He had put forward his theory of the "diminution of personal synthesis" (p. 246) in 1887, and again in 1889, in his influential *L'Automatisme Psychologique*, a work that, as Ellenberger remarked (1970), "was hailed from the start as a classic of the psychological sciences" (p. 361). The state of disintegration allows one part of the psychological system to become separated, or dissociated, from the rest. Janet put it this way:

> All the psychological phenomena that are produced in the brain are not brought together in one and the same personal perception; a portion remains independent under the form of sensations or elementary images, or else is grouped more or less completely and tends to from a new system.
>
> *(1901, p. 492)*

This second group of images separated from normal consciousness is the focus of what Janet called the "subconscious fixed idea." It is a system of unconscious traumatic memory in which is recorded the traumatizing event, or events, as a kind of "script." It is recorded in a state more disintegrated than the rest of consciousness. When triggered by circumstances in the environment that resemble the trauma, or by some internal trigger, the "script" is activated and played out, not as a coherent story, but often as fragments. Janet called these fragments *"mental accidents."* They were accidental to the diagnosis. They appear as if direct sensory imprints of aspects of the trauma on the mind–body–brain system. Particularly striking are those on the skin, perhaps as flaring or bruising. It is as if the brain has organized the vascular bed of the skin into the precise pattern of the traumatic insult; for example, apparently inexplicable parallel linear marks appear on the legs of a woman who, it later turns out, had been brutally caned as a child. These intriguing symptoms, which are very little reported in the literature, might be understood as an aspect of "dysautonomia" (see Meares, 2012c). Such phenomena caused Janet to call hysteria an "ensemble of maladies of representation" (1901, p. 488).

In some circumstances, the "subconscious fixed idea" invades and overthrows the remaining system of consciousness. Even, however, if it remains dormant, it continues to have an effect. Janet quotes Herzen (1887):

> An idea that disappears from consciousness does not, therefore, cease to exist; it may continue to act in a latent state, so to speak, below the level of consciousness ... in this subconscious state, it may still have motor effects and exercise its influence on other ideas.
>
> *(Janet, 1893a, p. 47)*

As evidenced by this citation, Janet did not claim for himself the role of discoverer of unconsciousness, as "the conquistador of entirely unexplored territories," as Freud was later to do (Van der Kolk & van der Hart, 1991, p. 433). Rather, he acknowledged not only that others before him had written of unconscious aspects of mental life but also of the pathogenic significance of trauma. He pointed out that Charcot had found "shock" (1901, p. 227), that is, trauma, to be a basis of psychogenic paralyses. A study of Janet's cases found that in 591 of these, trauma was reported in 257 (Crocq & De Verbizier, 1989). Janet, however, extended the notion of trauma beyond a single event to include cumulative trauma — a very modern concept. He wrote in later years that the "symptoms and fixed ideas that the subject presents in these cases" may be determined "by a succession of slight forgotten shocks," by "a gradual exhaustion brought on by a host of slight repeated fatigues, or even little emotions, each one insignificant in itself, which have left no distinct or dangerous memories" (1924, p. 275). Such a proposal has received confirmation in recent years by studies such as those of Giovanni Liotti (1999, 2000, 2004, 2006, 2009).

Janet had arrived at a theory that, he wrote, "is one of *subconsciousness through disintegration*. This dissociation, this migration of certain psychological phenomena into a special group, seemed to me connected with the exhaustion brought on by various causes, and in particular by emotion" (1924, p. 40). It should be noted that the disintegration, that is, *désagrégation*, is distinguished from the "dissociation" of the special group. It is, however, a common mistake to equate the two. As van der Hart and Dorahy (2006) point out, Janet used both terms. The latter cannot be regarded as a translation of the former.

The hierarchy of consciousness

Janet's theory implies a hierarchy decreed by the state of integration. States of high integration are associated with the experience of self, that is, higher-order consciousness. Indeed, we may say that integration *is* self. On the other hand, increasing degrees of disintegration are associated with corresponding states of unconsciousness. These conditions represent a lowering of the mental level – "*abaissement du niveau mental*" – an idea that Jung, who had studied with Janet in 1902–1903, found very useful and repeatedly referred to. The descent down the hierarchy on these occasions is a consequence of "exhaustion."

L'abaissement du niveau mental leads to the second main feature that Janet saw as an effect of trauma-induced exhaustion. Accompanying the "diminution of personal synthesis" is a contraction of consciousness. The number is reduced of the psychological phenomena that can be "brought together in one and the same personal perception" (1901, p. 492). Janet gave multiple examples of the simultaneous broken-up-ness and contraction of mental life in his patients: a woman who couldn't dance and look at the other dancer's clothes at the same time (p. 148), subjects whose "character is *mobile* and *contradictory*. The patient does not remain long in one of the same mental condition. She passes every moment from affection to indifference, from gladness to sadness, from hope to despair" (1901, p. 222).

In this state, attention, memory, voluntary effort, and the experience of time are all diminished. The disturbance of attention is central. The individual seems unable to concentrate and "attention is altogether the most difficult thing to fix" (1901, p. 22). The deficit can be demonstrated electrophysiologically. Those suffering "hysteria," as defined by Janet, but who are not dissociated at the time of testing, fail to habituate to meaningless and irrelevant stimuli (Meares & Horvath, 1972; Horvath, Friedman, & Meares, 1980). The authors explained this finding as the outcome of a relative failure of higher-order inhibitory control, an aspect of the "release phenomenon," to which we will soon come. It reflects a disability in the "screening out" of redundant stimuli not equaled in other forms of mental illness, with the exception of some forms of schizophrenia (Horvath & Meares, 1979).

Allied to the attentional deficit is a disturbance of memory. "What is it you asked?" the patient might say, or "What was I talking about?" (1901, p. 89). At this lower level of mental life a reduced form of memory is operative that we might call, using Tulving's terminology, semantic, a memory of facts. It may be even more primitive, repertoires of movement or simple and atomized perceptual representations (Tulving, 1983, 1985; Tulving & Schacter, 1990).

At the lower level, the capacity for voluntary action, for choice, and the operation of "will" is reduced, a condition Janet called "*abulia*." It is a kind of mental "laziness" (1901, p. 77). Actions tend to be automatic, manifest at an extreme in the wandering of fugue states and, to a lesser degree, the subject's telling the same monotonous story "day after day" (p. 201). They have no capacity for development.

The disturbance of the sense of time seems to involve all of the above deficits. In normal consciousness there is a certain freedom from the present, and the ability figuratively to roam about in places in one's past or even in spaces that have never existed, in the future. Janet's patients have no future. Time is static and repetitive: "How queer," she says, "two nights in succession! We have just had one night and now here is another night that begins" (1901, pp. 89–90). His patients, Janet said, "live from day to day" without "images of the future" or "remembrances of the past" (1901, p. 77).

A Jacksonian background?

Janet's theory resembles that of the great English neurologist John Hughlings Jackson (1835–1911). He, too, proposed a hierarchy of consciousness. In his formulation, it is determined by an organization of the brain decreed by evolutionary history.

Jackson put forward a notional three-tiered system; "notional" because, as he said, the brain does not work in tiers. It is a way of talking about something complex and not easily expressible. The "layers" can be called reflective, semantic, and sensorimotor. They correspond to the layering of memory conceived in recent years by Tulving (1983, 1985). The highest level is that of "self," a term that Jackson believed he introduced into the English language medical literature. "Self" is identified with, but not the same as, the reflective function, the capacity to be aware of inner events (Jackson, 1887).

Jackson considered that the hierarchy evolves not as a consequence of any new kind of tissue being tacked onto the nervous system at each "level" but as the outcome of increasing coordination between the fundamental elements of neural function. These, in his view, are not single neurons but sensorimotor units. "Self" is the manifestation of the highest level of coordination between brain systems. As his French follower Théodule Ribot put it, "*le moi est un coordination*" (Jackson, 1958, p. 82).

The process of coordination, or integration, is accompanied by increasing levels of differentiation, or specialization of function. This is dependent upon the emergence of a higher order of inhibitory function. Sherrington emphasized this element of Jacksonian theory in his Nobel lecture in which he used Jackson's "release phenomenon" as the starting point in his argument concerning "inhibition as a co-ordinative factor" (Sherrington, 1932). The "release phenomenon" comes into play when the system is upset by an insult, following which there is a "dissolution," a reversal of the trajectory of the hierarchy. The consequent "descent" results in disintegration, decreasing complexity and differentiation of function, and a reversion to states under diminished voluntary control, approaching automatism. The functions that evolved last are lost first. Lower-order functions previously under higher-order inhibitory control are "released," to become exaggerated.

Jackson's theory was based on meticulous observations of minor epileptic fits (*petit-mal*). He considered that the hyperactivity of nervous tissue during the fit is followed by "exhaustion" of these tissues. The symptomatology, which might include automatisms, is the result of such exhaustion. A brief consideration of his theory is helpful in giving greater shape and clarity to Janet's vision (Meares, 1999; Meares, Stevenson, & Gordon, 1999).

It is hard to believe that Janet was not influenced, indirectly, by Jacksonian theory. His two masters, he told his audience at Harvard, were Charcot and Ribot (Janet, 1907b, p. 3). Ribot had introduced Jackson's ideas into France (Ellenberger, 1970, p. 403). Janet even uses some of the same language as Jackson, for example, "exhaustion." Janet's use of this term is not metaphysical. It is implicitly understood, as it had been by Jackson, in electrochemical terms (Horton, 1924, p. 21). He extended, beyond Jackson, the list of those factors that might induce exhaustion – toxins, physical assault, epileptic disruption, and so forth – to include psychological trauma.

Janet fills out, provides the colouring of, the emotional and more human elements of "dissolution" not provided by the bare bones of Jackson's neurologically based scheme. For example, the loss of complexity in the *"abaissement du niveau mental"* is described in feeling terms. What are "quickly lost," Janet wrote, are "altruistic emotions, perhaps because they are the most complex of them all" (1901, p. 208). Emotions, in this condition, are "not very complicated" (p. 211), and "sad depressing emotions are the most frequent" (p. 213). Jackson's release phenomenon explains the fact that, as Janet observes: "Emotions are exaggerated" (p. 210).

Primary, secondary, and tertiary dissociation

Janet's ideas were swept aside during the twentieth century by the twin juggernauts of behaviourism and psychoanalysis. The consequence is that the term dissociation, despite a great deal of research on the subject, "continues to be vague, confusing, and even controversial" (Dell, 2009, p. 225). Janet's fundamental distinction between *désagrégation* and dissociation has been largely forgotten and the terms, at least in English, are regarded as meaning pretty much the same thing (Nemiah, 1989). Freud must take some of the blame.

Freud expressed his "absolute opposition" (Breuer & Freud, 1895, p. 173) to Janet's theory of the fundamental vulnerability of his patients, the diminution of personal synthesis. "The splitting of consciousness does not occur because the patients are weak minded," he claimed, "but the patients seem weak-minded since their psychic activity is divided" (p. 172). He never retracted his view, which became an "official" part of the Freudian doctrine. The eminent psycho-analyst, Charles Rycroft, explained:

> Janet believed that self is not a pristine unity but an entity achieved by integration. ... Contemporary psychoanalysis and psychiatry tend to take the opposite view: that self is a pristine unity but uses defense mechanisms, notably repression, which makes it unconscious of much of its total activity.
>
> *(2004, p. 254)*

The psychoanalytic view, as expressed here, ignores extensive developmental data suggesting that the course of maturation depends upon the parallel processes of integration and differentiation. Neurophysiological evidence also supports the idea that *désagrégation* is a vulnerability out of which dissociation, that is, split-ting, can arise. In borderline patients, for example, brain systems, which usually operate together to provide a unified and coordinated output, no longer do so (Meares et al., 2005; Meares, 2012a).

The fact that the Freudian viewpoint was accepted and that Janet's explana-tion of the trauma-induced syndrome is now little known is difficult to explain. Compared with Janet's careful and extensive observations of at least 120 cases, only five were presented in Breuer and Freud's *Studies on Hysteria*, which, as its original translator noted, became the "*fons et origo* of psychoanalysis" (Brill, 1937, pp. viii–ix).

Breuer and Freud's five patients were a heterogeneous group, Freud having rejected Janet's proposal concerning the diagnostic significance of the "stig-mata." It remained for Freud a protean disorder. For example, one of the cases, Miss Katharina, suffered panic attacks that seemed to be related to unpleasant sexually based incidents involving her uncle. She was not a patient but a girl who waited on Freud's table when he was holidaying in an Alpine hotel. After this brief encounter, he never saw her again.

Currently, the concept of dissociation is commonly confined to Freud's con-cept of an active splitting of consciousness, a "compartmentalization" (Holmes et al., 2005) for which numerous studies have demonstrated a neurophysiological basis (e.g. Lanius et al., 2002). Some writers, following this conception, believe the normal process of selective inattention to be dissociation. This mechanism, as Sullivan (1953) pointed out a long time ago, can be used for defensive pur-poses. It is not, however, dissociation. What is split off in selective inattention are those aspects of normal consciousness that are not relevant to the task at hand. Dissociated consciousness, as Janet understood it, is not normal. It is disintegrated.

The works of Ellenberger, in 1970, and Van der Kolk and van der Hart, in 1989 and subsequent publications, have stimulated a renewed interest in Janet. Another form of dissociation is now recognized beyond "compartmentalization." Holmes and her colleagues (2005) called it "detachment." This observation is consistent with the suggestion of Bremner (1999) that there might be two sub-types of response to trauma, one dissociative and the other of hyperarousal. This hypothesis was tested by Lanius and her colleagues (2002). They studied the effect of traumatic script-driven imagery in posttraumatic stress disorder (PTSD) patients. They found that 70 per cent showed an increase in heart rate, while 30 per cent had a "dissociative" response, typically involving "numbing out." The cerebral areas activated in this state included the medial frontal cortex (BA9), which "several studies have shown has inhibitory influences on the emotional limbic system' (Lanius et al., 2006, p. 714). The hyperarousal condition is predicted by Jackson's "release phenomenon." It might be called "primary dissociation." It is curious to find that, during this state, the subject typically does not appear to be in a state of relative excitation. It is as if there were a disconnection between the arousal system and that of expression (Meares, 2012a).

"Secondary dissociation," referring to that part of psychic life separated, or split off from consciousness, can be conceived as having two forms, one passive (Janet) and the other active (Freud). Important data from Felmingham and her colleagues (2008), suggest that the active form, involving ventral frontal activation, is likely to be associated with consciousness of threat, while the passive form is a response to unconsciously registered threat. The latter state is associated with amygdaloid activation (see for further details, Meares, 2012a, p. 144).

A tertiary form of dissociation was suggested by Janet. It is a relatively fixed state in which there is a split between "two groups of phenomena, one constituting the ordinary personality, the other being, besides, susceptible of subdivision, forming an abnormal personality different from the first and altogether unknown to it" (1901, p. 494). This psychopathology was also found by C. S. Myers, in his experience of treating the effects of First World War combat trauma (Myers, 1915, 1940). He spoke of an "apparently normal personality" and an "emotional personality" that was usually hidden. With a different understanding to the levels of dissociation, Onno van der Hart and his colleagues (2006) have elaborated further on the significance and complexity of this dissociative system in states of trauma (see also Chapter 11).

We believe that the distinction between primary, secondary, and tertiary dissociation (Van der Kolk, van der Hart, & Marmar, 1996, pp. 306–307; Meares, 2012d), derived from the writings of Janet, may be helpful in making less confused the current discourse involving the concept called, in English, dissociation.

9

THE HOLISTIC PROJECT OF PIERRE JANET

Part Two: Oscillations and becomings: From disintegration to integration

Cécile Barral and Russell Meares

A group of us white people are strolling in the Australian bush with aboriginal elder Uncle M. At one point, Uncle M stops, sits himself on a sandstone ledge, ponders for a few minutes before talking: "You, white mob, have got it wrong. Do you realize that? You think your ancestors are in the past, like behind you. Wrong. They are ahead of you ... they are the ones showing you the way." Uncle M's words resonate in my mind as I am reading Janet, encouraged to examine my perspective on this elder of my psychotherapist self. Yes, Janet was a pioneer in his own time. Was he also possibly showing us the way forward in our pursuit of the understanding and healing of the self, especially borderline conditions?

As a French native speaker living in Australia, one of us (CS) is fortunate to have access to Janet's later work that has not been translated into English and is therefore not accessible to non-French readers, as is his earlier work on hysteria, neurosis, and obsessions. After having dedicated his earlier work to the understanding of hysteria and the disintegration of the self as a consequence of trauma, Janet's attention, from 1909 till 1932 (the year *La Force et la Faiblesse Psychologiques* was published), shifted to deepening his understanding the self and the refining of his hierarchy of psychological functions, which we would argue became a hierarchy of self-states in constant oscillation from disintegration at the bottom of the hierarchy to integration/synthesis at the higher levels.

This long phase was followed, between 1935 and 1936, by Janet's exploration of "natural" psychological development, a necessity, he felt, to pursue and deepen his understanding of the conditions necessary for the self to move naturally towards higher functions, and for the self disintegrated by trauma to resume its development (Janet, 1935a, 1934).

Disorders of the self

While working at La Salpêtrière Hospital where the focus was on severe cases of hysteria (*aliénés*), Janet also had a private practice where he saw "*non-aliénés*" patients, patients who did not require hospitalization, but nevertheless presented with such complaints as feelings of emptiness (*sentiments du vide*), of inadequacy (*sentiments d'incomplétude*), shrinking of life (*rétrécissement de la vie*), derealization (*agir en rêve*), difficulty in finding a meaningful, effective way of living, feeling lost, not in the world, like an imposter (*de jouer la comédie*), incapacity to make decisions or to begin or end actions, self-doubt, agitation, anxiety and obsessions, tendency to compliance, addictions, and so forth. These were symptoms of what Janet called psychasthenia (Janet, 1903, 1909a, 1932a).

Janet was in fact describing symptoms of personality disorders, chronic, empty depression, and dysphoria, what we currently understand as disorders of the self. He described such symptoms as mental states (*états mentaux*) rather than illnesses (*maladies*). They are characteristically subject to gradual or dramatic ameliorations and worsenings (*oscillations*) (1909a).

Hierarchy of psychological functions

Janet, a philosopher and psychologist at heart on a mission to understand the human mind, felt the need to synthesize his vast clinical experience and spent 25 years, from 1905 to 1937, elaborating his central concept of a hierarchy of psychological functions.

By 1930, he had established a three-tiered hierarchy (see Appendix, Table 1), reminiscent of Paul MacLean's (1990) triune brain. It consisted of nine levels of functioning. At the bottom of the hierarchy we find reflexive pathological conducts, characterized by reactivity and a narrowing of the mind, rigidity of beliefs (*croyances asséritives*), black-and-white views (*tout ou rien*) (Janet, 1935a, p. 25), oversimplification, emotional instability, reactivity, confusion, lack of coherence, initiative, and persistence, and so forth. In the middle of the hierarchy is the reflective capacity (*croyances réflectives*), characterized by the capacity to tolerate difference and to modify one's views, to have one's own thoughts while allowing doubt. At the top of the hierarchy, Janet places progressive conducts, characterized by the achievement of a personal synthesis (1932a, p. 19), individualism as well as social conscience, altruism, efficacy, sustained attention, will, the capacity to deal skillfully with the present, to "time travel," to have a sense of continuity, and to act for the larger good. This is a state of vastness of the mind that stretches over space and time. It implies that "the more elementary an action, the smaller it is, and the more superior it is, the more it stretches over space and above all time" (p. 31).

Looking at Janet's hierarchy, we can see how he was elaborating on both William James's theory of the self and Hughlings Jackson's theory of disaggregation, clearly articulating an avant-garde psychology of the self understood as complex and dynamic states of consciousness.

It is interesting to note how the reflective capacity deemed by most contemporary therapies as one of the best markers of psychological maturity and health is situated midway on Janet's hierarchy. This suggests a direction for future developments for the psychologies of the self.

Oscillations: Self-states on a continuum

Based on his wealth of clinical observations, Janet concluded that "there is no fundamental difference between the conduct of a healthy person and the conduct of a sick one" (1932a, p. 295), with everyone functioning at, and shifting on, the dynamic continuum of psychological functioning, depending on circumstances. Falling down the hierarchy "can happen to any mind" (*cela peut arriver à tous les esprits*), wrote Janet (1932a, p. 25).

He was advocating a paradigm shift from the idea of symptoms and illnesses as clear-cut categorical illnesses to a new understanding of syndromes as complex and constantly shifting self-states, thereby confirming the idea of the mind/self as both structure and process.

From conducts to tendencies

Meanwhile, however, Janet was seeing limitations to his hierarchy of conducts. He wrote how "many of the higher psychological phenomena have an internal spiritual and moral aspect and appear entirely different from so-called actions" (1930a, p. 6). He saw the need to include consciousness, belief, memory, thought, and above all feelings in his hierarchy of the self:

> Feelings have always made psychologists uncomfortable, especially those who are above all interested in actions and conducts: In reality, consciousness is above all founded on the phenomenon of feelings. Consciousness is an ensemble of feelings that build one on the other (*qui s'ajoutent les uns aux autres*), and the loss of feelings is the beginning of a loss of consciousness.
>
> *(1932a, p. 111)*

William James comments how Janet was creating a new language for his time,

> to represent entirely other forms of thought: oscillations of the level of mental energy, differences of tension, splittings of consciousness, feelings of insufficiency and of unreality, substitutions, agitations, and anxieties, depersonalizations ... the conceptions that the total view of his patient's life imposes on this clinical observer ... nothing to do with the usual laboratory categories.
>
> *(1907, p. 322)*

Consequently, 1930 marked a significant shift from Janet's original hierarchy of conducts to a new hierarchy of tendencies, a tendency being, according to him, a living organism's disposition to accomplish a determined action (Janet, 1926a, p. 31).

One essential outcome of a hierarchy based on tendencies rather than conducts was that it "helps to distinguish individuals" (1932a, p. 324) and create a person's "dynamic balance sheet" (*bilan dynamique*) i.e. a picture of oscillating self-states constantly seeking equilibrium (p. 315). Isabelle Saillot (2005), a central figure in his revival, adds that it allows "for a good description of one's personality" (translate "self"). She hopes this will encourage practitioners to draw a dynamic "biographical hierarchy" for each individual rather than apply a categorical diagnosis.

La force psychologique: A new parameter

Janet had also become aware of the limitations of his original 1909 hierarchy that was based on the concept of "*tension psychologique*" (1932a, p. 76). "*Tension*" and its opposite "*détente*" had a different meaning for Janet from the contemporary one of unhealthy stress/anxiety and its opposite, relaxation. For Janet, *tension* meant the capacity to hold complexity, to create order and synthesis from the many, while détente had to do with the loss of such capacity.

Tension alone, although necessary to function at the higher level of the hierarchy, was not enough. "There exists in an action a quality that I call force," wrote Janet (1932a, p. 113). He described force as an overall "powerfulness" (*une puissance générale*, p. 311), which Ellenberger succinctly defined as "the quantity of elementary psychic energy, that is, the capacity to accomplish numerous, prolonged and rapid psychological acts" (1970, p. 378). Consequently, Janet felt the necessity to include a second parameter to his hierarchy – that of "*force psychologique*" (1932a), which he saw as "a measure of the effort a person was capable of" (p. 309).

Janet was noticing, for example, how some people, say an alcoholic, could have a capacity for higher functions – to reflect on the harm alcohol was doing to him and argue very reasonably as to why and how he was going to stop drinking, yet not be able to translate his decision into real healthier productive actions because he lacked a certain force to act. Tension requires force to translate thinking into action, while force without tension translates into pathological discharge of unusable energy, such as muscular discharge or acting out (p. 315).

Force makes one less suggestible and allows for a stronger personality (p. 309). It can be seen in an individual's capacity to engage in robust discussions and be consequently enriched by other minds, while *faiblesse* causes the individual to give into others' opinions (pp. 79–81). This capacity to engage other minds is one of the aims of models of psychotherapy like the Conversational Model created by Robert Hobson (1985) and Russell Meares, in which the therapist endeavours to create a resonance with his patient's states of mind with the purpose of gradually fostering a generative type of conversation.

Janet, however, struggled to explain his concept of "*force psychologique*," which he described as "a problem more than a solution" (1932a, p. 309). He saw in it "a very strange mix" (*un mélange extrêmement curieux*), a psycho-physiological phenomenon that combined "muscular force" (the body) with "moral force" (the mind) (p. 89). For him, "there are two ways of thinking and acting: the motor way and the verbal way" (p. 70). Janet, well ahead of his time, was tackling the concept of the self as a "bodybrainmind" system – addressed only much later by Damasio (1994, 2010).

La force psychologique: A form of energy

Energy was not a new concept in Janet's time; it was part of William James's psychology, and of Freud's theories. Nor was mental exhaustion, although Janet seemed unaware of the earlier work of George Beard on neurasthenia as a condition of physical and mental exhaustion (Ellenberger, 1970, p. 242). This left the idea of "psychological energy" or force unheard of at such a time of "laboratory psychology" (James, 1907, p. 2), and Janet was struggling to get the concept accepted.

He pointed out that psychological force or mental energy "was not a mysterious power" and "had nothing mystical to it." Energy was accepted in all other fields of science. Why not, then, by psychology (1932a, p. 310, 318)? Janet argued that energy is not the same as the physiological force (*force vitale*) that makes the embryo grow without requiring any psychological force. Nor is it simply a question of metabolism, brain, and nervous system (pp. 309–320). It is very complex as multiple functions need to come together in the building of psychological force (p. 323).

Janet foresaw that quantifying mental energy would be the object of future research (p. 324). He welcomed and encouraged experiments in the field of "psycho-physics." However, his wishes would become reality only in modern times with the developments of neuroscience.

This concept of energy seems to have been well reinstated by most respected modern theoreticians like Damasio (2010), Meares (2016), Porges (2016), Schore (1994), Siegel (1999), Stern (1985), Tronick (2016), van der Hart, Nijenhuis, and Steele (2006), and in the advances of neuropsychology that confirm that the electrical processes happening in the brain are one aspect of consciousness, of the brain–mind system. It has also been revived in the last decades with the attention given to the autonomic nervous system, the role of its formation and regulation in the development of the sense of self (Schore, 1994).

Meanwhile, Janet's grasp of the "*force psychologique*" had to come from his clinical observations (now recognized as a valid scientific approach): "though not concrete or measurable, it is qualitative and reveals itself in observable dynamic psychological phenomena" (1932a, pp. 117–118). Levels of energy were an experience expressed in his patients' everyday language as they described feeling low in energy and exhausted or being energized, having too much energy, their mind being foggy or clear, and so forth. Janet came to conceive of "psychasthenic states" as conditions of exhaustion and depletion (*maladies d'épuisement*) (p. 133), a "loss of the vital juices" (p. 125) causing an arrest in the natural development of the self.

Becomings and the human environment[1]

Having noticed how, "under certain circumstances, the activity of the mind can lower to an inferior level," while the fragile higher states of consciousness can only be maintained in "favourable circumstances" (Janet, 1932a), Janet's next questions became: Where does psychological force come from? What increases or diminishes force in an individual? How does the sense of self develop? And how to help those who have fallen to or are stuck at lower levels move up?

With his awareness that *force* and *faiblesse* are of the body and mind, Janet thought that rest could be an important part of treatment, showing his openness to consider a wide range of treatments best suited to the patient's specific "dynamic balance sheet" (*bilan dynamique*) (p. 315).

He had also noticed, and this is extremely important, that tendencies stay latent unless activated within the milieu in which the self develops (p. 314). This milieu is one of ongoing reciprocal relationships – one could say ongoing "conversations" in which each element contributes to the transformation of the other – for better or worse (Hobson, 1985; Meares, 2005).

Janet observed how "animals that show the least intelligence are those that live in isolation" (1935a), "how the conduct of thinking would not exist for a human being who had forever lived in isolation" (p. 54), and how a child plays more actively "if he is with friends" (p. 46). In a word, humans are social beings, and "social life increases force and enriches the mind" (1932a, p. 166).

Janet talked of the importance of "parental temperaments: parents who are calm, not too emotional seem to create their children's force" (p. 125), whereas "hostilities between a father and a mother … make children sick" (p. 177).

He understood the importance of being valued, an idea often left out of philosophy and psychology. He saw the consequences of habitual devalorization in depressions marked by a loss of interest (*à quoi bon?*, "What's the point?"), feelings of nonexistence and unreality or an "obsession to be loved" (pp. 38, 45).

In a similar vein, Janet saw how experiences of "triumph move us up the hierarchy" (1935a, p. 65). When "there is a success and a triumph, all our functions are better … a very good thing for humans" (1932a, p. 36). Janet's triumphs have nothing to do with grandiosity; they are victories over obstacles – for example, the student overcoming his block and managing to write an assignment. It requires effort and results in a sense of pride that is a form of joy and heals shame (1935a, pp. 64–65).

In brief, Janet came to see that the self develops through positive affective exchanges and in an intimacy that Janet called as "a conduct of feeling" (1932a, p. 170).

Inspired by Durkheim's theories that many intellectual operations are social in origin, and expanding from the family to society, Janet proposed that "our ideas, judgments, classifications, and principles of reason" are influenced by our complex yet essential relationship to society (1935a, p. 38). The relationship to the "socius" (Janet used Baldwin's term) is complex and necessary (p. 41). We need the socius to become conscious of ourselves; we constantly modify our behaviour to adapt to its actions, thus learning to collaborate, to develop a sense of the other, to read other minds and represent our own (p. 46).

Janet expanded even further to include a similar reciprocal relationship (p. 50) of the self to the culture it exists in, with ceremonies and rituals bringing people together in an experience of shared joy, "a good antidote to depression" (pp. 57–58). Again, this was a visionary view of the self, later taken up by Vytgovsky (Van der Veer & Valsiner, 1988), and recently by Trevarthen (2014) and Meares (2016).

Arrested becomings: Developmental trauma

Janet's elaboration of his developmental theory includes developmental trauma and arrest. He writes: "Pathologies caused by developmental arrests and regressions present themselves in all forms and levels of psychological maturation" (Janet, 1926–1928, in Saillot, 2008, p. 3).

A major source of drops (*chutes*) down the hierarchy are the "violent" (read traumatic) emotions (1932a, p. 158). "Emotions are a great output of force" (*une grande dépense*) (1932a, p. 162):

> No doubt that, faced with a very traumatizing (*émotionnant*) event, you would do well to tense up, have energy, and reflect on how to respond to these threatening circumstances and counteract them; no doubt you would be better off if, in such moments, you showed great intelligence. Then the huge amount of nervous energy released would not be a problem. However, it is very difficult to show intelligence in the face of surprises and dangerous circumstances, at a moment when you cannot see the way out.
>
> *(p. 315)*

Unresolved past traumas (*dettes*) are included in this: "events which had established a violent emotion and a destruction of the psychological system, [and] had left traces, ... they absorb a great deal of strength and play a part in the persistent weakening" (1930a, p. 4).

Janet translated his ideas into action. He rejected the blank screen method of his time and advocated a positive attitude towards patients to facilitate the building of the self. This, he knew from experience, was necessary before traumas could be resolved. In this way, he anticipated a central aspect of the Conversational Model in which a sense of "connection" between patient and therapist is necessary for the emergence of the self. This feeling of connection depends upon more than mere friendliness. The therapist must be aware of the patient's moment-to-moment states of mind.

Janet wrote of how clinicians need to enter their patients' world at their level on the hierarchy of functions, to listen to them deeply, believe them, and validate their experiences. He found that reasoning and explaining often did not help, thus radically distancing himself from Freud's fantasy theories and interpretative style (1932a, p. 18).

Connection is further enhanced by paying attention to the "minute particulars" of the conversation (Hobson, 1985) and to "what happens next" (Meares, 2000), that is, to any felt change in patients' oscillations up and down the hierarchy, to what has made them feel better (signs of vitalization) or worse, to the intrusion of traumatic memories (*émotions soudaines*), and by wondering what could have caused such changes – "an observation," Janet wrote, "that does not happen often enough in our clinical practices" (1932a, p. 204). In that vein, models of psychotherapy supervision that use video, or less intrusive audio recordings, allow for the development of such fine attention to details.

Becomings: Janet's perspective on development

Janet found that in order to understand pathology he needed to understand normal psychological development, thereby pointing the way to the necessity of combining developmental and trauma theories to create effective models of psychotherapy. As part of this project, he worked with and influenced the young Jean Piaget, who called Janet "my professor" for the rest of his life (Bringuier, 1989, p. 3). Freud, too, had realized the need to understand normal development. However, while Freud had focused on psychosexual development, Janet was interested in the development of "intelligence," as indicated by the title of his last two published books (1935a, 1934).

The word "intelligence" could be easily misunderstood. By intelligence Janet meant the capacity for new adaptations of conduct to "especially complex circumstances" (*présentification*) (1935a). It required a capacity to bring together multiple objects, including ideas, into a synthesis that allowed "greater efficiency," for example a scientific discovery that "will permit humans to live more, to live better and for longer."

This capacity to create new connections (*rapports*) starts with the infant's bodily experience and the formation of embodied schemas as the child engages with objects – first, concrete objects manipulated in the physical/external world, and later abstract conceptual objects (thoughts and language).

So, for example, Janet explores the development of the capacity for reciprocity. At a primitive level, an infant will first discover reciprocity through reaching out and pulling towards, coming and going, actions soon turning into what Janet called the "conduct of the basket" (*l'acte du panier*) (1934, p. 13). It is the act of gathering multiple objects in and out of the one container. This marks the beginnings of the capacity to synthesize. It later evolves into the putting together of words into sentences, and even later (around three years) into the child realizing that if he, Paul, has a brother Peter, then Peter also has a brother, Paul. The next stage in the development of the capacity for reciprocity comes with the mastery of time, which is more advanced than that of space (1935a). It is the capacity for complex and abstract reciprocal actions such as starting afresh, reparation, and remorse. The early conduct of the basket eventually grows into the experience of a unitary self, made up of multiplicity of selves in a constant process of mutual construction (1934).

In this example of the developmental line from the conduct of the basket to a unified self, we have one example among many of Janet's development of hierarchies within hierarchies, which has inspired a number of contemporary theorists: a hierarchy of engagement (Graham & Van Biene, 2007), a hierarchy of feelings (Meares, 2016). This is very much open to further developments.

Janet added that the integrated self is not absolute and remains fragile forever. We are bound, for example, to experience periods of hesitation, doubt, in which

> consciousness seems to become divided … Even slight mental troubles modify and suppress the sense of the unity of self … the unity of the self is an ideal … towards which the person leans … Our unity/integration, when it exists, is the result of a work of synthesis that is always incomplete and easily, even if temporarily, lost.
>
> *(1934, pp. 58 and 61)*

Becomings: From imitation to analogy

Janet's quest for evidence in the child's development that could be a basis for therapy culminates in an extremely interesting and, from our point of view, exciting proposal of a progression of conducts. It moves from the primitive "act of imitation" (*acte d'imitation*) (1935a, p. 41) to the "conduct of the portrait" (*conduite du portrait*) (1934, p. 28).

This progression begins in the first few weeks of life in which, for example, the baby replicates his mother's action of sticking out her tongue. The observation has been repeated in recent times, and quite famously, by Meltzoff and Moore (1977). The baby's "*acte d'imitation*" is unconscious and automatic. It is, as Janet believed, a manifestation of "a sort of confusion between the self and others" (Piaget, 1959, p. 28), an explanation repeatedly cited by Piaget. A behaviour that is more truly imitative emerges towards the end of the first year of life when the child, for example, imitates the gestures and body postures of those close to him. It is a "*double act*": the child exhibits the first form of the double consciousness that is a cardinal characteristic of selfness. The child is being two people, two states, or two things at the same time: he is simultaneously himself and something else.

The next step in this progression is crucial to the achievement of humanity. It is a move from simple copying, or imitation, the equivalent of "*trompe-l'oeil*" work in art, to use Janet's own words (1935a, p. 27), to resemblance (p. 23 ff). It is the first step towards the capacity for creativity. Something that resembles another thing, but is not a copy, is an analogue. An analogue is the representation of the shape or essence of a thing by resembling it. The child's "resembling" behaviour begins to be displayed in what Piaget called symbolic play. It is well developed in the third year of life. In this apparently solitary game, the child chooses objects in the environment that resemble the elements of the story the child is telling, apparently to itself, in a self-absorbed chatter. These objects have a "shape" similar to what they represent. For example, a stick is a man, a large leaf is a boat. The child is exhibiting analogical thought.

The analogue, it can be argued, is the origin of the symbol (Meares, 2016). Although analogue and symbol are not easily distinguished, it is important, in talking of the development of "mind," to establish the essential difference between them. An analogical resemblance is between things in the external world. A symbol, of which metaphor is the prime exemplar, serves to represent realities that cannot be seen or grasped, most notably feelings. Although more primitive feelings – rage, sadness, shame, and so forth – are expressed facially, those feelings that are complex, subtle, difficult, "*ineffable*" (1935a, p. 27). These "little emotions" (Meares, 2016) are not usually manifest in this way. They are, however, central to higher-order consciousness. They can only be "realized" by their representation in language, by the use of words that have a picturing function, for example by means of symbols. These symbols "portray" central features of an inner life.

The language of symbolization emerges with the achievement of the concept of "innerness," which is gained at about the age of four (Meares & Orlay, 1988) with the discovery of what Janet called the "act of secrecy" (1935a, p. 54). Janet ascribes to the "act of secrecy ... the utmost importance, since thought is the form taken by the act of the secret in its ultimate form" (p. 54). With the appearance of this milestone, doubleness of consciousness takes a step forward. The child now lives in two worlds, inner and outer, public and private. He or she can now hold in mind, at the same time, two models of reality – its own and that of others. This is demonstrated, in more recent times, in tests of "false belief" (Wimmer & Perner, 1983), which are the backbone of the so-called "theory of mind."

Symbolization goes on across a boundary between inner and outer. Things of the outer world are used to represent those of the inner. It is through this process that the "conduct of the portrait" is achieved. The symbolic act, Janet states, is in essence a relational act (1934, p. 58). It becomes lost when there is a lowering of the mental level to a state where the fundamental dualities are lost.

The conversation in which "the portrait" is painted is first of all between caregiver and child. The artist is the caregiver, performing "a conduct of the portrait of feelings" (1934, p. 57) through the use of symbols. This kind of portrait is very like a "form of feeling," as described by Hobson (1985) and central to the therapeutic practice of the Conversational Model.

It is here that we can return to the artistic approach of Matisse. The portrait is not a copy, like a photograph, but an abstraction, involving a sort of pruning of the real that is necessary to express the ineffable. An example is provided by Matisse's portrait of Yvonne Landsberg. Her brother watched as Matisse progressed through a number of versions of this portrait. He was "struck by how the less the painting came to resemble her physically, the better it conveyed her personality, i.e. her essence" (Flam, 2003, p. 100).

Following the achievement of the concept of "innerness" the child now begins to make its own "portraits." It can now enter into an interplay that, in some circumstances, can lead to the "act of intimacy," in which "pictures" of inner states can be shared by means of symbolic language. This behaviour is consistent with Janet's proposal that a new form of conduct, manifesting a state of mind higher on the hierarchy of consciousness, comes into being not as a consequence of some notional brain change, but through the "internalization" of a preceding form of social interaction that resembles it.

A further major expansion of the child's mental life occurs at this stage, manifest in memory and narrative. At about the age of four, two principal lines of development, underpinning logical and analogical processes, are brought together. Narrative is possible. One kind of thought, the logical and syntactical, becomes the vehicle for a second kind of thought that is analogical and symbolic (Meares, 1993, 2005). This coordination allows the development of "*le récit*," a narrative that is a form of intelligent representation (Janet, 1934, p. 129). This story has the capacity of showing a resemblance to an individual life, a larger kind of "portrait." It is an act of the narrative self. It is an expression of our "right to have a story, similar to our right to have a name (*un nom propre*)." Janet adds: "This personal biography becomes the starting point of what we call the identity of self (*l'identité de la personnalité*)" (p. 134). It should be noted, however, that Janet does not make clear in his writing that this narrative is not a mere chronicle (Meares, 1998), an account of a series of events. Rather, it is necessarily a resemblance, having the form of a personal myth (Meares, 2016).

Janet does make this clear in discussing another form of narrative, what has been called episodic memory (Tulving, 1983). Janet considered that this is the memory characteristic of humans. It is a story that is not "real" but is a reconstruction. Memory is another kind of a portrait, a picture. With it comes a realization of time, a subject beyond the scope of this essay.

An extremely important aspect of Janet's notion of the portrait is its relational and generative implications. Janet further comments on the impact of the "successful'" portrait (1935a, part 2, p. 35). A successful portrait brings "a particular form of joy" (1934, p. 160) jointly experienced by the maker and the viewer. Such joy comes with the experience of conveying the inner subtle experiences and knowing one has been understood. We recognize it in the transformative moments of therapy that move patient and therapist up the hierarchy when the patient feels met, understood, and recognized. It is the joy of synthesis (p. 27) or the joy of the self coming together (Meares, 2016). This feeling may be the origin of the positive feeling at the core of healthy selfhood that James called "warmth and intimacy," and which is lacking in the repetitively traumatized people who suffer instead a painful state of dysphoria.

Conclusion

Uncle M's words ring so true: Janet's thinking was remarkably far ahead of his time, and we can learn from him. He himself compared his work to the "exploration of the terrae incognitae of the human spirit" that starts "with following a small river through unknown territory and gradually gets to the bigger river" (1935a p. 17).

Janet's own personal journey exemplifies his hierarchy, the way he himself achieved his own singular synthesis of his multiple tendencies: Janet the philosopher, the psychologist, the scientist, the botanist, the mystic, the family man, to name the main ones (1932a, p. 1); the way he overcame his own traumas (his depression at age 15, when he lost his faith, three wars, and the Great Depression), and the force he gathered to reach and maintain himself at the higher levels of his hierarchy – a mind vast in space and time, working humbly and tirelessly to improve the human condition.

We may wonder how he could have spent so many years refining his hierarchy of psychological functions. But if we understand that he was pioneering a whole new psychology of the self – its healthy and its pathological development – we may appreciate the immensity of his enterprise and the courage and dedication it must have taken him in a time when classic analysis and behavioural psychology were the preferred theories. Janet's later work (1930–1936), although probably unfinished, may in time receive the same appreciation as his earlier more widely known texts.

The relevance of Janet's place in contemporary thinking deserves to be fully realized, as his work gives validation and solidity to emergent theories and contemporary theorists who are on similar journeys and, like Janet, may find it not easy to be heard – theories that integrate new scientific research as well as a philosophical approach to the understanding of the self and its pathologies, theories that integrate developmental and trauma science as well as a vast empirical experience to come to their conclusions, and theories that integrate the art and the science of psychotherapy in their clinical practices. Janet's work shows remarkable similarities to the main features of the Conversational Model, a form of generative therapy directed towards facilitation of the emergence of self. We have woven together salient elements of his descriptions to demonstrate this similarity.

Note

1 We are using "becoming" as a noun in its plural form, as is common use in French (un devenir (a becoming)/des devenirs (becomings). "Devenir" as a substantive is defined as "the passage of one state to another" (Le Petit Robert dictionary). Although the substantive becoming does not seem to be used anymore in English, it is also a noun defined as "any change involving realisation of potentialities, as a movement form the lower level of potentiality to the higher level of actuality" (Macquarie Dictionary).

Appendix

TABLE 1 *Janet's Hierarchies of Action Tendencies*

Janet's 1930 hierarchy of action tendencies

Conduites progressives	Progressive behaviours	Implying a synthesis of functions and individuality (sense of self)
		Reaching further into space and time (Janet, 1930b, p. 75)
Conduites experimentales	Experimental behaviours	Based on experience and facts
		Integrate past, present, and future
Stade rationnel ergétique	Rational-ergetic stage	Rational and action-based stage, with capacity to sustain work (*ergon* = activity)
Croyance réfléchie	Reflective beliefs	
Croyance asséritive	Assertive beliefs	Beliefs based on feelings (e.g. what one fears) rather than facts. Prone to suggestibility (Janet, 1930b, p. 76)
Actes intellectuels élémentaires	Elementary intellectual actions	Intelligence before language and beginning of language (Ellenberger, 1970, p. 390)
Conduites sociales	Social behaviours	The individual adjusts his own acts to the acts of the *socius* (Ellenberger, 1970, p. 388)
Conduites perceptives	Perceptive behaviours	Instinctive (Janet, 1930b, p. 74)
Conduites reflexes	Automatic/reflexive behaviours	Muscular discharge/no regulation

Janet's 1934 hierarchy

Tendances à des actes réflexes	Reflexive tendencies	
Tendances à des actes perceptifs ou suspensifs	Perceptive-suspensive tendencies	Require a two-step double stimulation with a period of suspense inbetween (Ellenberger, 1970, p. 388)
Tendances à des actes sociaux	Social tendencies	
Tendances à des actes intellectuels élémentaires	Elementary intellectual tendencies	
Tendances à des actes du plan verbal, actes asséritifs	Verbal and assertive actions	Verbal and bodily actions can be separated

Tendances à des actes réfléchis	Reflective actions
Tendances à des actes rationnels	Rational tendencies
Tendances à des actes expérimentaux	Experimental tendencies
Tendances à des actes progressifs	Progressive tendencies

10

PIERRE JANET ON HALLUCINATIONS, PARANOIA, AND SCHIZOPHRENIA[1]

Andrew Moskowitz, Gerhard Heim, Isabelle Saillot, and Vanessa Beavan

Pierre Janet is best known as the "father" of dissociation theory, and for his therapeutic approaches to hysterical and psychasthenic (obsessive) conditions (Pitman, 1987; Chapter 1). While he saw few psychotic patients in his practice, and probably did not read the works of Bleuler and Kraepelin (certainly not in their original German), Janet always had an abiding interest in psychotic symptoms. Indeed, his fascination with hallucinations entirely brackets his professional life – Janet's first impulse when he decided to study psychiatric patients in the early 1880s was to look for people experiencing hallucinations (Ellenberger, 1970), and in his last paper (Janet, 1947a), published posthumously, he returned to the topic. In between (particularly in his later years), Janet published close to 20 papers specifically addressing psychotic symptoms or the concept of schizophrenia. While this makes up only a small portion of his voluminous corpus, there are many riches to be found in these papers, which still have relevance today. As it is not possible to give a comprehensive overview of Janet's important ideas on psychosis within the short confines of this chapter, we have chosen to focus our discussion on Janet's important two-part 1932c paper, "L'Hallucination dans le délire de la persécution" ("Hallucinations in persecutory delusions"),[2] complemented by three shorter papers on hallucinations or schizophrenia, published between 1927 and 1947.

Historical overview

Placed in Le Havre, a small city in Normandy, to teach philosophy, Janet quickly expressed an interest in examining psychiatric patients. He was curious about hallucinations, which he wanted to study "in connection … with the mechanism of perception," and intended to produce a thesis on this topic (Janet, 1930a).

We do not know the reason for Janet's interest, but it appears very likely that he was aware of the ongoing debate about the nature of hallucinations, which had reached an apogee in Paris 30 years before (Berrios & Dening, 1996). However, when he approached a prominent physician in Le Havre, Dr. Gibert, he was instead directed to a woman known as "Léonie," who had reportedly demonstrated remarkable psychic abilities. Janet's careful studies of her, along with other patients in Le Havre, formed the basis for his doctoral thesis and first book, *L'Automatisme Psychologique* (Janet, 1889).

While Janet commented on hallucinations only briefly in several publications for the three decades following the publication of *L'Automatisme Psychologique* (during which time he developed his theories of hysteria and psychasthenia), his interest in hallucinations and delusions became renewed in the late 1920s. It is possible that this interest was stimulated by a visit to Zurich he made in late 1926, at the invitation of Eugen Bleuler,[3] or by Eugene Minkowski's book, *La Schizophrénie* (1927a), published in 1927. While little is known about this visit, Janet presented Bleuler with a personally inscribed copy of the first volume of his two-part book, *De L'Angoisse à L'Extase* (*From Anxiety to Ecstasy*; Janet, 1926a). A year later, Janet published a paper entitled "A propos de la schizophrénie" ("Concerning schizophrenia"), in which he examined a couple of case studies with regard to Bleuler's concept and the concept of dissociation. Then, in 1932, Janet published the important article, "L'Hallucination dans le délire de la persécution" ("Hallucinations in persecutory delusions") (Janet, 1932c), central to our discussion here, as well as several other papers that were apparently planned as part of the proposed book noted above. Subsequently, Janet wrote little on this subject until his important final contribution, published after his death in 1947, in which he returned to the topic of hallucinations in paranoid psychosis. Perhaps this paper was stimulated by another visit to Zurich, in late 1946, this time at the invitation of Carl Jung and Manfred Bleuler, Eugen Bleuler's son and at the time the head of the Burghölzi hospital (Ellenberger, 1970). Janet was apparently warmly welcomed by Bleuler; Ellenberger (1970) writes that Janet had been "well acquainted" with his father.

Important Janetian concepts

Janet's writings on schizophrenia, paranoia, and hallucinations occurred in the context of his general psychology of action (*la psychologie de la conduite*; cf. Janet, 1926a, 1938), developed while he was Professor of Comparative and Experimental Psychology at the Collège de France and through his psychotherapy practice. Janet followed the "pathological method" of Claude Bernard and Théodule Ribot (Brooks III, 1998; Nicolas, 2002), which he described as "using all available information from [normal] psychology for the classification and interpretation of psychopathological facts, and inversely by searching in the morbid alterations of the mind for observations and natural experiences with which to analyse [normal] human thinking" (Janet, 1903, p. vii).

Thus, in order to understand Janet's ideas about hallucinations, paranoia, and schizophrenia, one must first understand some of the basic psychological tenets of his general psychology of action. The concepts relevant to our discussion are those of *psychological force* and *psychological tension*, his hierarchies of *tendencies* and *levels of reality*, and his conception of feelings as *action regulators* and their relationship to *social division*.

Psychological "force" and "tension"

Janet's somewhat metaphorical terminology was influenced by the zeitgeist of the nineteenth century when electricity and advances in physical sciences, such as the "discovery" of the laws of "thermodynamics", had a fundamental impact on medicine and psychology (Rabinbach, 1990). In essence, he believed (as did Freud) that there was a form of mental or psychological energy, similar in many ways to physical energy, the perturbations of which had much to do with psychopathology. Janet's model contained several key concepts (1923b). *Psychological force* refers to an individual's psychological resources available for mobilization. Janet believed that people varied inherently in the levels of psychological force available to them, and that this level also varied within an individual depending on their circumstances. For example, physical illness or stress typically would lead to a reduced level of psychological force, which would make the person more susceptible to certain psychological conditions. As psychological force had to be applied appropriately in specific situations, Janet proposed a second concept or mechanism, *psychological tension*, to effect this. Adequate psychological tension allows an individual to make the most of the psychological resources (force) available to them, appropriately choosing from among potential actions and expending just the right amount of *force* (this characteristic has led van der Hart, Nijenhuis, and Steele (2006) to rename psychological tension *mental efficiency*).

In contrast, psychopathology involves insufficient force, inadequate tension, or a poor balance between the two, which often leads to the expression of actions inappropriate to a given situation (that is, too high or too low in Janet's *hierarchy of tendencies*, discussed later). For example, a surfeit of psychological force coupled with limited tension could lead to certain obsessions or compulsions, for example, or tics or mannerisms. Janet's therapeutic approaches involved directly assessing an individual's psychological force and tension, and proposing unique solutions.

The hierarchy of (action) tendencies

Janet (1926b, 1938) believed that all human behaviour could be conceptualized on a scale of tendencies. He uses the term *tendencies* to emphasize that not all of what he characterized on the scale would typical be seen as *actions*, that is – behaviours physically expressed towards other persons or objects. Thus, Janet considered many, if not all, mental or psychological activities to be *actions*, albeit *suspended* ones. To Janet, *thinking, remembering, contemplating*, etc., were best considered as actions because of their original social conception and relevance. For example, he believed that memories were stories about our lives constructed to be told to others, or told to ourselves as though we were *an other*, and that thought was largely internalized language. Importantly, Janet even believed that as basic a psychological function as "perception" was "a motor reaction," emphasizing that recognizing an object always implied a potential action (or "reaction") in relation to it (Janet, 1935a); such a position explains why different cultures have different ranges of words for concepts (Canadian Inuit have far more words for "snow," for example, than do Europeans, because relatively subtle differences in "snow" have action implications for them – i.e. in how the snow may be used – that do not exist for Europeans).

While it is not possible to discuss the hierarchy of tendencies in detail here (see for comprehensive overviews, Heim & Bühler, 2006; Saillot, 2005; van der Hart, Nijenhuis, & Steele, 2006), the points central to our discussion are that pathology often involves the substitutive expression of tendencies towards the lower end of the scale, and that mental activities are best conceptualized as actions.

Levels of the reality function

Janet also argued that humans ascribe a level of reality to internal or external events that could be conceptualized in terms of a hierarchy. He included on this hierarchy various concepts, including imagination, actions, and various states of the past, present, and future (Janet, 1928b; cf. van der Hart, Nijenhuis, & Steele, 2006). The highest level of the reality function involved what Janet called *presentification*, the capacity to act in a fully focused and meaningful way in the present, integrating one's past experiences and future plans. Janet argued that much of psychopathology could be conceptualized as a mixing up of levels of reality – for example, viewing the distant past as happening in the present, as occurs in posttraumatic disorders. However, this hierarchy can also be used to explain phenomena such as hearing voices as occurring when internal mental events are accorded an inappropriate level of reality ("The deluded patient is an individual who locates his speech badly on the hierarchy of the degrees of reality," Janet, 1932a, p. 25).

Feelings (sentiments) as action regulators and social division

Janet placed great emphasis in his theory on the importance of a wide range of internal states, which he called "sentiments," in regulating behaviour (Janet, 1928b). The English term "feelings" is a better translation of this term, but is a bit narrower than Janet's "sentiments," as some of these – that is, fatigue, effort – are more akin to what we might call "proprioceptive feedback." Janet further argued that feelings interacted with and modified "social division," that is, the process by which we attribute actions to others ("social objectification") or to ourselves ("social subjectification"), a distinction he suggests must be learned and is not always straightforward.

> All social behaviour requires complex representations in which there is, at the same time, both the representation of our action and the representation of others' actions. This behaviour always requires an operation of dividing-up, so that some of these complex representations are attributed to ourselves and some are attributed to others. This delicate and error-prone operation depends greatly on our feelings.
>
> *(Janet, 1936b, p. 385)*

Specifically, Janet argued that attributing actions to ourselves – *social subjectification* – was closely associated with the feelings of effort and fatigue that we experienced when the action was executed. *Social objectification*, in contrast, was most often determined by the less elementary feelings of failure and triumph, and the associated (respective) feelings of sadness and joy. We feel failure, for example, when an action occurs (or doesn't occur) despite our efforts (as though the action was independent of us). The obstacle is located within the object and resistance is linked to others. The action is objectified and thus becomes part of the social realm. The same thing occurs in a triumphant reaction. We triumph over an external resistance, but the action that accompanies our feelings of triumph is linked to the social realm.

Errors in social division may occur when strong feelings, *normally* associated with effort, fatigue, failure, or triumph, arise in their *absence*. Specifically, Janet argues that melancholia, occurring (by definition) in the absence of any genuine social failure, can distort social division so that a person's thoughts can be mistakenly attributed to the social realm.

Schizophrenia

In contrast to hallucinations, discussed below, few of Janet's writings directly address Bleuler's concept of schizophrenia; the primary exception is the 1927(b) paper, "Concerning schizophrenia." Indeed, when Janet discussed psychotic diagnoses besides paranoia at all, even after meeting Eugen Bleuler in 1926, he tended to use Kraeplin's "dementia praecox" rather than Bleuler's "schizophrenia."[4] Possible reasons for this are discussed below.

Janet appeared to understand schizophrenia as a severe form of psychological asthenia, a weakness of psychological force (Ellenberger, 1970) bordering on, but distinct from, psychasthenia (which he always saw as a form of neurosis; Janet, 1930a). He clearly placed the genesis for schizophrenia in the social realm; Ellenberger (1970, p. 379) quotes (but does not reference) Janet as regularly saying "dementia praecox is a social dementia" ("la démence précoce est une démence sociale").

His 1927 paper was stimulated by a presentation by Eugene Minkowski at the Parisian Société de Psychologie. Minkowski was a Russian-born psychiatrist who worked closely with Bleuler during the First World War, subsequently settling in Paris. Janet describes Minkowski's presentation as addressing "the theories of Monsieur Bleuler concerning psychological dissociation in schizophrenia" (Janet, 1927b), and notes that he planned to discuss how he would "interpret" this "dissociation." Though his presentation is not available, Minkowski published a book on schizophrenia in 1927 (Minkowski, 1927a), which has been described as an attempt to integrate the ideas of Eugen Bleuler and the philosopher Henri Bergson (Cutting & Shepherd, 1987).[5] In it, Minkowski focuses on the "loss of vital contact with reality" in schizophrenia, placing greater emphasis on Bleuler's concept of "autism" than on the "loosening of associations" that Bleuler considered to be the core deficit of the disorder (Minkowski, 1927b, in Cutting & Shepherd, 1987, p. 191).

Most of the paper consists of two case studies, Sonia and Claudine, whose presentation, Janet contends, matches that characterized by Bleuler (as conveyed by Minkowski) as "schizophrenic." They both experienced social withdrawal and a profound lack of interest in outside activities they had previously enjoyed (intellectual pursuits for Sonia and managerial/family responsibilities for Claudine). However, they differed in other respects. Sonia extensively engaged in what Janet called "reveries" of a grandiose and erotomanic nature (i.e. believing she was the author of famous works of literature, mother to children she met in the street, married to an important man), but did not describe particularly strong feelings of emptiness or unreality. While these "reveries" appeared delusional in many respects, Sonia recognized, at least at times, that they were fanciful. For example, she once asked Janet not to discuss her "stories" with her parents, as they would make her look "ridiculous." In contrast, Claudine, whose deterioration coincided with a profound physical exhaustion and melancholia, did not experience any such flights of imagination, but described profound and powerful feelings of emptiness and unreality (what would today likely be called "depersonalization" and "derealization").

Janet also questioned the appropriateness of the term "dissociation" with reference to Bleuler's schizophrenia. Janet's discussion appears to imply that Minkowski viewed Bleuler's "loosening of associations" as a dissociation of sorts, and cites the example (apparently proposed by Minkowski) of patients who respond to questions in vague and imprecise terms, not appropriate to the social context. Janet argues that this should not be considered "dissociation" because these patients only have "trouble constructing a new association, that is, they do not create a new synthesis easily, but the old associations are not destroyed, [therefore] they do not exhibit dissociation" (1927b, p. 487). Rather, Janet argues that the term "dissociation," in this context, should be reserved for: "the rupture of associations already constructed in the past, to the rupture of the association between a word and its meaning, between the consecutive movements of the same act, in a word, for the destruction of a primary tendency" (1927b, p. 487).

Janet appears to be using Bleuler's concept of "association" as equivalent to his concept of "synthesis," and insists that no such ruptures are seen in either of his case studies – which he believes Bleuler would have diagnosed as "schizophrenic." He sees his position as consistent with Bleuler's insistence that "no true destruction of a psychological function … (perception, language, memory, etc.)" occurs in schizophrenia (1927b, p. 487). Here Janet appears to equate "primary tendency" with "psychological function." Further, Janet goes on to argue that patients who claim not to feel, but who can be stimulated to express strong emotion, cannot be said to be dissociated, because the painful emotion itself is not "dissociated," but contains "the same elements grouped in the same manner." He concludes that one should not speak of dissociation when "the integrity of the primary tendencies and all the psychological systems" are conserved (1927b, p. 487).[6]

Janet's reluctance to see dissociation as playing a role in the concept of schizophrenia perhaps helps to explain why he continued to prefer the term "dementia praecox" to "schizophrenia." Indeed, he saw the "dementia" as central to these disturbed states, but viewed the disturbance as being primarily *social* instead of *intellectual*, as it was in these two clinical vignettes. "Social dementia" is very close indeed to Bleuler's concept of "autism," understood by Minkowski (1927b) as an attempted defence or buttress against psychological deterioration. Janet agreed, arguing in *La Force et la Faiblesse Psychologiques* (1932a) that these patients reduced their feelings and activities to a minimum, establishing an "inferior" equilibrium by autistic withdrawal to internal daydreams/reveries. Janet first stated this position in the concluding sentence of "Concerning schizophrenia" (1927b) – suggesting that schizophrenia be considered a form of "psychological asthenia" in which a "new equilibrium of forces" was produced with patients' "settling down comfortably into their illness" (1927b, p. 492).

Paranoia

Bleuler's concept of schizophrenia, unlike today's incarnation, did not emphasize delusions and hallucinations as central features. The disorder in which these symptoms featured most prominently, in the absence of signs of deterioration, was *paranoia*.

Janet's 1932(c) paper, "L'Hallucination dans le délire de la persécution," is translated most accurately as "Hallucinations in persecutory delusions"; clearly, his use of these terms differs from contemporary English nomenclature, where *hallucinations* and *delusions* are considered distinct psychopathological phenomena (which nonetheless, may closely relate to one another). In addition, Janet's final paper (1947a), which covers much of the same territory as his earlier one, is entitled "Caractères de l'hallucination du persécuté," which we have translated as "Characteristics of the paranoiac's hallucination." In these papers, Janet appeared to be discussing the nature of hallucinations in *paranoia*, as the term was used in the early part of the twentieth century. At that time, both Kraepelin and Bleuler considered paranoia to be a psychotic disorder distinct from schizo-phrenia, without the same level of dementia or deterioration, characterized by delusions (not only persecutory or paranoid delusions, but also grandiose, and other "non-bizarre" delusions) and also by hallucinations. As Janet clearly refers to both persecutory and grandiose delusions in this group, it appears most likely that he was referring to a group of people that Kraepelin and Bleuler would have considered *paranoid*, and not suffering from schizophrenia/dementia praecox.[7] In contemporary terms, it would be most consistent with the diagnosis of *delusional disorder* (though hallucinations are considered uncommon in it; APA, 2013).

Janet also seemed to recognize that these delusions could be "psychogeni-cally" caused. The following vignette, written by the American psychologist Ernest Harms (1959), illustrates this:

> When I asked Janet what his therapeutic approach here was, I received the strange reply: 'I believe these people, until it is proven to me what they tell is untrue.' I had just faced a young man who avoided stepping into any shadow because, in shadow, roamed Napoleon, who wanted to draft him into the army. Beside him was a woman of past 70 who feared persecution from the mayor of Paris, who wanted to make love to her. I found it dif-ficult to see any truth in such fixed ideas. Janet noticed my perplexity at his oracular words. He came over to me: 'You see, these people are persecuted by something, and you must investigate carefully to get to the root.'
>
> *(pp. 1036–1037)*

Janet's ideas on the genesis of delusions is discussed in the next section, as the mechanisms (involving social division and the reality function) were similar to those he posited for hallucinations; further, some of what he refers to below as *hallucinations* we would call *delusions*.

Hallucinations

Janet's lifelong interest in hallucinations may have been because analysis of the symptom could be seen as an ideal bridge between philosophy and psycho-pathology. His most comprehensive discourse on the topic, a 90-page paper, entitled "Hallucinations in persecutory delusions", was published in two parts (Janet, 1932c, 1932d) in an important French philosophical journal, the *Revue Philosophique de France et de l'Étranger*. In this paper, Janet set out to analyze the nature of hallucinations, distinguishing them from normal perceptions and also from what he called *illusions*, perceptual distortions. He disagreed with the long-held tenet, dating from Esquirol (1832), that hallucinations were best concep-tualized as perceptions lacking an (external) object. Janet begins his analysis by noting that different types of phenomena have been referred to as "hallucina-tions," and proposes to distinguish among them, focusing primarily on: (a) per-ceptual distortions, or *illusions*, experienced primarily in alcoholic or toxic states;

(b) disorders of memory, seen in traumatic flashbacks, or what he calls *halluci-nations-reminiscences*; and (c) the experience of auditory, and to a lesser extent visual, hallucinations, reported by persons experiencing paranoid or grandiose delusions.

Janet's understanding of hallucinations was based on a series of premises: (1) hallucinations were not related to perception but rather to a form of delusional belief, in contrast to illusions, which were due to a distortion of perception; (2) central to the experience of hallucinations were feelings or delusions of influence; and (3) such feelings of influence or imposition typically arose from melancholic feelings and led to distortions in social perception, such that internal experiences were attributed to others. Another way of conceptualizing this is that persons experiencing hallucinations accorded inner experiences (i.e. critical thoughts) a level of reality far above that which they deserved (Janet, 1932a).

Throughout the paper, Janet frequently contrasts the types of hallucinations, often visual, experienced in toxic psychoses with those that are experienced in delusional disorders – most often auditory in nature. He accepts that the former are best considered a distorted form of perception (*illusions*), but argues that the latter are not (though he does recognize that what he calls *illusions* others have called *true hallucinations*). Indeed, Janet questions whether voices heard in persons with delusional disorders are actually "heard" in any true sense, or are rather simply accorded the wrong level of reality – that of other persons and their acts as opposed to internal, private beliefs.

In contrast to illusions, which Janet relegates clearly to the domain of perception, he argues that the range of "faulty representations" he calls hallucinations are more complex, and relate primarily to issues of memory and belief. Janet begins his analysis by discussing traumatic flashbacks, in which individuals see and hear often complex stimuli from a past traumatizing event, reliving it as though it were occurring in the present. Here we clearly have an aberration in the reality function, as what was past is experienced (and treated) as though it were present. However, Janet (1932c) notes that flashbacks are not easily considered simply distortions in perception, as they lack characteristics of perception such as "irruptivity" (in contrast, genuine perceptions "invade our consciousness and transform, at least momentarily, our behaviour," p. 86). Janet appears to mean not only the intrusiveness of new perceptions, but also that they occur in a context of a stable, relatively unchanging background. This, he contends, is different from traumatic reexperiences, in which the true present context is lost and the past one reinstated. In an important foreshadowing of the concept of *peritraumatic dissociation*, Janet (1932d) contends that these *hallucinations-reminiscences*

> imply a problem at the time of the initial event that has not allowed the construction of the story following the laws of memory, which has left the situation unfinished, unsettled, and which caused the need to start it over and over again.
>
> (p. 290)

Janet contrasts hallucinations-reminiscences, which he considers disorders of memory, and illusions, with hallucinations experienced by patients suffering from delusions of influence (i.e. paranoia). He notes that, unlike the former two groups, there is no narrowing (constriction) of consciousness or confusion in the latter group, who experience their hallucinations as imbedded in the present context. In comparing hallucinations in paranoia with typical perceptions, Janet notes that they have certain characteristics in common, namely *immediacy, certainty*, and *exteriority* (though recognizing that some patients place voices within their own body – not externally).

Janet's conception of hallucinations includes much of what today would be considered delusions (indeed, he sometimes refers to them as "hallucinations-delusions"[8]); this can be seen most clearly in his discussion of visual hallucinations, among which he considers the phenomenon of "mistaken identities" (currently called "delusions of misidentification"), that is, Fregoli delusions, in which one mistakes strangers for friends of family members, and Capgras delusions, in which one becomes convinced that loved ones have been replaced by impostors. Janet notes, a position shared by contemporary psychopathologists (Christodoulou, 1986), that such beliefs do not typically involve any perceptual distortions – that is, people rarely claim that the features of strangers' faces are identical to the loved ones with whom they are confused – rather, they are convinced, because of a *feeling*, that they are the same, *despite* appearances. The same is true when loved ones are seen as impostors – their features do not change in any obvious way, but the feelings associated with them do.

Further, Janet also considered as hallucinations violent and aggressive attacks that patients reported happening to them in the immediate past, but never in the present, such as having their eyes scratched out, ears ripped off, etc. Indeed, Janet wondered whether this *past* placement was a core feature of hallucinations in paranoia, noting that he was never able to find a patient who reported having the experience *at the time* he was with them (i.e. "they're scratching my eyes out *right now!*"). Janet insisted that experiences that did not interfere with stimuli present in the current environment could not be considered perceptual in nature. Accordingly, he concluded that hallucinations of influenced (paranoid or grandiose) patients had much more to do with belief and with distortions in the reality function and social division than with perception. Indeed, he concluded that hallucinations in paranoia were due primarily to patients mistakenly according their thoughts and imaginings a higher level of reality than they deserved – that of other persons or objects. He believed that this mistake in social division could arise due to melancholia.[9]

Janet's narrow 1932 concept of hallucinations, the domain of which overlaps with much of what we might call "perceptual delusions" (i.e. believing that one's eyes have been scratched out), proposed that voices experienced in paranoid states were due to confusing levels of reality, and were not akin to perceptual distortions (which he called *illusions*). As such, Janet did not, in these articles, consider voices to be representing differentiated parts of the personality, such as is seen in hysteria or dissociative disorders (Moskowitz & Corstens, 2007). Interestingly, however, Janet explicitly takes this position in his last paper (Janet, 1947a; though insisting that it reflected his original position almost 60 years prior in *Psychological Automatisms*), describing the "objectified hallucinations" of delusional paranoia as "a fragmentation of the conscious personality," akin to the "divisions of personality and subconscious phenomena" seen in hysterical neuroses (pp. 251–252).

However, it is important that this "fragmentation of personality" not be viewed as a narrow psychological phenomenon, as Janet's focus was always on the social realm. Indeed, in the same late paper (Janet, 1947a) he wrote, "hallucinations are associated with the entire organization of personality, as much to the personality of the social realm as to the personality of the subject" (p. 252). This echoes a comment from his earlier (1932d) paper on the importance of social status and social position to both delusions and hallucinations. Janet distinguished hallucinations from illusions by noting that the former always involved the "malice or benevolence" of others, representing the patient's concerns about the place he holds in the social hierarchy, in contrast to illusions, which could be "completely indifferent in this regard" (1932d, p. 299).

Assessment and implications

Janet's discussion of the appropriateness of the term *dissociation* in schizophrenia is an important one, in which he makes crucial distinctions between the psychological processes underlying hysteria (dissociative disorders) and schizophrenia. In describing schizophrenia as a form of psychological *asthenia*, a disorder of psychological force, Janet is suggesting that it is similar to another important disorder, *psychasthenia*. Indeed, both he and Bleuler saw similarities between the concepts of psychasthenia and schizophrenia. The clinical implications of limited capacities to dissociate in persons diagnosed schizophrenic have also been explored elsewhere (Moskowitz, Barker-Collo, & Ellson, 2005; Moskowitz et al., 2009).

Janet's theory of hallucinations is essentially a descriptive one, which has its strengths and weaknesses. There are parallels with many cognitive-behavioural theories, which argue that voices are experienced when critical thoughts are mistaken for perceptions; some have recognized – as did Janet – that some people who hear voices experience slight and unrecognized movements of their vocal cords that can be measured – what has been called *subvocalizations*. This is also consistent with the position that voices are on a continuum with intrusive thoughts, and result from psychological defence and distancing against the unacceptable thought (Morrison, Haddock, & Tarrier, 1995). Further, Janet's emphasis on the *feelings of imposition* or *influence* that precede the experience of hallucinations is consistent with Schneiderian "made" feelings or thoughts, previously seen as pathognomic for schizophrenia but now found frequently in dissociative disorders, where they represent intrusions from one part of the personality into another. Such feelings do help to explain how one's own thoughts or imaginings can be taken as coming from an "other" instead of oneself. Further, Janet's emphasis on the importance of taking one's own body as an object, and how the continual experience of bodily sensations helps to build up the distinction between "others" (social objectification) and "oneself" (social subjectification), is also crucial here. Certainly, it helps to explain the frequent connection between sexual abuse, in which one's body is – by definition – experienced primarily or solely as an extension of another's needs, and auditory hallucinations (Read & Argyle, 1999; Ross, Anderson, & Clark, 1994), and suggests that social objectification may break down under such conditions.

What does not appear clear, at least from these papers, is why not all depressed persons hear voices (since melancholia drives the errors in social division that lead to the external attribution of one's thoughts),[10] and whether some "psychotic" persons literally do "hear" voices and not simply "believe" that they do. Certainly, in contrast to Janet's model, many apparently sincere psychotic patients report hearing voices in the presence of clinicians (though some, and perhaps most, could be considered dissociative instead of psychotic); nonetheless, the importance of distorted beliefs for both hallucinations and delusions cannot be underestimated. Accessing and impacting patients' beliefs about their voices has been the major focus of psychotherapeutic approaches over the last several decades (e.g., Chadwick, Birchwood, & Trower, 1996).

Finally, it is important to remember that Janet, like Bleuler, did not equate delusions and hallucinations with schizophrenia. Thus, he could contend, as is discussed above, that dissociation is as relevant to hallucinations in paranoia as it is to hysteria, without contradicting his position on schizophrenia. As contemporary researchers and clinicians are moving away from equating positive psychotic symptoms with schizophrenia, the wisdom of Janet's (and Bleuler's) position is becoming increasingly clear.

Notes

1 Originally published in *Psychosis, Trauma and Dissociation: Emerging Perspectives on Severe Psychopathology.* A. Moskowitz, I. Schafer, & M. J. Dorahy (Eds.). New York: Wiley (pp. 91–103). Most of the Janet translations for this chapter were completed by Vanessa Beavan; the 1927 paper, "Concerning schizophrenia," was translated by Paula Monahan.

2 In a footnote to the paper's title, Janet (1932c) indicates that it "forms a chapter of a book in preparation that will be entitled *Les Délires d'Influence et les Sentiments Sociaux* (p. 61; *Delusions of Influence and Social Emotions*), based on two series of lectures he gave at the Collège de France in the mid-1920s, and early 1930s. For unknown reasons, the book was never published. Even so, the fact that such a book was planned and prepared indicates that Janet attributed considerable significance to his developing ideas on delusions and hallucinations. The second part of the paper (1932d) is entitled "Les croyances et les hallucinations" ("Beliefs and hallucinations"), and was published later in the same issue of the journal.

3 Janet's letter in response is held at the Bleuler archives in Burghölzi Hospital.

4 Janet also always recognized a psychotic form of hysteria (cf., van der Hart, Witzum, & Friedman, 1993).

5 Bergson, a friend of Janet's since his youth, is considered to have strongly influenced many aspects of Janet's thinking (Ellenberger, 1970).

6 Janet was clearly using the term "dissociation" in this discussion in a narrow sense, as essentially the opposite of "association," which he rarely did elsewhere. His more usual use of the term was to describe a pathological separation of personality subsystems (Janet, 1889). It appears likely that he was stimulated to stick to a narrow use of *dissociation* by Minkowski's focus on *associations* and lack of emphasis on "splitting" (*Spaltung*). The latter term is not only central to Bleuler's concept of schizophrenia, indeed, the justification for its name (see Chapter 3), but is often translated as "dissociation" in French discussions of Bleuler's work (for example, Garrabé, 1997). Janet may have been unaware of Bleuler's emphasis on "splitting" in schizophrenia.

7 "There are persecuted who have disorders of intelligence that lead to dementia. These are the delusions of persecution in the praecox-demented [*déments précoces*] ... [but] three quarters of the persecuted are not demented" (Janet, 1932a, p. 237).

8 As such, it appears quite likely that Janet would not include among this group persons who experience auditory hallucinations *with insight* – that is, persons who recognize the voices as coming from themselves and do not come up with delusional explanations for them.

9 "(T)his form of belief is caused by the particular, already abnormal, feelings that preceded it, feelings of influence. These feelings add to action an impression of failure and embarrassment, and feelings of being enslaved ... The paranoiac does not actually hear the words 'cow, pig, slut' in the same way that you or I would hear them with elementary auditory reactions. She feels them vaguely in her thoughts, but at the same time experiences the regulatory feelings that usually accompany external auditions. The addition of this regulation to her thoughts is already abnormal and paves the way for the delusions" (Janet, 1932d, p. 330).

10 Though it could be argued that the distorted, critical beliefs central to depression – and the associated feelings of guilt and failure – could be on a continuum with voices. Certainly, as Janet sees the hallucinations in these conditions as a form of belief, he would probably find no difficulty here.

PART III

Janet's influence on current psychotherapy

11

THE HYPNOTHERAPEUTIC RELATIONSHIP WITH TRAUMATIZED PATIENTS

Pierre Janet's contributions to current treatment

Kathy Steele and Onno van der Hart

In 1897 Pierre Janet publicized his important contribution on the trauma patient's relationship with the therapist in the context of hypnotherapy. For those readers who may be unfamiliar, a brief definition of terms can be found in the appendix. These terms are asterisked in the text. Janet noted that the patient develops intense feelings toward the therapist, termed *la passion somnambulique*. During this period of *passion* Janet noted that the patient experiences intense dependency upon the therapist. At the time, little was understood about attachment and how dependency is related to, and differs from, attachment. We will describe and critique Janet's approach, and integrate his approach to the hypnotherapeutic relationship with a more current understanding of attachment and dependence in the phase-oriented treatment of trauma. Case examples from Janet, as well as contemporary ones, will be included. It is important to note that Janet's use of certain terms may be quite different from the way in which we currently use them.

Janet's meticulously recorded clinical and experimental observations serve as an extensive database regarding the nature and course of the therapeutic relationship with traumatized patients. These notes documented his observations of cases at the psychiatric hospitals of Le Havre and the Salpêtrière in Paris. They offer intriguing insights into transference, attachment, and dependency issues in trauma, hypnosis, and dissociation, and the manifestations of suggestibility, all salient issues in the current treatment of trauma patients.

Other authors, notably Haule (1986) and Brown (1994), have previously commented on Janet's observations regarding the hypnotherapeutic relationship and early transference phenomena described in his publication, "L'influence somnambulique et la besoin de direction" ["Somnambulistic influence and the need for direction"] (Janet, 1897/1898a). Of course, it is essential to note that hypnotherapy is only one treatment technique used with traumatized patients; there are many other approaches commonly employed in contemporary treatment. Thus, although Janet discussed the therapeutic relationship primarily within the context of hypnotherapy – a treatment technique in heavy use during his time at Le Havre and the Salpêtrière – some of his observations are relevant for all treatment approaches to traumatized individuals. As we discuss below, *la passion somnambulique* is likely a manifestation of insecure attachment that may be heightened by hypnosis, rather than an expression of hypnosis per se.

Janet's patients at the Salpêtrière were highly symptomatic and unable to function. The women of Salpêtrière were typically rather young, highly impoverished and illiterate, severely and chronically traumatized, often abandoned as children and passed around or grew up in a harsh religious setting, lived in terrible, exploitative conditions, and had little to look forward to in life (Walusinski, 2014). While there have been recent critiques of patriarchal exploitation of these women at the Salpêtrière, it is also clear that clinicians like Janet made compassionate efforts to better the lot of these women, who were essentially rejected by society. While some of Janet's treatment approaches may seem unorthodox in the present, it is essential to understand them in the context of his times and not make one-to-one comparisons of treatment then and now. So, while there is much we understand now and many things we may do differently, there is much to learn from Janet. Indeed, his idea of *rapport* was the precedent for understanding transference, as defined by Freud.

As Janet has already observed, and others have noted later, many trauma patients have a distressing *intolerance for aloneness* that creates an atmosphere of crisis and excessive dependency needs for the therapist (Adler & Buie, 1979; Bornstein, 1995, 1998; Gunderson, 1996; Janet, 1897, 1898a; Linehan, 1993, 2014; Modell, 1963; Steele, van der Hart, & Nijenhuis, 2001; Steele, Boon, & van der Hart, 2017). Janet emphasized that the nature of the alliance should follow a particular course over the stages of treatment: (1) symptom reduction and stabilization, (2) treatment of traumatic memory, and (3) integration and rehabilitation (see Chapter 11; Janet, 1898b; van der Hart, Nijenhuis, & Steele, 2006; van der Hart et al., 1993). He described the therapist as needing to be quite active early in therapy, particularly in helping the patient understand and regulate feelings of aloneness and dependency, and gradually becomes less so over time. Eventually intolerance of aloneness and dependency issues are resolved and the patient becomes increasingly more active and autonomous in treatment and in life. Of course, clinically we see that treatment of chronically traumatized individuals is not necessarily quick or straightforward, so the degree of activity of the therapist, and the particular ways in which the therapist is active, are important to monitor.

While we tend to make interpretations of the therapeutic relationship from the perspective of various theories – e.g. attachment or psychodynamic theory – Janet's goal was to make precise observations of the subjective experience of his patients without always including interpretation (Haule, 1986; Schwartz, 1951).

The concept of transference was only just developing during this time (Kravis, 1992; Makari, 1992), although hypnotic rapport had been a focus of interest for some time, and indeed was the basis for the concept of transference. Janet, Breuer, Freud, and, later, Ferenczi were on the earliest cusp of movement towards a more sophisticated conceptualization of transference and alliance problems. During this period, there was not much clarity that negative transference having to do with early traumatic conflicts should be expected, especially with trauma. Nor were there particular ways to manage it (Bokanowski, 1996). Instead, the focus was on the positive idealized transference and dependency on the therapist. This rather limited view may have been influenced by the culture at the time, with women viewed as needing and appreciative of the guidance of authoritative male figures. However, Janet was known to have encouraged his female patients eventually to develop their own independent will and action.

Janet begins his chapter, "L'influence somnambulique" (1897/1898a, p. 423), with a comment that abnormal sentiments emerge in the hypnotic process. He understood the hypnotic relationship to be an attachment relationship (as defined at that time), and that exaggerated elements of natural human dependency were natural as part of the relationship. Dependency, and its larger context of attachment and collaboration, are currently important themes in the conceptualization of trauma and dissociation (Barach, 1991; Bokanowski, 1996; Brown & Elliott, 2016; Davies & Frawley, 1994; Deitz, 1992; Hill, Gold, & Bornstein, 2000; Liotti, 1992, 1999; Olio & Cornell, 1993; Steele, van der Hart, & Nijenhuis, 2001, 2017; Van der Kolk & Fisler, 1994; Van Sweden, 1994; Walant, 1995).

Rapport magnétique

The early magnetizers, such as Puységur, Bertrand, Dupotet, Charpignon, Noizet, and Despine, noted the special characteristics of the hypnotic relationship (Crabtree, 1993), and this formed the basis for Janet's observations on the *rapport magnétique* (1897/1898a, 1919/1925). There are three characteristics of this relationship: (1) the hypnotic subject tolerates touch only from his or her magnetizer and suffers if touched by another; (2) the subject obeys only the suggestions of the one who hypnotizes; and (3) in extreme cases, the subject only perceives the magnetizer and negatively hallucinates all others as if they do not exist (1897/1898a, p. 424).

Janet determined that it was posttraumatic dissociation of the personality, feelings of helplessness, a severe narrowing of attention, and absorption with the therapist that together created these negative hallucinatory experiences and the inability to work with other hypnotists (see Chapter 12). He referred to this absorption as an "act of adoption" in which patients became convinced that their therapists are the only ones who fully understand them (Janet, 1919/1925, p. 1154). The manifestations of the *rapport* depended upon the suggestions of the magnetizer along with the experiences of the patient. That is, what the patient brings of him or herself to therapy will inevitably interact with therapeutic interventions. The sentiments expressed by the patient disappear on awakening from trance. *Rapport* was viewed a function of the frequency and duration of the hypnosis; thus, sessions were long and frequent.

L'influence somnambulique and la passion somnambulique

Janet observed a predictable succession of psychological states following hypnotic sessions in which significant symptom alleviation eventually occurs. These states include fatigue, somnambulistic influence, and passion. This process involves micro-iterations of Janet's much longer phase-oriented treatment of trauma over a few days or weeks: symptom reduction and stabilization, treatment of traumatic memory, and integration and rehabilitation (see Chapter 12, van der Hart et al., 1993; van der Hart, Nijenhuis, & Steele, 2006). The immediate post-hypnotic period is characterized by marked lethargy and fatigue, usually only lasting a few minutes up to one or two hours. This lethargy does not appear to be related to the phenomenon of somnambulistic influence, but is merely an indication that the patient had entered very deep trance and is highly hypnotizable.

Second, following this lethargic episode is a period of relative health and sense of well-being – *l'influence somnambulique* – with variable durations, usually hours to months, and very rarely years, as in the case of Léonie, whose cure lasted 30 years (Janet, 1897/1898a, p. 441, 1919/1925). This initial and *temporary* symptom abatement is the result of efforts in early treatment to provide symptom relief and stabilization for the patient, and composes the first phase of treatment: symptom reduction and stabilization. For example, Janet's patient Gu, who had a hysterical contracture of her arm, went for two days after a session with normal arm movement (Janet, 1897/1898a, p. 426). Lz, who entered spontaneous and lengthy somnambulistic states, did not fall asleep during the day for eight days following treatment (Janet, 1897/1898a, p. 426). Marguerite, who regularly had one or two hysterical attacks a day, was able to be symptom-free for 8 to 12 days following a hypnotic session (Janet 1897/1898a, p. 426). Another patient, M., had a history of chronic vomiting (quite possibly bulimia), and after hypnotic sessions could eat without vomiting for up to three weeks at a time. For days, Janet's patient Justine did not think of cholera on which she had been previously fixated, nor did she have any secondary fixed ideas (*idées fixes*) related to it (1894c/1898a, 1897/1898a, p. 427).

This improvement is due to a state of *somnambulistic influence*. During this time the patient approaches a normal state, and fixed ideas disappear. Memory, attention, motivation, will, and intellectual functioning improve. During this period, the patient does not seem interested in further hypnotic sessions, and although she or he may think about the therapist, these thoughts are not experienced with any emotional intensity. These improvements are temporary and eventually the patient's symptoms return. However, these episodes of higher integrative capacity gradually link together over time and become more extended, as we see in contemporary treatments.

Following a stressful event or emotional upset, the patient relapsed into a full hysterical state again, in which there was a return of *original (primary) fixed ideas*, as well as additional secondary ones, and he or she experienced a state of helplessness and despair involving a very low integrative capacity (Brown, 1994). At this point, reactivated traumatic memories cannot be integrated due to the very low mental level of the patient. Rather, they should be contained for the time being. The full return of symptoms was accompanied by an intense yearning to see the hypnotist and to be hypnotized. Janet compared the urgency of this need with "*morphinomanie*," an addiction to morphine, describing the drive toward hypnosis and the hypnotist as an addiction (1897/1898a p. 429). We might also understand this resurgence of symptoms as a distress cry for help, with desperate attachment-seeking behaviour, as is common in insecurely attached trauma survivors. The patient's dependency has become activated. In our view, it is not an addiction, but a desperate attempt to keep the therapist engaged and close.

This intense need for the therapist, the *somnambulistic passion*, follows rapport and somnambulistic influence. The need for, and the relationship with, the therapist became paramount. We could perhaps consider Janet's observations on *somnambulistic passion* as the root of Freud's concept of the transference neurosis. Thus, this intense dependency is no mere aberration. Janet emphasized that this *passion* was a critical and natural component of the patient's process that *must* occur in order for the patient fully to heal, despite the symptom exacerbation with which it was accompanied. He seemed to understand what we now know explicitly – that the early attachment void of the patient must be brought into the therapeutic relationship in order to be resolved.

The therapist's effective understanding and management of the *passion* over the course of treatment is critical. Janet believed that the *passion* was not only a symptom in and of itself, but also the means by which cure took place (see Chapter 12). He noted that the therapist must not position him or herself in the role of surrogate parent or caretaker, but instead, be a skilled agent of change, while still acknowledging the *passion* was inevitable and necessary (Janet, 1919/1925, p. 1112; see Chapter 12).

According to Janet, there are two simultaneous and contradictory activities in which the therapist must engage in order to balance the therapy. The patient learns to trust the collaborative guidance of the therapist, and the therapist must continually minimize control over the patient (Haule, 1986; Janet, 1897/1898a; see Chapter 12). Every action of the therapist must be directed towards using the patient's dependency as a vehicle for the patient's increasing control over his or her own life. This is no small feat and a difficult challenge. Over-reliance on the therapist can lead to regressive (maladaptive) dependency and only temporary improvements, and sometimes decompensation and a failure to improve (see Chapter 1; Gunderson, 1996; Modell, 1963; Modestin, 1987; Steele, van der Hart, & Nijenhuis, 2001, 2017; see Chapter 12, van der Hart, Nijenhuis, & Steele, 2006). The patient's intense sentiments do not mean it is necessary to enact such feelings behaviourally in the therapy, but rather to modulate them within a secure attachment.

Janet described a patient who experienced somnambulistic passion to such a degree that she felt the therapist was no mere human, and nothing could balance this extreme idealization:

> The patient waits in agony for my arrival, shakes when one talks about me, imagines to see me enter, begins to write me a letter in order to disclose to me details of her life which I hadn't asked her.
>
> *(1897/1898a, p. 431)*

The awe the patient feels also may be mixed with fear for a being much more powerful than she or he is. However, if the patient is not hypnotized, she or he gradually forgets the hypnotizer and resorts mainly to the pre-treatment condition, with some patients becoming a little worse, and some a little better. Thus, the original symptom abatement during the period of somnambulistic influence is entirely temporary without the appearance and resolution of the *passion*. While many, if not most, patients do not experience this intense obsession with the hypnotist and the need to be hypnotized, readers should be reminded of the extremely low level of functioning of most patients treated by Janet. They likely had severe insecure attachments and a strong need for support and guidance.

Janet also commented on the amnesia that occurred between the somnambulism (hypnotic state) and awakening. This amnesia for the somnambulistic state must be resolved for healing to occur (1889, p. 344). This is consistent with Janet's phase-oriented treatment of trauma, in which the amnesia for the trauma must be alleviated as part of the integrative process (see Chapter 1; van der Hart et al., 1993, van der Hart, Nijenhuis, & Steele, 2006).

In Janet's (formally or spontaneously) hypnotized patients the onset of somnambulistic passion was variable, sometimes gradual and sometimes sudden. As the passion developed, an occasional form of serious relapse sometimes occurred in which the patient deteriorated to complete mental confusion. We would hypothesize that this might have indicated dorsal vagal activation in reaction to being overwhelmed, and perhaps involved a collapse of attachment strategy in disorganized attachment. Clearly, these patients were far outside their window of tolerance and had few skills to regulate themselves and to reflect on their experience.

Janet believed this was an extreme form of somnambulistic passion rather than a more serious mental disorder because it was temporary. The *passion* is apparently manifested in the following current example, which involved a highly hypnotizable patient who developed intense and unremitting attachment to her therapist. That particular therapist was unable to resolve the intensity of the patient's feelings and transferred her to one of the authors. The patient spoke of nothing but the former therapist for four months after the transfer and later described her mental condition during that time as a complete grey fog ... I couldn't think, see, feel, or do ... couldn't recognize my own husband, forgot how to drive the car ... it was as if nothing in my mind worked ... the simplest task was completely confusing.

(Unpublished)

According to Janet, the duration of influence (as opposed to intensity) was also important, and determined the frequency of need for hypnosis. In some cases, the duration was very short, so as apparently to require daily sessions, from his perspective. For example, in 1850/1851, Dr. Andries Hoek's trauma patient, Rika van B., suffered from dissociative amnesia, depression, suicidal urges, pseudoseizures, and mania. He provided daily hypnotic sessions for 11 months, when her symptoms finally abated (van der Hart & Van der Velden, 1987).

Janet commented on the frustration of intensively working several hours each morning with a patient called T., only to have her symptoms fully remit by the next morning (Janet 1897/1898a, p. 439). Today, we can understand that symptoms are often chronic and enduring with patients who have very low integrative capacity, and thus take much time. This symptom rebound can be understood as a symptom of phobic avoidance of some realization the patient cannot (yet) tolerate (Steele, Boon, & van der Hart, 2017; van der Hart, Nijenhuis, & Steele, 2006). In such cases, patience and curiosity about the "resistance" can be helpful.

The therapist attempts to extend gradually the duration between symptom flare-ups so that less frequent interventions are required. Today, we might explore and help the patient resolve resistances before continuing to target refractory symptoms, and help patients learn more adaptive relational and regulatory skills. We currently understand that patients experiencing passion actually need a *secure* attachment, i.e. a sense of *felt security*, rather than a *constant* attachment (e.g., Ainsworth, 1989; Bowlby, 1988; Steele, van der Hart, & Nijenhuis, 2001). The earlier therapists did not have our current appreciation of attachment issues in traumatized patients, and thus did not fully understand the implications of increased contact with the therapist and its potential positive and negative impact on secure attachment. On the other hand, we must recall the terrible state of these patients who were admitted to the Salpêtrière; it might be understandable that their treatment needed to be more intense in some ways than usual.

Several key components of somnambulistic influence and passion as described by Janet – the influence of suggestion, the persistent thought of the hypnotist, the need for direction, and the illness of isolation – will be discussed in more detail below.

The influence of suggestion

Janet believed that hypnosis and the extent of influence depended on neurophysiological modifications, in contradistinction to the Nancy School of Hypnosis, which proposed that hypnosis was a purely psychological phenomenon related to suggestion (see Chapter 1; Ellenberger, 1970). He was convinced that somnambulisms involved "cerebral modifications" and that some of these modifications continued during awakening. It followed that the end of the period of influence and the somnambulistic passion and need for direction were also driven physiologically as well as psychologically. This belief now fits well with our increasing understanding of the physiological basis of attachment (Bowlby, 1969, 1973; Deitz, 1992; Holmes, 1993; Reite & Fields, 1985; Van der Kolk, 1987, 1996).

Suggestion and influence appear and disappear at the same time, Janet observed. They are intimately related in that suggestion gives a command for cure. However, the duration of the posthypnotic suggestion is indefinite and variable. Prolonged influence is a function of highly hypnotizable patients, and is not the general rule. But for the duration of influence, healing may extend to the whole character, including behavioural issues that were not addressed with hypnosis. Thus, symptom reduction occurs in areas in which hypnosis and influence have not been applied. These are perhaps related to autosuggestion. Conversely, there is a limitation to the duration of suggestions, so they must be repeated again and again, sometimes without cure. Janet did not believe this was related to mistakes made by the therapist in most cases, but again was a function of lack of influence. In our current understanding, it is related to resistance, which we consider to be a phobic avoidance of what is intolerable, particularly in those whose integrative capacity is very low (Steele, Boon, & van der Hart, 2017). Often the therapist expects more of the patient than he or she can do at a given time (Steele, Boon, & van der Hart, 2017).

The patient may be susceptible to the influence of one hypnotist, but not to others; thus, the influence is selective and therapist-dependent. If there is a succession of different hypnotists, the patient does not develop an attachment to any one therapist, and becomes immune to suggestion. Janet was convinced that hysterical somnambulism (i.e. dissociated states) was synonymous with hypnotism. He stated that "the hypnotic state has never any character that cannot be found in natural hysteric somnambulisms" (1907b, p. 114). However, he also noted that the relationship of suggestion and hypnosis was not simple. Suggestion could occur without hypnosis, and hypnosis does not always confer suggestibility. He concluded: "The phenomenon of suggestion is independent of the hypnotic state; outspoken suggestibility can be completely outside artificial somnambulism, and suggestibility can be completely absent in somebody who is in a state of complete somnambulism" (1889, p. 171).

The persistent thought of the therapist

Janet observed that the patient has a natural inclination towards developing positive feelings for the hypnotist, given the nature of the influence of the therapist. We would add that both positive and negative transference are also emerging from the patient's history, traumatic and otherwise. Janet acknowledged that some sentiments may be intense or negative as well, as we typically experience in highly traumatized individuals. Some patients will think of the therapist as a parent, some as a sibling, some a friend, some merely with great respect. Janet noted that the somnambulistic influence will mix with these various sentiments to provide a "cure." He believed it was crucial that the therapist understand the nuances of these sentiments and their meanings to the patient. If a patient needed to be transferred to another hypnotist, the thought of the former hypnotist must also be transferred to the new therapist. Some patients will feel intense affection; this is the most common sentiment. But some will feel terror or fear; some feel humiliated at being controlled; a few will eroticize the feeling. Here we note that traumatic transference is endemic to interpersonally traumatized patients, in which they experience the therapist as the abuser from the past. The positive and negative aspects of the relationship may blend: fear, awe, love, hatred, admiration, envy, humiliation, and gratitude form convoluted and complex sentiments about the therapist, today easily recognized as the complex transference pattern of the traumatized patient (e.g., 1994; Dalenberg, 2000; Loewenstein, 1993; Steele, Boon, & van der Hart, 2017).

The patient may have dreams in which the therapist watches and judges him or her. Hallucinations of seeing and speaking with the therapist commonly occur, and arise spontaneously from the patient without suggestion from the therapist. Janet described several patients who believed he was near them all day (though he was not), and they talked softly to him. They felt Janet spoke back to them although they could not precisely hear his voice (Janet, 1897/1898a, p. 448). These auto-suggestive hallucinations may, in some patients, take the form of persecutory delusions, in which the patient believes the therapist has the overt intent to harm. The subconscious fixed idea may be related to trauma and the traumatic transference.

The intense rumination about the therapist directs the patient's behaviour. Following initial obsessive thoughts of the therapist, further symptoms manifest. When the period of influence ends, whatever positive sentiments existed now change to negative ones. The hypnotist, ever present in the patient's thoughts, dreams, and hallucinations, now disappears. The patient feels abandoned, neglected, and alone, marking oscillations between the need for attachment and the fear of attachment loss. The thought of the hypnotist is now painful rather than curative. Once these sentiments have changed, all negative symptoms return, until once again the therapist intervenes. We believe that these negative sentiments do not develop sequentially after the positive ones, but instead have been submerged beneath the positive transference. These patients had severe attachment disruptions and losses, so abandonment would have been a major issue for them.

The need for direction

Janet noted that the sentiments regarding the hypnotist are analogous to both adaptive and maladaptive sentiments in other relationships, except the therapeutic sentiments develop more quickly and more intensely. Neither somnambulism nor suggestion determines the need for affirmation and the fear of isolation: These are attachment issues found in everyone. Janet found that somnambulistic passion was similar to falling in love in its intensity, need, and expression. Within the sentiments of somnambulistic passion there exists an intense need of the therapist. This is not dissimilar to what nonhypnotized patients experience towards their therapists. The need for the therapist to soothe and cure is paramount. At times the patient completely regresses without the therapist on whom to depend.

Janet commented on patients who exhibit this dependency:

> They show themselves to be extremely demanding; they want their physician to be everything for them, and for the physician not to confer with anyone else, to see them every moment, to remain a long time with them and take their smallest preoccupations to heart.
>
> *(1897/1898a, p. 447)*

Janet also observed that dependency on institutionalization is a related phenomenon, a common struggle for contemporary therapists who work with severe borderline and other extremely dependent patients. He relates the case of Am, who behaved quite normally on the ward, but as soon as she was given leave for a day or two, she engaged in "absurd and delirious acts" to be readmitted, and was thus confined to the Salpêtrière for 30 years. She reported that she desperately needed "a rule, a domination" to control her own behaviour (Janet, 1897/1898a, p. 460). Contemporary therapists might help the patient explore the need to be institutionalized while setting compassionate limits and helping develop more effective emotion regulation skills.

The illness of isolation

What is remarkable about the need for direction described by Janet is the intensity and persevering nature of the dependency. In one case reported by Janet, a 45-year-old man insisted his wife accompany him wherever he went, even to the toilet. He could only be reassured and calmed by her, only directed by her. The need for another to care, to love, is evident, and *intolerance of aloneness* is striking (Gunderson, 1996). Janet referred to this as "the illness of isolation." The psychological symptoms related to experiencing a desperate need for the other when alone (1897/1898a, p. 462). Intolerance of aloneness has been identified as a core borderline characteristic (Gunderson, 1996) and is common in seriously traumatized individuals (Steele, Boon, & van der Hart, 2017). It is the precipitant of many therapy crises, such as self-harm gestures, suicidality, unhealthy or dangerous relationships, and substance abuse, among others. One of Janet's patients, Zy, poignantly explained her promiscuous behaviour in this way: "It must be that somebody takes care of me, is interested in me, no matter how …" (Janet, 1897/1898a, p. 463). Another patient, Qe, described her unbearable aloneness and accompanying derealization: "I feel myself alone like a big emptiness, as if the world does not exist. I have only an automatic life, I dream while completely awake" (Janet, 1897/1898a, p. 465).

Again, Janet made it clear that dependency (need for direction) and intolerance of aloneness (illness of isolation) are not a function of hypnosis or suggestion, but exist apart from them as more universal psychological dynamics in certain people, hypnotizable or not. Today we may understand these in terms of attachment disorders that manifest themselves in particular symptom constellations common in chronic developmental trauma. However, hypnosis and suggestion give a specific intensity and precision to these dynamics, and in many cases they can be utilized in the service of treatment.

In order to manage and direct dependency in a therapeutic manner, Janet believed the therapist must initially provide the outside influence that directs the patient's mental process, which she or he is unable to manage alone. The patient has a hallucinatory or imaginative image of the therapist that urges, supports, threatens, or encourages. The image of the therapist has the potential to provide a secure base for attachment and somewhat alleviate the intolerance of being alone. However, for long periods, this beginning internalization is unstable and unpredictable, and may only serve to evoke unbearable yearning. Thus, the patient needs more but different kinds of help. For example, the therapist can explore how and when a mental representation of the therapist (and others) is available to the patient or not, and whether the patient experiences it as helpful or not (Steele, Boon, & van der Hart, 2017). The therapist might also introduce a hypnotic image of an ideal figure that supports the patient (Brown & Elliott, 2016; Steele, Boon, & van der Hart, 2017).

Janet believed that vehement emotions destroy or suppress therapeutic work. These emotions, particularly of a traumatic nature, are endowed with a capacity for disorganization and dissociation rather than synthesis (Janet, 1889, 1907b, 1909b; cf. Van der Kolk & van der Hart, 1989; van der Hart, Nijenhuis, & Steele, 2006). In contrast, will and attention create synthesis, a new construction of complex systems constructed with elements of thought, feeling, sensation, and image. These systems form beliefs, perceptions, and judgements, as well as memory and personal consciousness. Through appropriate direction, the therapist facilitates synthesis. She or he helps collaboratively to organize solutions, beliefs, and emotions, and supports the patient in integrating what is dissociated.

Such work, by necessity, involves the resolution of traumatic memory. Janet noted that following personality integration – including trauma resolution – all the symptoms of hysteria disappear, including suggestibility and the ability to go into deep hypnotic trance with amnesia. This perhaps implies that the *somnabulistic passion* – a hypnotic phenomenon – resolves along with symptoms of traumatic memory, and that the middle and last stages of treatment are necessary in the final cure of the *passion*.

In summary, Janet's conception of the therapist's work with traumatized patients contains many seeds of contemporary treatment. He believed that hypnosis, suggestion, and psychological treatment are almost always of long duration in cases of chronic trauma because they consist of a methodical and precise focus on the many challenges of the patient. During the course of treatment therapists need to work towards two simultaneous and seemingly contradictory goals: (1) the therapist must be willing to be more active than usual, helping the patient to cope adequately with dependency, and supporting the patient to accept at least some input from the therapist; and (2) the therapist must gradually reduce his or her active stance and support the competence of the patient in directing daily life.

Early in the course of therapy, when symptom reduction and stabilization are the focus and when the *passion* has intensified, the therapist must be especially active, for example, helping the patient focus on what is important, encouraging small forays into experiences that are avoided. But this active stance still has definite boundaries and limits. Janet was clear that the therapist should not attempt to reparent, but was to be a facilitator of the patient's agency to change, and to provide a stable relationship for the patient. As a function of increasing the patient's ego strength (psychological tension) and sense of mastery, the therapist must pace the therapy, constantly gauging when to intervene and when to encourage the patient's autonomy. The therapist should constantly promote a synthesis of emotion and thought, with the expectation of increasing awareness and agency on the part of the patient. In order to facilitate these capacities, the therapist must assist the patient in at least temporarily simplifying his or her life in order to diminish the effort of adaptation and provide increasing psychological tension toward healing. If and when the patient has achieved an adequate degree of psychological tension and stabilization, the second stage of treatment may then proceed to alleviate traumatic dissociated memory. The patient may then begin the long process of realization and integration for a more complete healing than temporary symptom reduction alone may give.

Discussion

Traumatized patients are generally highly hypnotizable, therefore transference (and countertransference) will be produced within the hypnotic surround, whether formal hypnosis is utilized or not (Diamond, 1984; Loewenstein, 1991; Peebles-Kleiger, 1989; Spiegel, 1990). What we observe in Janet's patients suffering from hysteria is the oscillation between, or coexistence of, an apparently normal part of the personality (ANP), dedicated to daily life functioning, and an emotional part of the personality (EP) fixated in trauma and thus being in a state of autohypnosis. Janet (1894b, 1910; cf. Chapter 1) used the term *hémisomnambulisme* to denote the coexistence of one dissociative part of the personality oriented to the present and one in a state of autohypnosis. We have called this dissociative organization *primary (structural) dissociation of the personality* (van der Hart, Nijenhuis, & Steele, 2006). This oscillation, or coexistence, can also exist between one ANP and two or more EPs, which we have called *secondary dissociation of the personality*. Finally, in more complex cases there is an oscillation between two or more ANPs and two or more EP that alternate and coexist; this is labelled *tertiary dissociation of the personality*. In other words, these patterns exist in the context of dissociation of the personality and high hypnotizability (cf., Myers, 1940; Nijenhuis & van der Hart, 1999; Nijenhuis, van der Hart, & Steele, 2004, 2002; Steele, van der Hart, & Nijenhuis, 2001, 2016; van der Hart, Van der Kolk, & Boon, 1998; van der Hart et al., 2000; 2006). Thus, the relationship of Janet with his patients would have been developed within a strong hypnotic context. The hypnotic qualities of therapy with trauma patients should not be underestimated or neglected, and play an important role in the transference/countertransference process. And the more complex the dissociation of the personality, the more complicated the hypnotic transference and the counter-transference may be.

It is clear that Janet's writings are replete with observations that hypnosis enhances the transference process as well as fosters transference regression, although expressed in other words (1897/1898a, 1919/1925). Twentieth-century clinicians have noted the same (Brown & Fromm, 1986; Gill & Brenman, 1959; Kubie & Margolin, 1944; Smith, 1984). Hypnotic effects on the transference can create a primary-process world in which the patient freely interacts with hallucinatory and imaginative perceptions of the therapist. In this state the experiences psychic equivalence, in which there may be limited distinctions between internal and external reality, past and present, thought and action. The patient may perceive conversations with the therapist that have never occurred, and may act on these imaginary conversations, and develop whole belief systems in relation to them. For example, a patient of one of the authors insisted that she had had a phone conversation the prior evening in which the therapist had told her not to visit her parents. In fact, the therapist had not talked with the patient at all, and had never suggested the patient stop seeing her parents. The patient was able to avoid her own inner conflicts about her parents by projecting onto therapist a "solution." The patient developed a strong belief that the therapist was "protecting" her by forbidding her to visit her parents, and she subsequently avoided contact with her parents for many months thereafter, all based on an imagined conversation. Janet's observations of such phenomena indicate he was well aware of the fact that these hallucinations were not a function of the therapist's suggestion, but seem to emanate entirely from the patient's unresolved conflicts and wishes.

The therapist may possibly suggest imaginative experiences as a therapeutic intervention. For example, the therapist may ask a patient to imagine what the therapist or an imagined ideal figure might say in regard to a difficulty the patient is experiencing. However, therapists are cautioned that the use of intense imagery in highly hypnotizable patients may further deepen their trance and make active mindfulness and being present even more challenging.

As noted earlier, the idea of transference was in its early conceptual stages during Janet's time. However, much of his observation regarded the feelings, thoughts, and experiences of the patient that were directed toward the therapist. Janet's ideas about the *rapport magnétique* parallel the basic trusting transference given little heed by Freud, but later explored as the "primordial transference" (Greenacre, 1954), the "basic transference" (Stone, 1967), the "narcissistic trans-ference" (Kohut, 1966), and the "background transference" (Modell, 1990). The dialectical tension for the therapist is to lend sufficient ego support to the patient when needed, but not to evoke overwhelming dependency. Janet hinted at this by noting that the therapist "must reduce his or her influence to a minimum and little by little teach the patient to do without it" (Janet, 1897/1898a, p. 478). He was clear that a balance of direction must occur.

It is interesting to note that Janet found that symptom exacerbation occurred simultaneously along with the patient's shift from an initial idealization of the therapist to a feeling of abandonment and neglect. It is possible that the very attachment to the therapist is a trigger for the unmitigated pain of traumatic (or past disrupted) attachment, and this distress exacerbates symptoms. Thus, the patient would consciously experience missing the therapist, and feel the therapist was perhaps uncaring. A classic transference in trauma patients is one in which the intensity of the patient's need creates internal shame, disgust, and fear, and is subsequently projected onto the therapist. In addition, the patient is often enacting early scenes of abandonment. It cannot be emphasized enough that the therapist should attend not only to symptoms and their appropriate alleviation, but also to the attachment process (including transference and countertransfer-ence) that is occurring simultaneously (Olio & Cornell, 1993; c.f. Davies & Frawley, 1994). The therapist should note that many symptoms and exacerba-tions of symptoms have a relational context.

Perhaps Janet's patients would have further benefited if he had thoroughly processed their need for him as part of the therapeutic process in the treatment of their symptoms. However, some of his patients were so dysfunctional and exhausted that symptom reduction and stabilization were perhaps the only option. One current patient described her years of remitting symptoms in retrospect:

> They were real, I definitely wasn't faking, or doing it just to get attention. But now I know they were also the bridges to you that I didn't know how to make otherwise. I was so far gone from human connection that they were the only things that held me to you.

The therapist must provide a relationship that can be verbally processed as it develops and meaningfully connected to the context of treatment.

Janet was well aware that when working with dependency, therapeutic safe-guards must be taken to prevent malignant regression. He suggested that the therapist employ certain safeguards, such as minimizing suggestions, carefully monitoring the interval between and the length of sessions, and stimulating the patient to raise his or her level of mental tension (1897/1898a, p. 478). He also mentioned techniques that parallel the enhancement of mindfulness, an important skill needed for the development of affect regulation and distress tolerance (Janet, 1897/1898a; Linehan, 1993, 2014; Steele, Boon, & van der Hart, 2017; van der Hart, Nijenhuis, & Steele, 2006).

The therapist needs to be mindful of the difference between *gratifying* the patients' wishes and *compassionately exploring and grieving that needs were not met sufficiently*. Yet, there is evidence that *some* flexible meeting of the patient's needs within a proscribed range of limits can be helpful in some cases, such as giving an extra session from time to time and offering predictable (not constant) availability (Bornstein & Bowen, 1995; Gunderson, 1996; Laub & Auerhahn, 1989; Linehan, 1993; Steele, van der Hart, & Nijenhuis, 2001; Van Sweden, 1994; Walant, 1995). It should go without saying that any deviation from the usual therapeutic frame can be a complex and precarious process that ought to be thought out thoroughly and be theoretically sound. Therapists are encouraged to seek consultation before changing the therapy frame.

Integrating Janet's works with modern treatment approaches, we have observed that intense dependency in trauma patients may arise from four distinct underlying problems. Each problem must be addressed with specific therapeutic interventions:

1. *The patient has genuine ego deficits and dissociative lacunae regarding critical thinking, interpretation of perceptions, affect tolerance, tolerance of aloneness, impulse control, internal integration of mental contents, and general coping skills*. The therapist must support affective regulation and cognitive work, as well as other ego-strengthening techniques early in therapy (e.g., Linehan, 1993, 2014; McCann & Pearlman, 1990). The therapist should be active in establishing coping skills early in therapy, occasionally serving as an "auxiliary ego" for the patient.

2. *Emotional/physical need and literal survival become inextricably linked in the psyche during neglect and trauma such that "wishes" becomes confused with "biological need" and both are experienced as a life-and-death issue* (Cohen, 1985; Krystal, 1988; Laub & Auerhahn, 1989). Janet (1897/1898a) determined that the need for the therapist was paramount in cure, and that it was necessary for the therapist to be directive and engaged. The gratification of need becomes synonymous with a secure attachment, and the therapist's failure to meet needs is experienced as abandonment and annihilation (Cohen & Sherwood, 1991). The patient gradually must be assisted to differentiate needs and wishes, and to disentangle intolerable affect from needs. The therapist must become a constant object (attachment figure) and provide a secure base for exploration, one who provides structure and can tolerate becoming an object of intense affects without losing therapeutic boundaries (Cohen & Sherwood, 1991; Farber, Lippert, & Nevas, 1995). Simultaneously, the therapist must be careful to attend to the patient who becomes overwhelmed by dependency

yearnings, and help to contain and process them within the capacity of the patient.

3. *The patient has a chronic tendency to reenact helplessness, confusion, and chaos of the trauma in which her or his synthetic and organizing capacities* (mental tension) *are lost. In addition, her or his development may be arrested or significantly impaired at the time of trauma.* Janet noted that dissociated traumatic memories continued as subconscious fixed ideas and sometimes emerged as behaviours, thoughts, feelings, and impulses that were a repetition of the past trauma, and unrelated to the present time (see Chapters 1 & 11; van der Hart et al., 1993, van der Hart, Nijenhuis, & Steele, 2006). Janet also observed that trauma patients seemed unable to assimilate new experiences because "it is … as if their personality, which definitely stopped at a certain point, cannot enlarge any more by the addition or assimilation of new elements" (Janet, 1919/1925, p. 660). A complete working-through of the trauma, though a mid-phase treatment, is inevitably necessary to reduce such enactment entirely. Until such time as that difficult work can be undertaken, the therapist must provide constant counterpoint to the reenactment with directives toward critical thinking, impulse control, stability, consistency, predictability, boundaries, and containment.

4. *The emergence of the patient's experience of previous traumatic deprivation and pain activates a powerful resistance to painful grief that the past can be remediated by current gratification.* Janet described the trauma patient's fear and avoidance of the trauma as a *phobia of the traumatic memory* (1904). This is indicative of the extreme nature of the avoidance, and the intensity of the fear of the pain of loss. But confronting the loss is absolutely necessary in order to heal. We have stated elsewhere that

> integration and realization involve confronting enormous loss. … The patient must learn to grieve deeply … the loneliness and pain that have been and must continue to be endured. … Yet grief … enables the survivor to relinquish unrealistic expectations … and therefore, to move fully into the present with new clarity and purpose.
>
> *(van der Hart et al., 1993, p. 172)*

The therapist must engage in much preparatory work early in therapy. Then in the mid-phase treatment, the alleviation of the dissociation and the subsequent process of realization can gradually move the patient towards grief work. Much resistance is directed towards avoiding it, and the patient must gradually come to terms with the fact that the therapist (or anyone else) cannot, will not, does not, and should not meet every need; thus, the losses must be endured and grieved (Stark, 1994).

The illness of isolation described by Janet – what we would now term *intolerance of aloneness* (Gunderson, 1996) – is an integral part of insecure attachment and dependency issues. Traumatized patients feel entirely unable to meet any of their own needs, and acutely feel the depth of their lack of internal ego resources (although this cannot usually be verbalized). They often feel terrified of their own mysterious and powerful internal process that includes intense traumatic material, unrelenting affects, and frightening impulses and needs. In addition, they lack both object constancy of a soothing external other and an internal soothing introject, so that when alone they cannot remember human contact and are unable to soothe themselves or modulate themselves. One patient reported that her experience of being profoundly alone was one of

> absolute certainty that I am the last person on earth and you [the therapist] have gone into the great abyss along with the rest of the human population. I am sure I will walk out my door and the street will be empty, just like a science fiction novel, but only real. I do walk out and it's not empty, but as soon as I come in and close the door it starts again.

It is quite understandable that patients struggling with such enormous and difficult issues would feel and behave dependently. The therapist's struggle will be to accept the patient's need for dependency while setting clear limits on behavioural enactments of dependency, and gradually to help the patient gain enough ego strength to verbalize and master the process.

Gunderson (1996) has suggested that the therapist must understand the underlying attachment difficulties of the patient, then proceed to create a consistent but "nonintensive" availability. This is consistent with the idea of pacing treatment and limiting sessions, as we do today. Contact between session should be limited. When contact does occur, it should be explored and processed with the patient in the next session. He went on to suggest that all intersession contacts or use of transitional objects be initiated by the patient rather than the therapist, that decreasing use of contacts was an indication of improvement, and that it was crucial to process all the patient's responses to the therapist's absences or unavailability (Gunderson, 1996, p. 757).

Conclusion

Janet clearly endorsed the therapist's steady provision of a consistent, active, and supportive relationship that offered the patient opportunities to reestablish attachment, to eradicate symptoms, to develop internal capacities to soothe, modulate, and control impulses and affects, to alleviate and realize traumatic memories, and to explore increasing autonomy and self-initiated activities. Working in a hospital during the period he wrote this study, he was perhaps less aware of the therapeutic pitfalls of dependency, but he had a keen sense of balancing the patient's dependency on the therapist with a continual activation of their own self-agency. His masterful use of the hypnotic rapport is a rich learning opportunity for those clinicians who work with the most challenging trauma patients.

Appendix

Definitions

Idées fixes: "Fixed ideas" (*idées fixes*) are thoughts or mental images that take on exaggerated proportions, have a high emotional charge, and, in hysterical patients, become isolated from the habitual personality, or personal consciousness. When dominating consciousness, they serve as the basis for behaviour (see Chapter 1). *A primary fixed idea* is "the total system or complex if images of a particular traumatizing event plus the corresponding emotions and behaviours" (see Chapter 1, pp. 16). *Secondary fixed ideas* have similar characteristics of primary fixed ideas, but are present after the successful treatment of the primary ideas. They may derive from the original trauma *(derivative fixed ideas)*, be related to an earlier or different trauma *(stratified fixed ideas)*, or may be absolutely new and related to something in present day life *(accidental fixed ideas)* (see Chapter 1, p. 17).

La passion somnambulique: "The patient's overpowering need to be hypnotized by his own therapist" (see Chapter 1, p. 19). The patient is obsessed with thoughts of the hypnotist, may hallucinate suggestions or conversations with the hypnotist, and the obsession can become a dangerous addiction, analogous to "morphinomanie" or morphine addiction (Haule, 1986).

Mental (psychological) tension: An individual's capacity to utilize his psychic energy at a more or less high level in the hierarchy of tendencies [the hierarchy of more simple, automatic actions to very complicated and creative actions – or the tendencies towards these various actions] as described by Janet. The greater the number of operations synthesized, the more novel the synthesis, and thus the higher the corresponding psychological tension. (Ellenberger, 1970, p. 380)

Janet insisted that in order to act calmly, one must preserve a *certain proportion between the psychological force and the tension* (Janet, 1903, 1919/1925).

Rapport magnétique: "The hypnotic phenomenon in which the subject responds only to suggestions from the hypnotist and from no one else unless the hypnotist so directs" (Udolf, 1987, p. 361).

Sentiments (as opposed to emotions): "Sentiments are above all *regulations* of action, which action can be increased in strength, diminished, modified, or arrested in different ways" (Janet, 1937, p. 67). Emotions, on the other hand, are the expenditures of a surplus of energy. Actions are regulated by sentiments (feelings), which also give them some degree of activation (Janet, 1937).

Somnambulism: "A phenomenon whereby two or more states of consciousness, dissociated by a cleft of amnesia, operate with seeming independence of one another" (Haule, 1986, p. 88). This may include a broad range of processes, including hysteria, hypnosis (artificial somnambulism), multiple personality, spiritualism, and the more narrow definition of the word as we use it today – sleepwalking (see Chapter 1).

Suggestion: "The complete and automatic development of an idea which takes place outside the will and personal perception of the subject" (Janet, 1893a, p. 251). As such, suggestion is considered to be a psychological process. Suggestion should not be confused with other forms of influence, such as persuasion.

Will: "The faculty of deciding in advance and having it result in a (goal-directed) action" (Janet, 1891/1898a, p. 11). The ability to decide adaptively based on changing circumstances.

12

PIERRE JANET'S TREATMENT OF POSTTRAUMATIC STRESS

Onno van der Hart, Paul Brown, and Bessel A. van der Kolk

Pierre Janet was probably the first psychologist to formulate a systematic therapeutic approach to posttraumatic psychopathology and to recognize that treatment needs to be adapted to the different stages of the evolution of posttraumatic
stress reactions. Starting in the early 1880s, Janet developed an eclectic treatment approach based on his clinical experience with many severely traumatized
patients with either hysterical (dissociative) or psychasthenic (obsessive-compulsive) posttraumatic features. Our review of Janet's psychotherapy of posttraumatic syndromes covers publications written over a period of 50 years (1888,
1889, 1898a, 1898b, 1903, 1904, 1911, 1919, 1923a, 1932a, 1935b). However,
throughout this paper we shall refer mainly to his *magnum opus* on psychotherapy,
Les Médications Psychologiques (Janet, 1919), translated into English as *Psychological
Healing* (Janet, 1925).

The stages of posttraumatic adaptation

Janet considered the inability to integrate traumatic memories to be the core
issue in posttraumatic syndromes: treatment of psychological trauma always
entailed an attempt to recover and integrate the memories of the trauma into the
totality of people's identities. He never developed a nosology for a posttraumatic
stress disorder (PTSD) as such, but he clearly recognized the fundamental bipha-
sic nature of the trauma response, and he described all the contemporary *DSM-5*
criteria for PTSD in great detail in both his case histories and in his theoretical
works (see Van der Kolk, Brown, & van der Hart, 1989; van der Hart, Nijenhuis,
& Steele, 2006).

He divided the trauma response into three stages. The first consists of a mixture of dissociative (hysterical) reactions, obsessional ruminations, and generalized agitation precipitated by a traumatizing event. The second stage of delayed

posttraumatic symptomatology consists of a blend of hysterical, obsessional, and anxiety symptoms in which it often is difficult to recognize the traumatic etiology of the symptoms. The third and last stage is characterized by what modern authors call posttraumatic decline (Titchener, 1986) and includes somatization disorders, depersonalization, and melancholia, ending in apathy and social withdrawal. Like modern writers, Janet recognized that in chronic cases complete recovery is rare, even when the patient is capable of recounting the trauma in detail.

Therapeutic rapport and moral guidance

Janet was very much aware of the need to establish a special, safe patient–therapist relationship before attempting to deal with traumatic memories. He considered "rapport" between patient and therapist indispensable for resolution of the trauma, but recognized that severely traumatized patients are prone to idealization, which can develop into intense "somnambulistic passion" (1897, 1935b; cf. Chapter 11). "Rapport" was not only what we would today call a therapeutic alliance, but also a specific method for reducing symptoms and increasing mental energy. True to his times, Janet thought that moral guidance was an essential element of the doctor–patient relationship at all phases of treatment (1925, p. 1112). This was based on the notion of the late eighteenth-century hypnotists, the *magnetizeurs,* of *rapport magnétique;* the notion of "rapport" also was the ancestor of the psychoanalytic concept of *transference.* Like Freud, who later declared that "transference is a resistance" (1911), Janet considered *rapport* both a symptom of illness in its own right and a vehicle for cure (Janet, 1897; Haule, 1986). In the hypnotic rapport, the traumatized patient was prone to develop a pathological fixation on the therapist that Janet called "the somnambulistic influence" (Janet, 1897). He thought that "this strange illusion" (1925, p. 1156) was related to posttraumatic dissociation, narrowing of consciousness, and feelings of helplessness. The intensity of this somnambulistic influence bore no apparent relationship to the therapist's competence. The pathological need for guidance built up between treatment sessions and reached a crescendo – the somnambulistic passion – early in the therapy. Janet claimed that it usually was a transient phenomenon that decreased when patients became ashamed about the intensity of their dependence. The real motivation for therapy came from the patients' despair and their hope for improvement. Janet called their settling down to talk seriously about what troubled them "the act of adoption" (1925, p. 1154; Janet, 1929a).

Personality characteristics of the therapist also played an important role in the nature of the therapeutic relationship. He was not to position himself as a parent surrogate or as an omnipotent protector, but as a skilled agent of therapeutic change (1925, p. 1112). Janet advocated two apparently contradictory attitudes for the therapist: on the one hand the patient must accept his authority and guidance; on the other, the therapist needs to minimize his control over the patient (Janet, 1897; cf. Haule, 1986). Relying too much on the doctor's authority would lead only to temporary cures – Freud, (1914) was to warn later also about the danger of transference cures; while ignoring the need to keep patients fundamentally in control over their own lives led to excessive "somnambulistic influence" (today we would call this transference psychosis), which made treatment impossible. Like many contemporary therapists, Janet learned the hard way that if one neglects the dimension of control, passion is likely to get out of hand. In several case reports he tried to demonstrate how "rapport" could be used even with severely disturbed patients to foster independent action rather than excessive dependency and misdirected passion.

"Psychological force" and "psychological tension"

While most of Janet's concepts are readily understandable in contemporary terms, his notion of *psychological force* and *psychological tension* (see Chapters 1, 8, and 12) are not easily translated into contemporary concepts. Psychological *force* referred to the total amount of psychic energy available, and psychological *tension* to the level of organization of this energy and the capacity for competent, creative, and reflective action. Janet thought that a person's psychological tension largely determined whether one could deal with potentially traumatizing experiences. Once traumatized, the degree of remaining psychological tension also influenced the severity of the patient's impairment and determined what treatment would work. The patient's mental resources must be carefully assessed; in acute and simple posttraumatic reactions there usually are enough mental energy reserves to do the work of integrating the traumatic memories successfully. However, chronic and complex traumatization decreases psychological tension, causing mental energy to be wasted on compulsive repetitions, psychosomatic symptoms, agitations, crises, and impulsive and purposeless acts. The end result is mental exhaustion and disorganization:

> the subject is unable to recite the events as they occurred and yet, he remains confronted with a painful situation in which he was unable to play a satisfactory role and make a successful adaptation. The struggle to repeat continually this situation leads to fatigue and exhaustion which have a considerable impact on his emotions.
>
> *(1925, p. 663)*

Janet organized the treatment of this mental exhaustion around three economic principles: increase psychological income by promoting sleep and diet; reduce expenses by curing coexisting medical conditions and relieving crises and agitation; and liquidate debts, by resolving traumatic memories. Janet advocated two strategies for treating mental disorganization: channeling energies that would otherwise be wasted on agitations constructively; and stimulating the mental-energy level by such methods as performing progressively more difficult tasks (Ellenberger, 1950; Schwartz, 1951).

Janet's phase-oriented model for the treatment of posttraumatic stress

Janet's psychotherapeutic approach to posttraumatic stress consisted of the following phases:

1. Stabilization, symptom-oriented treatment, and preparation for liquidation of traumatic memories.
2. Identification, exploration, and modification of traumatic memories.
3. Relapse prevention, relief of residual symptomatology, personality reintegration, and rehabilitation.

In all phases, some degree of retrieval, exploration, and modification of traumatic memories were indicated. Taking charge of one's life also needs to be fostered during all stages of posttraumatic stress, within the limits of the patient's capacity. Janet's phase-oriented model is very similar to modern models of treatment for posttraumatic stress disorder (PTSD) and dissociative disorders (Braun, 1986a, 1986b; Brende, 1984; Brown & Fromm, 1986; Brown, Scheflin, & Hammond, 1998; Chu, 2011; Courtois, 1999; Herman, 1992; ISSTD, 2011; Parson, 1984; Kluft, 1987; van der Hart, Nijenhuis, & Steele, 2006; Steele, Boon, & van der Hart, 2017). Brown and Fromm (1986) identified five phases: (1) stabilization; (2) integration, with the subphases of (a) controlled uncovering, (b) integrating introjects, and new personality states; (3) development of self; (4) drive integration; and (5) dealing with enduring biological sensitivity. Each of these phases requires different therapeutic techniques. Similarly, in multiple personality disorder (MPD), now known as dissociative identity disorder (DID), a condition with a well-established childhood traumatic etiology, Sachs et al. (1988) have identified five phases: (1) making and sharing the diagnosis; (2) identifying the various personality states and understanding their purpose and function; (3) sharing with the therapist and other personality states the specific traumata associated with each personality state; (4) integrating the various personality states into a single functioning whole; and (5) learning new coping mechanisms that will enable functioning of the unified personality and prevent future division of the personality. However, since then, most phase-oriented treatment models distinguish, in harmony with Janet, three treatment phases.

Phase-oriented treatment models such as these can only provide broad therapeutic guidelines; they must be modified to fit individual cases. Janet varied the sequence and methods according to the stage of the disorder and the status of the patient's mental economy. Certain issues, such as working through the traumatic memories, must be addressed over and over again during the course of treatment. Janet was well aware that systematized treatment approaches without solid scientific verification had serious limitations (1925, p. 1210). He therefore offered his phase-oriented treatment model only as an heuristic approach.

Phase 1: Stabilization and symptom reduction

People with acute posttraumatic reactions, or with exacerbations of chronic pathology, first of all needed stabilization of symptoms. This consisted mostly of rest (including hospitalization), simplification of lifestyle, and forming a therapeutic relationship. In uncomplicated, generally acute, cases these procedures usually were sufficient to allow for retrieval and integration (*liquidation*) of the traumatic memories. Because of their low level of psychological tension, chronic and complex cases first required mental stimulation and reeducation in preparation for liquidation of the traumatic memories.

Rest, isolation, and simplification of lifestyle

Rest was meant to restore energy and build up reserves and was particularly suitable for patients who were too exhausted by repeated failures to overcome the vicissitudes of the trauma (1925, p. 466). Traumatized patients often had great difficulty achieving a modicum of calm; acute patients often were delirious, while chronic patients sometimes were so agitated that they could not even lie down. Janet did not have much faith in sedatives such as bromides (1925, p. 693). Hence, even in these agitated energy-wasting conditions and in depletion states Janet advocated more active remedies.

In many cases, a simplification of lifestyle was necessary to get treatment underway (1925, p. 473). Janet believed in protecting patients from their social obligations and family pressures. He regularly utilized hospitalization and called this "isolation" (1925, p. 485). Initially, little was expected of the patient beyond automatic (as opposed to complex) activity. The therapist made all the decisions, solved the problems, and made the necessary changes in the environment. Hospitalization was used as an opportunity to effect changes in family organization (1925, p. 587). He thought that younger patients with recent trauma histories benefited most from hospitalization, but it often was beneficial for more chronic cases as well. Janet recognized that institutionalization had serious drawbacks, but he felt that when there was too much disruption in the patient's life, short-term asylum allowed for a more specific focus on the treatment of the psychological trauma (1925, p. 581). For example, his patient Irène twice attempted suicide and became progressively worse until she was hospitalized at the Salpêtrière (Janet, 1904). Sometimes, readmission was necessary; for example, Irène returned three months after discharge, following the death of her father (Janet, 1904; cf., Van der Kolk & van der Hart, 1991).

Stimulation and reeducation

For patients suffering from low psychological energy Janet prescribed stimulation in order to get treatment going (1925, p. 942). This included education to enable patients with posttraumatic reactions to perform elementary daily functions such as eating and sleeping, and to make social contact, particularly in the doctor–patient relationship, where they could begin to face traumatic issues. These methods, to be described more fully under Phase 3, ranged from simple focused self-disclosure (1925, p. 969) to awareness exercises (1925, p. 972). The risks of these treatments, including agitation and fatigue, could be balanced by varying the exercises (1925, p. 982 ff), or by stopping them altogether.

Hypnosis for the stabilization phase

Hypnosis for symptom relief was commonly used at the end of the nineteenth century. Janet used hypnosis in the stabilization phase to produce relaxation, to modify symptoms, and to alleviate life-threatening conditions (1898b; cf. Chapter 11). In some posttraumatic psychasthenias, it could increase the patient's energy level and strengthen the therapeutic rapport. Sometimes Janet used extended hypnosis, for days or even weeks, without offering any specific suggestions (Wetterstrand, 1892). Hypnosis could provide relief from insomnia, conversion reactions, and amnestic states; intractable motor paralyses or life-threatening anorexia could be approached directly; patients could exercise their limbs, eat, or drink, and thereby protect their physical wellbeing (1925, p. 457). Success at this stage improved the "rapport" and facilitated later hypnotic retrieval of traumatic memories (Barrucand, 1967).

Symptom-oriented suggestions during this phase might address such minor symptoms as headaches or such debilitating conditions as epileptic pseudoseizures. Janet recognized the limitations of this approach. Sometimes, patients were able to accept suggestions unrelated to the trauma, while trauma-related material met with stiff resistance. In some cases, this produced an exacerbation of symptoms or the development of new complaints. Janet felt that these failures were the result of emotional states related to subconscious trauma-related fixed ideas that could only be resolved when the underlying traumatic memories were successfully liquidated (van der Hart & Horst, 1989; Van der Kolk & Ducey, 1989).

Phase 2: The modification of traumatic memories

For Janet, liquidation of traumatic memories was the key to resolution of post-traumatic stress. Dissociated traumatic memories continued as subconscious fixed ideas and emerged periodically out of personal and conscious control as behaviours, feeling states, somatic sensations, and dreams without relevance to current experience, but appropriate to the original trauma (1893c). The lack of integration of the traumatic memories led to arrested personality development:

> unable to integrate the traumatic memories, they seem to have lost their capacity to assimilate new experiences as well. It is … as if their personality which definitely stopped at a certain point cannot enlarge any more by the addition or assimilation of new elements: all [traumatized] patients seem to have had the evolution of their lives checked; they are attached to an insurmountable obstacle.

(1925, p. 660)

In uncomplicated cases, traumatic memories and the psychological charge associated with them were "near the surface" and often available to nontrance interventions. Simply discussing their experiences and sometimes sharing a diary with the therapist could lead to resolution. Usually, posttraumatic patients were more complicated, requiring technical modifications for trance induction, uncovering traumatic memories and transforming them. Controlled emotional expression of traumatic memories was later taken up by Breuer and Freud (1895) as the cathartic method.

Uncovering traumatic memories

Janet pioneered the use of hypnosis and automatic writing in the therapy of posttraumatic patients who suffered mainly from dissociative symptoms (1888, 1889, 1898a, 1898b, 1904). He believed that even in the most complicated and chronic cases, memories had to be traced back to the first significant traumatizing event. Patients frequently expressed surprise and relief to discover that their symptoms were not physical, but due to psychological trauma. In many patients, trance induction itself was the first obstacle; some took weeks or months before they could successfully enter into a hypnotic state. Janet thought that these patients often were trying to hide traumatic secrets. Modern explanations of this resistance to trance-induction would also include a fear or phobia of reexperiencing trauma-related emotions (Brown & Fromm, 1986; van der Hart, Nijenhuis, & Steele, 2006).

Janet employed a variety of visual imaging techniques to uncover traumatic memories, ranging from direct hypnotic suggestions to automatic writing, and fantasy and dream production. In floridly symptomatic or highly resistant patients, suggestion by distraction eased uncovering techniques. Once traumatic memories had been uncovered, Janet drew upon three treatment approaches: (1) direct reduction, using a technique called neutralization; (2) the substitution method, in which traumatic memories were replaced by neutral or even positive images; and (3) therapeutic reframing. Janet frequently used only hypnotic suggestion to transform traumatic memories. An example of this was Zy, a woman who was admitted to the Salpêtrière suffering from depression, insomnia and night terrors (Janet, 1897). Trance-induction revealed that her dreams dealt with her son's death three years earlier, and that of her father and brother before that. Through hypnotic suggestion, Janet first transformed the dream contents and then eliminated them completely. In a similar case, the hypnotic suggestion to "dream aloud" uncovered traumatic memories in his patient Co (Janet, 1895). This 33-year-old woman had become ill four years earlier. She had experienced a series of psychological shocks that included witnessing her father's economic ruin, a man crushed by a street-carriage, and the death agony of a close friend. Co suffered from insomnia and she had no conscious recollection of the traumas. After her admission to the Salpêtrière, Janet produced hypnotic sleep and instructed Co to dream aloud. She was thereby able to recover the traumatic dreams of the funeral of her friend.

Janet uncovered Lucie's traumatic memories using automatic writing (1888, 1889). Lucie was one of Janet's earliest patients who suffered from DID. She had hallucinatory episodes consisting of feelings that scary men were hiding nearby. Lucie was unable to recall an earlier experience related to this phenomenon either awake or under hypnosis. After Janet encouraged her to use automatic writing under hypnosis, her alter-personality, Adrienne, described how, at age seven, two men had frightened her while playing at her grandmother's home. In this case, posttraumatic dissociation was responsible for the development of a hidden dissociative identity or dissociative part of the personality based on the primary fixed idea. A modern author, Summit (1987), has called such parts "the hidden child phenomenon." Following Myers (1940), other authors labeled them "emotional parts of the personality (EPs)" (van der Hart, Nijenhuis, & Steele, 2006).

Neutralization of traumatic memories

Hypnotic liquidation of traumatic memories was Janet's most direct and venturous treatment approach (1925, p. 670). It consisted of a stepwise process of reexperiencing and verbalizing traumatic memories, starting with the least threatening and working towards assimilation of the most traumatizing events. For many traumatized patients, however, it was too painful and demanding actually to relive and verbalize the trauma. They simply could not manage to transform the traumatizing event into a neutral narrative. Putting pressure on them to do so could lead to increased resistance and produce more unbidden intrusions of traumatic memories; this procedure clearly was not without its risks. However, when cautiously applied in suitably prepared patients traumatic memories often could be successfully assimilated. Janet's most famous example of this approach was Irène (Janet, 1904).

Irène was a 20-year-old Parisienne with an intensely dependent relationship on her mother, who had fallen dead from her bed in front of the patient after a long illness that had exhausted them both. Irène entered a fugue state and was amnestic for the loss. Her posttraumatic symptoms included somnambulistic crises occurring several times per week. During these episodes Irène dramatically reenacted the sequences of her mother's death and funeral. Janet used hypnosis to uncover the traumatic memories and to liquidate them. At first, attempts to induce hypnosis met with resistance. Trance states frequently resulted in delirious crises, in which Irène would mimic her mother's death. Over several months, Irène's memories slowly came into consciousness: "After much labor," Janet reported, "I was able to construct a verbal memory of her mother's death. From that moment ... the assimilated event ceased to be traumatic" (1925, p. 681; cf. Van der Kolk & van der Hart, 1991).

The substitution method

For many patients, symptom-oriented hypnotic approaches were too superficial, and neutralization too potentially traumatizing. Sometimes Janet substituted neutral or even positive imagery for the traumatic memories (1889, 1894, 1894/5, 1898a, 1898b). He either changed the cognitive interpretation of the traumatizing events or the patients' emotional reactions. Changing the content of the imagery helped Janet's patient Cam to integrate the memory of the death of her two children. Janet successfully replaced the hallucinated traumatic images with a picture of blossoming flowers (Raymond & Janet, 1898).

Another example of changing traumatic memories is Marie, one of Janet's early patients (1889). Marie had severe anxiety attacks, seizures, and spasms during her menses. Under hypnosis, she recovered the memory of her first menstrual period: she had been totally unprepared, and was deeply shocked. To stop the blood flow she jumped into a cold tub. After this she fell ill and didn't menstruate for five years. Subsequently she experienced her periods as episodes of reliving the original drama, for which she had total amnesia afterwards. Janet's initial attempts to influence Marie's traumatic memories were fruitless. Using hypnotic age regression to the time before her menarche, suggestion of normal periods led to cessation of the monthly crises. However, her anxiety attacks persisted until their relationships to another trauma were uncovered. At age 16 Marie had seen an old woman fall down the stairs and die. Since then, just hearing the word "blood" was enough to trigger the somatic sensations related to this traumatizing event. The anxiety attacks disappeared when Janet suggested the woman had only tripped and not died. Marie had yet another hysterical symptom: she was blind in her left eye. Initially she was opposed to exploration of this blindness and said she was born with it. Hypnotic age regression to five years, however, revealed normal vision. At age six, Marie had been forced to share a bed with a child suffering from impetigo on the left side of her face. The hypnotic suggestion that this child had not had impetigo and was really a nice person relieved Marie's blindness. The improvements were maintained at five months' follow-up, and Janet thought that Marie had benefited in her physical appearance as well.

While Janet's hypnotic substitution techniques worked fairly well for patients with predominantly hysterical, that is, dissociative, posttraumatic symptomatology, technical modifications were required for patients with predominantly psychasthenic features. These patients dealt with their traumatic memories with excessive scrupulosity and obsessions (1903). They were plagued by guilt and preoccupied with how they should have behaved differently. Janet thought that these "mental manias of perfection" were attempts to restore their pretraumatic harmony (1935b).

Under these conditions, Janet focused purely on the verbal memories, rather than on traumatic imagery, and sought to reframe the narrative account in terms acceptable to the patient. Instead of hypnotic substitution of imagery, he used reassurance and restoration of morale. An example was Janet's treatment of Nicole, a 37-year-old married woman whose posttraumatic psychasthenic illness developed over a period of 12 years (1935b). Nicole was obsessed with the traumatic ending of a love affair several years prior to her marriage. Following this rejection, she became depressed whenever she thought about her former lover, during which she experienced terrible feelings of anxiety, abandonment, and guilt. Nicole's subsequent recovery barely concealed the continuing lack of resolution of her psychological trauma. She was silent about the affair, but she continued to suffer from agoraphobia and was beset with fears of dying or fears of throwing herself from a window. She married six years later and never wondered whether she should tell her husband about the affair. After her third delivery, which coincided with an anniversary reaction, a radical change occurred: there was a recurrence of the posttraumatic psychasthenic reaction along with all the memories of the affair and its termination. Nicole confessed to her husband, overwhelming him with interminable and insoluble questions, "How come I didn't offer any resistance? How come I didn't feel any shame after I had been thrown out, no regret? Am I thus not worthy to live? Is the past irreparable? Can I continue as if nothing has happened?"

Janet thought that Nicole functioned at a higher mental level during this second crisis than during the first. She was better able to put her unhappy story into words, but was still ill-equipped to deal with the moral issues over which she was brooding. He helped her to reinterpret her past conduct as pathological rather than immoral. Although still difficult to accept, it was easier to see herself as a patient than as a criminal. In modern terms, Janet substituted Nicole's "patient myth" for a "therapeutic myth" (Frank, 1973; van der Hart, 1988), which made the traumatizing event acceptable, and promoted its integration.

Phase 3: Personality reintegration and rehabilitation

Integration of traumatic fixed ideas was necessary but insufficient for complete resolution of posttraumatic stress. Three further clinical issues had to be addressed: prevention of relapse, reintegration of the personality, and management of the residual symptoms of the posttraumatic pan-neurosis. All three conditions were associated with psychological instability and a lowering of psychological tension. Janet described how continued reliance on dissociation in the face of threat made these patients vulnerable to repeated relapses. He tried to deal with this problem by trying to stabilize the patient and to consolidate the gains made in the first two treatment stages (1893c). Psychological trauma often had not only caused an arrest in the capacity to integrate new experiences (Janet, 1904), but sometimes led to a regression to earlier developmental stages as well (1893c).

Specific posttraumatic personality defects included poor attention and concentration; suggestibility; inability to initiate, maintain, follow-through, and complete acts; constricted affect; and hypochondria. Each of these personality deficits could coexist with residual symptoms of the posttraumatic pan-neurosis. These might include functional somatic complaints, motor contractures, psychasthenic doubts, ruminations, and scrupulosity. All patients were likely to experience residual apathy, boredom, and depression. Janet addressed his therapy to these symptoms of the pan-neurosis. Treatment for each of these conditions – relapse prevention, symptom relief, and personality reintegration and rehabilitation – included education, stimulation, and moral guidance. Janet tried to integrate these various therapeutic approaches in order to increase patients' mental energy, recover lost functions, and acquire new skills.

Education

Janet's educational approach was based on a learning model, and was aimed at reducing symptoms and restoring personality functions (1898b, 1903; 1925, p. 710). Posttraumatic patients with residual psychasthenic (obsessional) symptoms, for example, were taught techniques similar to contemporary thought-stopping and response prevention (1903). Education was used to restore attention and concentration, motor functions, and contact with reality. Aesthesiogeny was a specific technique for recovery of the awareness for physical sensations (1893c; 1898b; 1925, p. 788). Janet also described behavioural methods for more complex and purposeful acts. The graduated treatment sequence started by performing simple actions; these were first modelled by the therapist and then carried out by the patient. Simple tasks were repeated until they came naturally, and finally the patient was urged to get involved in spontaneous activities without supervision. Janet remarked that it was not always clear how this could be accomplished; often, he met with resistance regardless of whether he coaxed firmly or gently (1925, p. 741). Treatment failures might develop either recurrences of old symptoms or symptom substitution (1925, pp. 743, 745).

Excitation

Although educational activities, hypnosis, and psychological treatment were meant to be psychologically stimulating, most posttraumatic patients required further therapeutic excitation to foster positive emotions, motivation, and a sense of mastery (1925, p. 858). Stimulating activities included awareness exercises (1925, p. 972) and graduated performances of familiar but neglected activities (1925, p. 967). Patients were encouraged to work on their social phobias, residual psychological and external conflicts, procrastination, and unresolved problems. Janet thought that repeated courses of stimulating educational treatment had a cumulative beneficial effect (1925, p. 1022). There was an ever-present risk of fatigue or exhaustion, and a need to channel agitation into creative pursuits. Janet encouraged patients to take pride in their own successes and urged them to overlook failures (1925, p. 986). However, he advocated being truthful when patients asked for feedback about the quality of their performance.

Drug treatment

Janet saw sedatives, such as bromides, and stimulants as a necessary evil (1925, p. 1030). He made the astute observation that psychological symptoms were often less troublesome when the patient's general health was worse (1925, p. 1064). Nevertheless, he did employ pharmacological agents such as tea, coffee, alcohol, opium, and strychnine to increase psychological tension and used physiotherapy, hydrotherapy, and electrical stimulation as well. He also experimented with newly discovered endocrine preparations such as adrenaline, pituitary extract, and thyroxine (Janet, 1904).

Termination

Janet used the hypnotic rapport in the second treatment phase to "liquidate," that is, integrate the traumatic memories, and in the third phase to stimulate growth and assist in rehabilitation. Reduction of the therapeutic influence signaled the beginnings of termination (1925, p. 1194; cf. Chapter 11). The patient developed a quieter attitude, was more open to positive influences, and relapses were less severe and of shorter duration. Janet regarded ingratitude as the best sign of recovery. When the patient started to forget appointments, he was on the road to recovery (1925, pp. 1198–1199). He lengthened the gap between sessions at this phase, and in severe and complicated cases infrequent appointments maintained the therapeutic influence over time; for example, Janet stayed in touch with Irène for 16 years (1925, p. 1202).

Discussion

Janet's treatment model anticipated modern approaches to therapeutic integration. He was well aware that psychotherapy still was at a prescientific stage and that it was less specific than drug treatment in medicine (1925, pp. 1208, 1210). However, his own data showed that his patients improved more by psychotherapy than was predicted by chance or likely to be due to spontaneous remission (1925, p. 340 ff, p. 1211). He advocated the need to define specific treatment techniques for specified conditions (1925, p. 146) and repeatedly warned against therapeutic panaceas (e.g. 1925, pp. 132, 464, 490). Janet's approach to psychotherapy was a theoretically informed eclecticism applied to both traditional nosological categories and his own unique model of mental economy. It was truly prescriptive in that characteristics of the disorder, its stages, and the vicissitudes of mental economy dictated treatment, rather than vice versa. Janet utilized both traditional methods and his own innovations, but always embedded treatment within the frame of the therapeutic alliance.

Janet was a flexible clinician who viewed the different stages of posttraumatic syndromes as constantly shifting and returning, requiring different treatment approaches at different times.

Sometimes, restoration of personality functioning was required before all of the traumatic memories could be integrated; at other times, retrieval of a traumatic memory could stabilize a patient's mental state (1894/5). In patients with dissociative disorders Janet emphasized integration of traumatic memories more than integration of various dissociative parts of the personality. He was impressed by how "liquidation" of traumatic memories could bring about personal integration and he frequently saw these two processes occurring simultaneously (1893c). Modern authors are more outspoken about the need to distinguish a separate treatment phase for the integration of dissociative parts of the personality, even though a return to previous treatment phases is often needed.

Traumatic memories were often difficult to resolve completely because they tended to contain multiple layers: just when the therapist felt that all of the memories had been explored, a new layer might emerge (Janet, 1894c). Janet attributed his failure to help some of his patients with a pathological dependence to his inability to reach inaccessible traumatic memories. He reported relatively few examples of liquidation of traumatic memories from before age six. Contemporary studies of patients with DID have revealed severe physical and sexual abuse in some patients during infancy (e.g., Boon & Draijer, 1993; Coons & Milstein, 1986; Putnam et al., 1986; Kluft, 1987; Lewis et al., 1997; see Brand & Frewen, 2017, for an overview).

The substitution technique is one of Janet's most original contributions to psychotherapy. The same technique later shows up in the work of Breukink (1923), Erickson (Erickson & Rossi, 1979), and during the 1980s (Eichelman, 1985; Lamb, 1982, 1985; Miller, 1986; Waxman, 1982). In Janet's and Erickson's approaches the therapist was the operator, but some modern clinicians encourage their patients to be self-directive and to construct and enact their own revisions of the original traumatizing event. The question whether such approaches lead to further dissociation of traumatic memories – as Janet thought – or to their implicit integration remains unanswered. Contemporary authors (Kluft, personal communication) have warned that in patients with a history of incest where the child was denied validation of the trauma because of threats by the perpetrator, the substitution technique could easily be misunderstood by the patient as an extension of the process of negation of the trauma.

One of Janet's pioneering concepts that has fallen into disuse and has not been retrieved for contemporary psychiatry is his model of mental economy (cf. Chapters 8, 12; Ellenberger, 1970; van der Hart, Nijenhuis, & Steele, 2006). This model proposed that trauma causes an instability in patients' psychological energy levels and always interferes with psychological tension, the capacity to organize energy into focused and creative action. Recent research has again supported the validity of these concepts. Van der Kolk and Ducey (1989), analyzing the Rorschachs of people with PTSD, stated that the lack of integration of the traumatic experience causes extreme reactivity to environmental stimuli: the initially overwhelming external event, through lack of assimilation, is perpetuated internally and continues to exert disorganizing effects on the psyche.

This research concluded that the effort to keep memories of the trauma at bay interferes with the capacity to sublimate and fantasize, preventing thought as experimental action. This interferes with the ability to grieve and to work through ordinary everyday conflict and to accumulate restitutive, gratifying experiences. Hence, they are deprived of precisely those psychological mechanisms that allow people to cope with the injuries of daily life. Janet's recognition of this unfocused and ineffectual psychological energy provided the rationale for his system of psychotherapy that divided treatment into those methods that encouraged conservation of mental economy (psychological restitution) and methods to enhance economic augmentation (aimed at psychological growth). Concluding a tribute to the broad scope of Janet's vision, Ellenberger (1950, p. 482) remarked that Janet's psychotherapy is not a partial and exclusive method: "Not only does it not exclude other methods, but if often enables us to understand them better and to specify their domain of application. It is less a special therapy than a general economy of psychotherapy."

13

PIERRE JANET'S VIEWS ON THE ETIOLOGY, PATHOGENESIS, AND THERAPY OF DISSOCIATIVE DISORDERS[1]

Gerhard Heim and Karl-Ernst Bühler

In the last few decades, the formation of theories concerning dissociative disorders was mainly determined by Freudian thought or its derivatives, whereas Pierre Janet's works had fallen into oblivion (though Janet took up his scientific career as philosopher, psychologist, and psychotherapist before Freud and continued to practice it longer than Freud did). The reason for this disuse may be that Janet's scientific endeavours – like scientific theories in general – were not the point of departure for a wider movement. His works were less speculatively conceived than Freud's, which is why they now are appropriate as a starting point from which to reformulate the scientific explanation and treatment of dissociative disorders (Bühler & Heim, 2001; Fitzgerald, 2017).

Janet's intellectual background and his place in French psychiatry and medical psychology

Janet's intellectual background is marked, first, by his training in the tradition of French spiritualistic philosophy. This school had an enormous influence on nineteenth-century France and the politics of science. The principal exponent was Maine de Biran (1766–1824), who stressed – in his "subjective" conception of psychology – emotional and volitional aspects of mental life in contradistinction to contemporary sensualistic conceptions of this science (Carroy, Ohayon, & Plas, 2006; Sjövall, 1967).

Second, positivism, represented by philosophers such as Hippolyte Taine and Théodule Ribot, had the strongest influence on Janet's practice of "objective psychology." In particular, Ribot's contributions, his treatises on British psychology from 1870, German psychology from between 1874 and 1879, as well as his monographs on disorders of memory, willpower, personality, and attention between 1881 and 1889 founded the new French psychology and strengthened its "pathopsychological" orientation (Nicolas & Gounden, 2017; Nicolas & Makowski, 2017). Ribot believed that Claude Bernard's approach to research in pathophysiology was the model for this objective psychology. In addition, Ribot made G. H. Spencer's evolutionistic philosophy public in France (Brooks III, 1998).

Third, Janet belonged to the medical-psychological school of thought, or the School of the Salpêtrière, whose descriptive psychopathological approach had been, since Esquirol, the dominant trend in psychiatry. This school, however, did not exclude psychological topics of the spiritualistic tradition discussed by scholars of subjective philosophy. Until nearly the middle of the twentieth century, eminent French psychiatrists often had, like Janet, a double qualification as philosophers and physicians and were called *médecin-philosophes* (Bogousslavsky, 2011; Pichot, 1996; Postel & Quetel, 2004).

Janet's philosophical dissertation of 1889, entitled *L'Automatisme Psychologique*, was a series of pathopsychological investigations concerning psychiatric inpatients. These famous studies – carried out between 1885 and 1900 – qualified Janet as a leading representative of objective psychology. He was supported by his uncle Paul Janet, one of the most influential spiritualistic philosophers, by Charles Richet, a subsequent Nobel-Prize winner of medicine, by Théodule Ribot, holder of the chair in pathological psychology at the respected Collège de France, and, above all, by Jean-Martin Charcot, the famous neurologist who treated the – at the time – despised hysterical patients with a disapproved method – hypnosis. Janet, who meanwhile studied medicine, was appointed by Charcot as head of the psychological laboratory of the Salpêtrière, and remained head of this department until he finally followed Ribot as holder of the chair of psychology at the Collège de France in 1902 (Brooks III, 1993; Ellenberger, 1970; cf. Chapter 1).

Etiology of dissociative disorders: Basic disturbances and fixed ideas

Janet proposed a diathesis-stress model of dissociative disorders and presumed as causes, first, basic disturbances – "stigmata" – as symptoms reflecting a fundamental vulnerability, and, second, accessory disorders like "fixed ideas" as effects of traumatic experiences. Heim and Bühler (2006) have attempted to relate Janet's earlier ideas on dissociation to his later dynamic psychology of tension and conduct, already evident in his case report on Irène (1904; cf., Chapters 1, 11) after his two-volume study on *Les Obsessions et la Psychasthénie* (*Obsessions and Psychasthenia*) (1903). The fixed ideas are highly variable and depend on the particular circumstances – including the biography – of the patient but not the basic disturbances, stigmata, or dispositional disorders. Fixed ideas are defined as psychological states and processes that autonomously and in a natural way develop in the psyche outside the will, as well as outside the personal consciousness of the subject, but occur experimentally by suggestions during hypnosis.

This disentanglement (*désagrégation*) of ideas from a wider context is very unusual in healthy psychological conditions; fixed ideas are frequently the result of a psychological trauma. Indeed, they may – to a certain extent – be known to the subject, but often they are so isolated from the rest of the subject's ideas that they must be called subconscious. Unlike normal ideas, fixed ideas develop unhindered, which Janet put down to their being disentangled from the system of other ideas that carry out a control function.

Janet conceived the development of fixed ideas as follows: the trauma-induced emotion is a pathological phenomenon that leads to an exhaustion of the individual; that is, to a weakening of her or his psychological energies, or mental tension and force. This weakening of tension and force causes a diminution of psychological synthesis, thereby facilitating the formation of fixed ideas. For a person with the corresponding disposition, the traumatic experience often serves as a trigger leading to an exhaustion of psychological energy. As a consequence, synthetic processes are weakened and fixed ideas can emerge. Fixed ideas develop only when they become isolated from other thoughts or, in other words, when synthesis is weakened. This process is called "*désagrégation*" or dissociation.

In the simplest case, fixed ideas are the clinical symptom, that is, the reexperiencing of a life-event by the individual, and they bear a close relation to an unequivocally stressful event. However, very frequently, the causality is more complicated, because the clinical symptom or the fixed idea has no recognizable relation to any stressful event that can be assumed to be its cause. In this case, the current event did not cause the fixed idea, but weakens psychological tension and force so that a former fixed idea can reappear. Moreover, the reverse may occur when the original experience has left a memory with no inherent traumatic quality. The memory in question only acquires its traumatic quality through a later experience that causes the above-mentioned exhaustion. In this case, the fixed idea was qualified by Janet (1898b, p.149) as secondary, being only a symptom of the weakening of the psychological constitution that should not be treated in the same way as a (primary) fixed idea based on a preexisting traumatic memory. These more complex constellations appear frequently, and may well explain the apparent incongruence between the trigger event and the observed symptom.

Because basic disturbances (stigmata) as symptoms of dispositional disorders and fixed ideas constitute different factors in the causal network of dissociative disorders, the one may prevail over the other concerning the beginning and development of the illness. If basic disturbances prevail, a "weakened psychic constitution" is the main cause for the beginning and the development of the illness (see Figure 13.1). Compared with normal subjects, those with basic disturbances have dispositions to cognitive or mental dissociation. This typically leads to a weakening of the ability to perform mental synthesis, a narrowing of the field of personal consciousness, absent-mindedness, impairment of attention, cognitive or psychic instability, suggestibility, reduction of sensibility. It can also lead to an increased influence of cognitive or mental factors on bodily processes,

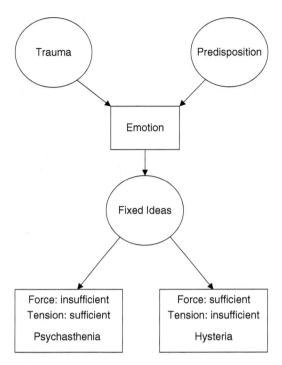

FIGURE 13.1 Pathogenesis of neuroses.

resulting in "somatoform" dissociative symptoms in contrast to "psychoform" dissociation (Nijenhuis, 2004; van der Hart, Nijenhuis, & Steele, 2006; cf., Epilogue).

The main or most basic disturbance of dissociative disorders is a weakening in the ability to perform mental synthesis. This is the cause of the narrowing of the field of personal consciousness. Therefore, in dissociative disorders, personal consciousness is impaired. These patients are able to synthesize only a small part of mental states or processes in a single personal consciousness. As Janet explained in his Harvard lectures from 1907 on hysteria:

> this notion of the retraction of the field of consciousness summarizes the preceding stigmata, and we may say that their fundamental mental state is characterized by a special moral weakness, consisting in the lack of power, on the part of the feeble subject, to gather, to condense his psychological phenomena, and assimilate them to his personality.
>
> *(1929b, p. 311)*

This impairment of personal consciousness explains the occurrence of dissociative amnesia because some psychic content may not be remembered by a particular personal consciousness. It also explains the occurrence of dissociative fugue, dissociative stupor, dissociative trance, dissociative identity or depersonalization disorders, as well as impairment of sensorimotor functions.

The second (or the other) existence(s) in dissociative fugue, dissociative stupor, dissociative trance, and dissociative identity or depersonalization disorders is but of a rudimentary form, being able to encompass only a limited number of sensations and ideas and, therefore, less able to control itself. This is why fixed ideas may develop without restriction in the rudimentary consciousness(es) and why they are even more powerful than in normal consciousness.

The impairment of personal consciousness is also the cause of dissociative anesthesia. Dissociative anesthesia, however, is not a real anesthesia – an extinction of sensations – but a dissociation of psychic phenomena. The sensations that have left the normal personal consciousness continue to exist as part or parts of a different consciousness(es) and may be rediscovered there. Janet (1889, p. 314) explained this as follows: "The systematized or even general anesthesia is like a lesion, a weakening not of the sensation but of the faculty to synthesize the sensations in a personal perception that leads to a real disaggregation of psychic phenomena."

Elsewhere he remarked:

> Because the psychic phenomena may not be completely united in hysteria, they clearly separate themselves in several more or less independently existing groups. The subject is not able to perceive all the phenomena and definitely sacrifices some of them; this is a sort of autonomy and these abandoned phenomena develop in isolation without the subject having knowledge of their activity.
>
> *(1911, p. 443)*

Because of the restriction of the field of consciousness, the patients are unable to unite all the sensations in one and the same personal perception over time. Therefore, in order to be able to perceive, they must select, and they select one or the other content of consciousness. This is the origin of unstable personal perception.

Janet described dissociative processes as manifesting in a second personality originally in his case-reports on Lucie (1886a, 1887).[2] In addition to disturbances in sensation, disturbances of voluntary motor functions are also caused by the restriction of the field of consciousness. The patients behave as if they were disturbed only in the voluntary, conscious, and attentively performed movements, not in habitual and automatic movements, such as those performed in an absentminded manner. It seems that psychic automatisms are even more pronounced. In general, these movements are slower and coarser in manner; they are not performed as a reflex.

As such, the patients are not aware of the basic disturbances. These are negatively characterized as a toning down or even suppression of sensations, memories, and movements. For Janet, these disturbances are proof of a weakening and exhaustion of central-nervous-system functions. Strictly speaking, these phenomena should be valued neither negatively nor positively, but according to the circumstances. If dissociation develops in an uncontrolled manner it is disturbing and, therefore, valued as a negative.

The basic disturbances are based on hereditary dispositions or an acquired biological vulnerability.

Personality presentation in dissociative disorders

The personality in these disorders, in modern parlance (see next section), is affected, theatrical, or histrionic, and dramatizing. The subjects work themselves into affects and emotions, or they abandon themselves to them. Janet connected the personality of patients with dissociative disorders with the basic disturbances, mainly weakening in the ability to perform mental synthesis and restriction in the field of consciousness. He argued as follows:

> Their passing enthusiasm, their exaggerated and so easily consolable despair, their unreasonable convictions, their impulsiveness, their whims, in a word their excessive and unstable character, seems to depend for us on this fundamental fact that they wholly abandon themselves to the present idea without any of these nuances, reserves or restrictions which give to the thought its moderation, its equilibrium, and its changes.
>
> *(Janet, 1909a, p. 339)*

Additionally, Janet described supplementary personality features of dissociative disorders, which, however, partially overlap with those of psychasthenic disorders (see Janet, 1903) and are listed in Table 13.1 (Benhima, 2010, p. 86ff). They are not pathognomic for both kinds of disorders. Some features are common to several disorders and thus characterize a psychically vulnerable personality. Histrionic personality features on the one hand and dissociative disorders on the other were originally believed to be causally connected only with subjects whose features seem tricky, complex, and ambiguous enough to explain sufficiently these polymorphous disorders. In fact, the psychic strain by the particular personality itself is the connecting link between personality on the one hand and the disorder on the other. The personality features mentioned by Janet are factors of psychic vulnerability because they contradict the principle of psychic economy, that is, they highly waste "psychic energy" (i.e. tension or force).

The metaphorical concepts of "force" and "tension" are taken from the language of electricity or maybe even mechanics and transferred to psychology and, therefore, need some explanation. We propose that "force" is explained as potential rate and extent of the activation of "latent energy" (so that it is the counterpart of a reaction triggered by the activation of "latent energy"), and "tension" is viewed as potential or latent energy (as opposed to actual, manifest energy).

Janet assumed that "mental force" and "mental tension" are impaired differently in dissociative disorders in contrast to psychasthenia. In psychasthenia the

TABLE 13.1 Comparison of hysterical *vs.* psychasthenic personality traits

Hysterical personality	*Psychasthenic personality*

Apathy – indifference, tendency to boredom
Asthenia – weakness of will, lethargy, lack of stamina, monotonous behaviour

• suggestibility, dependence, submissiveness	• inability to make decisions, fearful of decision making,
• unfocused (need for guidance)	• submissiveness
• inferiority	• inferiority, feelings of failure
• incompleteness, helplessness	• incompleteness, helplessness
• restlessness	• restlessness
• stubbornness, obstinacy	• irritability, excitability
• absent-mindedness, inattentiveness	• anhedonia, dejection
• fickleness (need for change)	• feelings of an inner void
• instability, conflicted, exaggerated	• dissatisfaction, disgruntlement
• emotionality	• inability to enjoy
• histrionic-dramatization, affected nature, unbridled enthusiasm	• self-contempt
	• feelings of insecurity
• unchecked despair and desperation	• pessimism
• inappropriate and unexpected behaviour	• catastrophizing
• inconsistent nature	• worries, grief
• loss of social feelings and social competence	• moral self-deprecation
	• guiltiness
• egoism	• self-accusation
• need for attention and affection	• perfectionism
• need for moral support	• miserliness
• insincerity, shiftiness	• social retreat
• jealousy	• introversion

"psychic tension" may be sufficient but not the "psychic force," that is, the activation of "latent energy" or tension, which is why the subjects quickly become exhausted. Feelings of incompleteness, doubt, weakness of decision, and other symptoms result from this imbalance of "psychic tension" and "psychic force" (1903, p. 675, p. 784). With dissociative disorders, the relation between "psychic tension" and "psychic force" is inverse: "psychic force," i.e. the potential rate and extent of the activation of "latent energy," is sufficient, but "psychic tension," that is, potential or latent energy, is not. This is the cause why the field of consciousness is restricted and limited to a few psychic states and processes.

The metaphors of "mental tension" and "mental force" need further clarification through neurophysiological and neurochemical factors, which, then, may explain the specificity of the disorders.

Traumata

Charcot, and later Janet, took additional causes concerning psychic disorders (besides organic and hereditary predispositions) into consideration – psychic traumata in the sense of psychologically impressing events. In his lectures during 1884 and 1885, Charcot was able to prove convincingly the influence of these traumatizing events on the genesis and the development of "hysterical" attacks and symptoms. Psychic traumata are conceived as life events triggering over-whelming affects. Janet (1925) wrote:

> The memory has only become traumatic because the reaction to the hap-pening has been badly affected. Either because of a weakness already induced by other causes, or else because of a depression induced then and there by the emotion aroused by the incident, the subject has been unable to achieve, or has but partially achieved, the assimilation that is the internal adaptation of the person to the event.
>
> *(p. 678)*

In addition, chronic weakness increases the effects of psychic traumata because, according to Janet, they are pathological phenomena, that is, maladaptations of behaviour to particular situations. So, affects are indispensable parts of psychic traumata.

Charcot showed that in some cases of "hysterical" paralysis caused by an acci-dent, the emotion immediately originated by the accident is not the only cause of the disorder. The memories, the ideas, and the images of the accident, combined with the accompanying emotions and worries about the accident, are as influ-ential on the disorder as the accident itself. Here, the causes are mediate and not immediate ones (Janet, 1923a, p. 23 and p. 39).

Concerning the diagnosis of disorders caused by traumata, Janet was a very cautious scientist. He preferred to explain the genesis of the symptoms of a disor-der through their conformity to natural laws, not primarily through accidental painful memories. Janet (1919, p. 208) explained:

> Both for the explanation and for the treatment of certain neuroses, every effort must be made to discover such memories should they exist. On the other hand, seeing that traumatic memories might be absent in other cases of neurosis (which would then have to be explained and treated in a differ-ent way), great care must be taken to avoid discovering traumatic memo-ries when they do not really exist.
>
> *(Janet, 1925, p. 593)*

Symptoms should be considered as caused by accidental biographical events only if such a consideration is indispensable, and taking the clinical context into account. Janet warned psychiatrists against abandoning themselves to speculative thinking. They have to carefully examine if the disorders necessarily take place in combination with the particular event, if there exists a relationship between the disorders and the memories, and if both terms of the assumed causal relation are actually connected with each other, so that it is possible to change one by changing the other. To assert a causal relation between an event and a disorder, the influence must exist in the present; it is not sufficient that an event has had an influence in the past. All these precautions did not stop Janet from carefully looking at the patient's biography if an explanation for the disorders was not forthcoming in present findings. However, traumatic memories should be taken into account only if they recur in the present and if they convincingly cause enduring strain that causes exhaustion. As a link between traumata and disorder, Janet assumed a proneness or predisposition, that is, diathesis, for overwhelming affects. The psychic traumata make the predisposition manifest and thus occasion a progressive loss of psychic energies.

Pathogenesis of dissociative disorders: Fixed ideas

Basic disturbances and psychic traumata are but partial causes of dissociative disorders. The fixed idea is an additional cause. It results from an enduring loss of psychic energy (force or tension) caused by traumatic affects. Janet connected his theory of psychic traumata to his overall nosology of dissociative disorders. According to this hybrid theory, a patient is unable successfully to integrate an awkward and painful experience of a traumatic life event by coping with it and by fitting it as a coherent part into present life. On the contrary, the memory of the event and the efforts to assimilate it continue persistently because the problems connected with it remain unsolved. There never exists a feeling of triumph that normally takes place after overcoming difficulties (1919, p. 280; 1925, p. 669).

The repetition of the particular situation, or the reexperience of it through intruding traumatic memories as well as its reenactment, and the incessant endeavour to adapt or assimilate it into life, leads to a decrease of psychic energy (force or tension), to tiredness, to exhaustion, and to the origination of symptoms of sickness. These cause further effects.

Patients with fixed ideas of a former event do not really remember it. Janet called this particular kind of memory "traumatic memory" of unassimilated life events. Therefore, patients are often unable to talk about this event in a regular conversation, as is the case with common memory. Instead, the traumatic memory has to be inferred by psychological analysis of clues and hints.

The fixed idea refers to something unsettled, that is, something uncompleted, which Viktor von Gebsattel called "presentification of the past" or "inhibition of becoming" (see Bühler & Rother, 1999). Therefore, it is not surprising that fixed ideas, being closed to cognitive influences, resist changes, which Freud called "resistance"; and that resistance influences one's conception of the world, of oneself, and of the formation of interpersonal relations, which were named "transference" by Freud (Janet, 1897; Haule, 1986; see Chapter 11).

Vehement affects being themselves attached to the senses are of utmost importance in the genesis and development of fixed ideas. These affects disconnect the overall structure of ideas and thus weaken the control of ideas by the person.

Normally, ideas do not exist in isolation from each other but build up complexes as effects of a synthesis. In subjects with a sound psychic constitution, these complexes nest together to become a superordinate system. That is, they become the system of the whole consciousness of a person. Traumatic memories that have become fixed ideas, however, primarily develop in isolation from other psychic states or processes and without the knowledge or control of the person. They act in a way comparable to autosuggestions. The ideas become fixed and develop themselves autonomously and stay outside the personal consciousness and will of the patient (Janet, 1893a, 1907c). Therefore, fixed ideas may be characterized as being subconscious (Bühler & Heim, 2009). Charcot and Janet compared such fixed ideas to parasites. Nowadays they could be likened to computer programs, computer viruses, or computer worms.

Vulnerability

Psychic traumata are not the only immediate causes of developing fixed ideas. Often traumata are caused by a hereditary predisposition or an acquired weak psychic constitution. Exposure to an external traumatizing event or even events further weakens the already frail psychic constitution, which itself is the source of increased affects, and thus continues the existence of fixed ideas. The result is more damage to the psychic constitution and a vicious circle among affects and fixed ideas so that psychic disturbances ensue. Janet (1921) described this vicious circle as follows: "The preexisting depression paves the way for enhanced emotionality, which, of course, is increased even more by a new emotion in such a way that the nervous and mental troubles of the depression accelerate like an avalanche" (p. 221).

Janet conceived his diathesis–stress model on this basis: if the initial life event was very stressful, then it caused severe emotions. In this case, the emotionally originated fixed idea is very important for the genesis and development of the disorder. In other cases, there is only a minor emotional reaction at the beginning of the disorder. Here, the psychological weakness (*faiblesse psychologique*) is of utmost importance. It conditions an unstable psychic equilibrium, a loss of the ability to perform psychic synthesis, a paralysis of the association centres, and an impaired function of the sensory centers (1911, p. 636). Occasionally Janet compared mental disorders to infectious diseases, the symptoms of which partly persist even if the infectious agent has already disappeared, so that a subsequent disinfection no longer has any influence on the processing of the sickness or the cure. Therefore, a mental disorder does not always disappear if a traumatically conditioned fixed idea has been removed. A proneness or vulnerability to psychic traumata remains, causing multiple relapses. This proneness or vulnerability may be the reason why new or secondary fixed ideas, of which Janet distinguished several kinds (1894c, p. 133), emerge, grow in strength, and engender a new appearance of the disorder.

According to Janet, the causal processes of psychic traumata may be summed up as follows. In the case of an already weakened psychic constitution, the trauma originates marked affects. Because of maladaptive patterns of reactions, the individuals are unable to cope with the difficult situation. They continue with their coping efforts. These repeated efforts occasion an exhaustion of psychic energy (tension or force), resulting in different types of mental disorders. In case of sufficient tension but insufficient force, the ideas do not become subconscious but cause disorders that Janet called "psychasthenia." In case of insufficient tension but sufficient force, the ideas weaken the psychic synthesis and, thereby, the connection of consciousness. The ideas become fixed as well as subconscious, the field of consciousness restricted, and the suggestibility increased. Janet labeled the disorders resulting from this process "hysteria." These energetic conceptions of the etiology of mental disorders permit the possibility of the summed-up causal effects of similar but also of different traumata to function as causes.

Therapy of conversion disorders and dissociative disorders

Charcot noted that the success of a therapy depends to a considerable extent on mental hygiene, and that it has as an aim, among others, to eliminate pathogenic thoughts, images, or presentations. In this vein, Janet developed numerous therapeutic procedures. These procedures are presented here proceeding from the particular to the general.

Uncovering and influencing fixed ideas through psychological analysis

Generally speaking, the method of "psychological analysis" (Janet, 1930b) is appropriate not only for the treatment of dissociative disorders but also for the therapy of psychasthenia, because both maladaptation disorders cause a weakening in the psychic constitution (i.e. a weakening of force and tension, in Janet's language). This psychic constitution should be strengthened through the liquidation of unresolved experiences. If the causes of a disorder are not found in the present life of a patient, it is justified to seek them in the past. This is done through analysis of the deeper layers of consciousness. Janet discussed this kind of treatment of traumatic disorders in his book *Les Médications Psychologiques* (Janet, 1919, pp. 204–307 and pp. 589–698) under the heading "Treatment by mental liquidation." He proposed an interesting kind of "catharsis," that is, abreaction (*décharge*), using the force of strong emotional reaction to reestablish higher mental levels after dysfunctional adaptive responses to traumatic experiences.

Psychological analysis in Janet's sense of the term is apt to uncover traumatic subconscious memories. In therapy, a subconscious fixed idea that wastes psychic energy (force or tension) is reintegrated into the whole of personal consciousness, so that the loss of psychic energy (force or tension) is reduced. The reduction of these losses through the "liquidation" of fixed ideas explains the successes of psychological analysis. Janet (1924) elucidated this effect "after this liquidation, sometimes to be sure, painful and costly, the mind stops making the efforts at adaptation that were being indefinitely repeated" (p. 196).

In many cases, he recommends hypnosis and automatic writing as appropriate methods of psychological analysis, because by activating tendencies that are latent in the waking state it is possible to retrieve memories. Janet also accepted dreams for this purpose. Dreams may indicate traumatic experiences that may stay in direct connection to psychic disorders, because they are connected with latent (i.e. subconscious) tendencies. These latent tendencies may trigger dreams that are wholly or partly remembered on awakening. In such cases the traumatic experiences are manifested in dreams. The distortions of the dream contents are the result of the way that the nature of dream consciousness differs from waking consciousness (Janet, 1909a, p. 31). For Janet, a dream had no meaning other than its manifest content. He rejected every symbolic interpretation of dreams. The analysis of dreams has to confine itself to recognizing the automatic and recurrent processes in dreaming.

We propose the following procedure: the recognition of automatic and recurrent processes in dreams may become easier by using more abstract categories for description, thus enabling an optimal grasp of dream content and a more comprehensive discovery of recurrent processes. The use of more abstract categories for description is not, however, an interpretation of dreams in the Freudian sense, that is, it is not an amplification, but a reduction of the manifold of dream contents.

A sample of the most conspicuous similar themes of dreams may clarify this proposal. These themes are only part of a more complex treatment of a patient with a longer lasting depression Janet would have called "neurasthenia." The patient dreamed recurrently that she searched for her parental home but could not find it. Or she searched for her classroom but could not find it. Or she wandered around a town to look for her hotel but could not find it. Or she wandered around to look for a place to sleep but could not find it. Or she wandered around to find her room in a conference site but could not find it. These are only the most salient dreams of a more complex sequence.

The so-called common denominator of these recurrent dreams gained by abstraction could be that the patient has not yet found her place in life. As a consequence of this abstraction, the patient was advised not to seek her place in real, but in spiritual, life. This advice covered only a partial but decisive aspect of the overall and successful treatment of the patient. Presumably as a consequence, the reported themes diminished in appropriate time and gradually vanished.

In particular cases, Janet was able to show that discovering the subconscious fixed idea and rendering it conscious is sufficient either to diminish symptoms of sicknesses or to heal them completely. The healing process is accomplished by reducing the strength of a fixed idea that has become conscious through other conscious ideas, thus strengthening the psychic constitution through inhibiting losses of psychic energy (force or tension). Discovering subconscious traumatic memories through psychological analysis is – apart from rare exceptions – but a first step in healing, because not all psychic disorders vanish by making a sub-conscious fixed idea conscious. In some cases, a pathogenic fixed idea has to be removed and replaced by a different nonpathogenic idea. Janet called these quasi-surgical interventions "extraction," "substitution," "isolation," or "dissociation." Besides other techniques, for example, persuasion or explanation, hypnotic sug-gestions are helpful for these purposes. They are given while the patient is in a subconscious state, and are either induced by suggestions or occur spontaneously. Patients awaken from this subconscious state and have no memories of the pro-cesses that occurred. Another way to neutralize a fixed idea is to tone down the pathogenic nature of it through making positive aspects apparent.

Influencing fixed ideas through treatment by suggestion

Because there is a disturbance in the natural suggestibility of patients with dis-sociative disorders, treatment through suggestion is very important. Diminished ability for psychic synthesis, restriction of the field of consciousness, and, thus, increased dissociation are the causes of this natural suggestibility. Janet (1893a) saw a similarity between (hypnotic or artificial) suggestions and fixed ideas: "The knowledge of these suggestions, artificially called forth, seems us the nec-essary introduction to the study of fixed ideas, naturally developed" (p. 5). He continued: "We consider the typical cases of suggestion to be those complete and automatic developments of an idea which take place outside the will and personal perception of the subject" (p. 30).

The exaggerated development of an idea occurs when it is isolated from other psychic states or processes. Suggestions are, therefore, due to activation of a single tendency that is not corrected or completed by other tendencies. Suggestible per-sons rarely have more than a single idea in their restricted field of consciousness. This is why they are unable to unite several ideas in a single, personal conscious-ness. Janet (1909a) explained:

> In a word, with what is called suggestion, an idea completely develops even to its transformation into an action, a perception, and an emotion, but it seems to develop for itself and in isolation without the involvement of the will or the personal consciousness of the subject.
>
> *(p. 302)*

The suggested idea develops as it does because it is isolated and does not counter ideas in the field of consciousness that oppose or are able to modify it. Acceptance of the suggestion takes place immediately and involuntarily without reflection or rational consideration. It happens like an impulse. Janet commented as fol-lows: "To evoke an impulse, which is the essential of suggestion, is not, indeed, any more than the activation of a tendency under a lower form, with a lesser degree of perfection in the place of a higher form of activation" (1924, p. 138). The automatic association of psychic elements must be possible to accomplish a suggestion, but the actual synthesis of these elements is altered or restricted. A preexisting illness is a prerequisite for such an alternation of mental synthesis, since psychically well persons maintain the ability for synthesis.

Janet tried to influence fixed ideas through suggestions. If such an influence is not immediately possible, then a fixed idea should likewise be replaced through suggestions and transformed into a more harmless idea, or dissected into its elements, which will be suggestively dissolved one by one. Janet himself described this procedure:

> For us the fixed idea seemed to be a construction, a synthesis of a great number of images; instead of attacking it as a whole, one should try to dissect it into single parts, to destroy or to transform its elements; then it is probable that the whole will not persist any more.
>
> *(1894d, p. 128)*

Treatment through plain ordinary suggestion is complemented by hypnosis through activation of automatic rather than higher cognitive tendencies. This complement is very helpful because the natural suggestibility of patients with dissociative disorders is increased during the hypnotic state. Through these procedures lower-level tendencies are freed from the control of higher ones, and this occasions an immediate (*asséritif*) consent rather than a reflected (*réfléchi*) one. Janet's concept of hypnosis is connected with his overall psychological view of psychic tendencies (see Heim & Bühler, 2006). The low level of the middle tendencies or patterns of behaviour (*conduites moyennes*), that is, the pithiatic or assertive (automatic consent or affirmation) stage with its suggestible imitation or unreflected consent, is very important for treatment through suggestion. The shortcomings of this stage are obvious: some steps leading to reflected beliefs (*croyances réfléchies*) are skipped and substitutions in the patient's beliefs go unchecked. Janet believed that the phenomenon of suggestibility and suggestion may not be understood without in-depth knowledge of the pithiatic state of consciousness.

However, treatment through suggestion, and especially through hypnotic suggestions, is limited. First, it would be a wholly wrong understanding of a psychic image or presentation to restrict the cause of such disorders to a single fixed idea, and to think that it would be sufficient to remove it through suggestions. Secondary fixed ideas must not be overlooked. To do this would be to misunderstand essential elements of these disorders and to have an incorrect conception of psychic images or presentations.

Second, the ease with which the suggestions relieve a patient's suffering is simultaneously a symptom of a deep dissociation of the personality. The more easily the cure is accomplished, the deeper the psychic condition is bound. Therefore, Janet regarded the treatment of dissociative disorders through suggestions, and through hypnotic suggestions, as problematic because these procedures replace "one evil with another." If one symptom is removed through suggestions, another may emerge. The basic disturbances of patients with dissociative disorders (their increased suggestibility) would not be improved by suggestions or hypnotic suggestions, but rather made worse. In addition to these considerations, it is not certain if the fundamental fixed idea is actually removed through the suggestive elimination of symptoms. These objections do not imply, however, that treatment through suggestions or hypnotic suggestions is not effective in particular cases (though it may fail in many others). Therefore, a trial of treatment through suggestions or hypnotic suggestions is always indicated.

Like every drug, suggestions are, according to Janet, useful in some cases and harmful in others. They are useful in weakening or suppressing subconscious fixed ideas that individuals cannot influence, and this enables the patients to recover from the loss of psychic energy (force and tension).

Apart from these cases, Janet considered treatment through suggestion or hypnotic suggestion as harmful because it increases psychic dissociation, which is the cause of all dissociative symptoms. Janet remarked:

> From the moment that it is possible to heal a subject through suggestion, he is still sick. Apart from very rare cases, it seems to me that it is not possible to heal through suggestion the condition of psychic misery which is an essential condition for suggestions to be effective.
>
> *(1889, p. 456)*

Janet even compared the craving to be hypnotized with morphine addiction and makes it responsible for a part of the disturbances of these patients. He argued:

> Many times, these relapses seem to become even more complicated by a very strong desire of the patient to get hypnotized, led, and suggested by the person having cured them before. This craving which I have investigated using the expression "somnambulic passion" is comparable in many respects with morphine addiction.
>
> *(1911, p. 664; see Janet, 1897; Chapter 11)*

All in all, treatment through suggestion is a symptomatic therapy with many limitations, such as patient resistance to suggestions, transient relief, or the generation of additional symptoms, including dependence or even addiction. In addition, if fixed ideas influence interpersonal relations (or are triggered by them), an immediate effect on fixed ideas through suggestion or hypnotic suggestion is hardly possible, but a mediated one is possible through implicit shaping of interpersonal relations or explicit reinterpretation of them.

Influencing fixed ideas by rational treatments

Antagonistic ideas, which are opposed to the pathological fixed ideas, trigger deep emotions or affects so that a new equilibrium is effected in the whole system of consciousness. Janet recommended the concrete procedures of common counselling, words of encouragement, incentives, and specialized exercises with strengthening or constructive cognitions. He summed up the procedures of his times in treating traumatic disorders: "The best methods are those that cause the assimilation of the exciting emotion, that bring the subject to comprehend through inducing the subject to comprehend it by reflection, to react against it correctly and to resign himself to it" (1924, p. 196).

However, Janet viewed these methods as only being applicable in a limited way because of their shortcomings: high rates of relapse, fast habituation, high variability concerning persons and situations, and low transferability to other cases. In addition, fixed ideas are not fundamentally changed by these procedures because the fixed ideas do not depend on the will and the rational susceptibility of the patients.

Janet, cognitive therapy, and other current behavioural therapies

It is not our intent to demonstrate that many ideas in modern psychotherapy were anticipated by Janet, because psychotherapy has many "parents." But Janet may be called a precursor of behaviour and cognitive therapies. We can appreciate Janet's holistic approach, including his model of personality, as paradigmatic in that it was engendered by extensive, careful clinical descriptions and only a few cautious, theoretical "top-down" as well as "bottom-up" hypotheses, which were open to modifications by empirical research. Considering the relevance of Bandura's (1977) "self-efficacy" model or Kanfer's (1991) "self-management" model for the cognitive-behavioural therapies, as well as the recent shift to constructivist and dynamic conceptions ("third wave") in cognitive therapies, the actuality of Janet's conception of the mind becomes evident.

In general, Janet's methods resemble today's cognitive-behavioural procedures for treating dysfunctional and affectively tinted thoughts and cognitive complexes. His methods correspond with the principles of cognitive-behavioural therapy that a therapeutically structured reexperiencing of traumata to neutralize phobic behaviour will oppose fixed ideas and integrate the traumatic experience, thus allowing an appropriate reappraisal of the trauma. For instance, the cognitive-behavioural "narrative" method for treating posttraumatic stress disorders (PTSD) is implicitly based on Janet's conception of subconsciousness (Janet, 1907c; Bühler & Heim, 2009; Fiedler, 2008). It consists of reintegrating dissociated emotional memories of traumata, conceived as temporarily unrelated elements that are context-free, though reactivated by trauma–associated stimuli, into a chronological autobiographical context. Most modern approaches (see Kennerley, 1996) are congruent with Janet's views that during traumatic experience there is a lowering of "mental strength," that is, pathogenic associative learning processes prevent the synthetic processing of the trauma. Traumatic memories return because they are dissociated (or disintegrated) fixed ideas evoked by stimulation. Later Janet (1928b, p. 214) explicitly distinguished memories (*souvenirs*) from reminiscences (*réminiscences*). The latter are automatic responses to stimuli representing the circumstances of the traumatizing events (for instance a bed, which may have played a significant role in the trauma). Janet referred to his important case report on Irène, where he discussed several modifications of the personal consciousness and behaviour in traumatic experience, including the role of peritraumatic stimulation: "The events that were involved in the modification are those that have been the occasion of a violent emotion, those that attach themselves there by association, or those that precede it immediately in time" (1904, p. 440). In other words, deficient inhibitory processes (rather than voluntary recall) in autobiographical memory lead to involuntary reexperiencing (reminiscence) of the event.

Janet already proposed a three-phase therapeutic strategy in PTSD: stabilization of the patient, synthesis of memory, including the effortful increase of mental tension, and integration into daily life (see Chapter 12). Janet's approach resembles neo-behaviourism because of his reference to covert processes as well as overt behaviour. His concept may be understood as a dynamic resource-allocation model, which implies a functional model of psychological disorders. His blueprint of a sociogenetic hierarchy of behavioural "tendencies" might represent a stimulating elaboration of the concept of behaviour. Janet also made systematic descriptions of psychotherapeutic interventions (Janet, 1919, 1923a) which have similar differential-therapeutic objectives similar to present endeavours to integrate empirically supported therapies into a common psychological framework (see Grawe, 2002).

Nowadays, there exist a multitude of new cognitive-behavioural (or other somewhat related) approaches that focus on concepts like "schema," "mindfulness," and "emotional regulation and processing." They use narrative, imagery, and body-related procedures to promote assimilative processes in the treatment of traumatic disorders. They seem to confirm Janet's prediction made in 1907, summarizing his lessons about "Psychological analysis and the critics of psychotherapeutic methods" at the Collège de France:

> Finally, the education of attention, the treatment of emotionality, the various excitations that intend to raise the mental level form methods that are already applied a bit by chance, but which will play a more and more important role in education and in the treatment of the mind.
>
> *(Janet, 1907d, p. 710)*

Such plausible links to current cognitive-behavioural therapies exist for the treatment of posttraumatic stress disorder (PTSD), obsessive-compulsive disorder (OCD), and depression as well as to behavioural therapy in general (see Heim & Bühler, 2003, 2006). Usually, almost no explicit references are made to Janet by authors of cognitive-behavioural therapy manuals. One exception is Hoffmann (1998), who has developed an OCD treatment program based on Janet's key concept of "feeling of incompleteness," which was further elaborated by Ecker and Gönner (2008). Additionally, Greenberg's (2004) "emotion-focused therapy" conceives of emotions or feelings in a manner that resembles Janet's notion of feelings as secondary actions that regulate primary ones. For example, in Janet's terminology, fear helps in avoiding dangerous ventures, thus preventing harm; fatigue assists by resigning oneself from endless efforts, thus preventing exhaustion; effort assists in reaching a goal; and joy helps in finishing the action. All these feelings contain bodily sensations that bestow meaning on acting in concrete situations and these become part of autobiographical storytelling. In Janet's (1929b) view, they confer a substantial momentum to the evolution of personality. Greenberg's "dialectical-constructivist" concept regards such a bottom-up process as essential in changing automatic emotional responding. His approach (including training in emotional awareness, regulation, and transformation) is a paradigm of Janet's above-mentioned vision of "treatment of emotionality," which is perceived as one important element of modern psychotherapy. It should be mentioned that Janet's pioneering role for those body-oriented therapies was recognized by Boadella (1997) and inspired Ogden, Minton, and Pain (2006) to develop sensorimotor psychotherapy for trauma-generated disorders (see also Ogden & Fisher, 2015; Chapter 14).

In the tradition of cognitive and hypnotherapeutic approaches, a group of Dutch and American researchers and therapists (van der Hart, Nijenhuis, & Steele, 2006) has designed a comprehensive multimodal conception for treating chronic, severe traumatic disorders. The authors explicitly refer to Janet's model of a dynamic personality, with its key concepts of action and its adaptive regulation by feelings. The authors conceive of dissociation of the personality as the manifestation of a disturbed interaction between adaptive action-systems of the person (i.e. the relation between actions directed to the demands of daily needs and the action systems necessary for extraordinary situations like defences against danger). Their comprehensive multimodal idea for treatment fosters harmony between the apparently normal part of the personality (ANP) and the emotional part of the personality (EP), dissociated from each other, which causes secondary dissociations within the defensive systems of the EP and tertiary dissociations within the action systems of the ANP.

Another form of intervention in cognitive restructuring is clinical logagogy (Bühler, 2003, 2015). It is a demanding type of psycho-philosophical intervention aimed at the spiritual sphere, insight, and reasoning of human beings to influence emotions and affects by means of verbal interventions and dialogue. It also includes written instructions such as aphorisms, epigrams, proverbs, or sayings. The aim of clinical logagogy is the conduct of one's life and the prevention of, as well as guidance for and support in, hopeless-seeming life crises or in insoluble-seeming conflicts. It is directed at thoughtful persons who are open to education and culture and willing to grasp their particular situation and to attempt to tone down the problems and conflicts by fitting them into general considerations. In his textbook of psychotherapy, Janet (1919, pp. 54–97) dedicated a chapter, "Philosophical psychotherapy," to forms of psycho-philosophical intervention. However, he was sceptical about such interventions because he felt that they depended too much on the particular therapist and that training could not be generalized. We do not share. his scepticism, though we acknowledge the limits of logagogy.

Additional interventions

According to Janet's diathesis–stress–model of dissociative disorders, therapy for fixed ideas is more important than the treatment procedures of basic disturbances or stigmata. However, in cases of high vulnerability, this principle demands that they receive equal treatment.

Treatment of dissociative stigmata (basic disturbances)

In the case of a still severely disturbed psychic constitution, a cure after having treated fixed ideas is not always lasting. In addition to the therapy for fixed ideas, basic disturbances or stigmata have to be treated because the general mental constitution is a collateral cause of suggestibility and the fixed ideas themselves. Therefore, treatment has to cure the basic disturbances in, for example, mental synthesis. All general treatment procedures help the mental constitution in preventing or minimizing unnecessary expenditures of mental force and tension.

Physical or psychophysical therapies

Janet recommended general treatment procedures like physiotherapy, hydrotherapy, a course of treatment at a spa, and medical treatment by means of diets, for example, to enhance the mental constitution. According to Janet, physical or psychophysical as well as dietetic procedures are very helpful because they strengthen health in general and the nervous system or the ability of mental synthesis in particular. They prevent relapses after a treatment through psychological analysis or through suggestion.

Psychoeducation

In addition to the other methods, Janet (1911, 1919, 1925) recommended psychoeducation as a therapeutic procedure. In order to overcome the effects of unsuccessful adaptation, patients have to find new coping strategies that foster the ability to solve problems or to learn to live with the inevitable. Psychoeducative methods range from the uncomplicated method of "economizing" energy, for example, by treatment through rest or isolation and by strengthening resilience. Training of attention (*l'éducation de l'attention*) is especially worth mentioning here. Comparable to pedagogy, it is a kind of mental gymnastics that improves the patient's ability to perform mental synthesis through exercises. In turn, the increased ability to perform mental synthesis prevents suggestibility and fixed ideas. Janet described the training of attention as follows: "[It is] a method of treatment which consists in getting them [the hysterics] to do regular mental work like children in school" (1911, p. 675).

Here, modern cognitive and hypnotherapeutic procedures for treating histrionic personality disorders should be mentioned. In this connection, "ego state" is a core concept. Watkins and Watkins (1997), for example, define it as an organized system of experiences and behaviours connected by a common principle and separated by somewhat permeable borderline from different "ego-states." As a psychotherapeutic approach for histrionic personality disorders, these authors propose a multi-level description of situations (encompassing thoughts, emotions and affects, bodily sensations, tendencies of behaviour, and feedback information of the social environment) activating mostly conflicting "ego-states" (Janet, 1904, p. 431). This approach can be combined with cognitive therapy connected with behaviour modification. The patients learn to be aware of and to distinguish their ego states by means of analyses of cognitive experiences and behaviours. As a consequence, they learn to prevent, moderate, or adaptively change the effects of these mostly conflicting "ego states."

Janet also proposed work therapy (a modification of it nowadays is called ergotherapy). The basic idea of such a therapy is to train higher tendencies, to broaden the field of consciousness, and to enable it to take in several ideas simultaneously as well as to synthesize them or oppose one another. Therefore, automatic activities that may be carried out with low attention should be avoided. Rather, activities should be graded according to the attention required and the number of elements to be synthesized, that is, according to their complexity. The tasks must neither be too undemanding nor too demanding. Here, parallels to Morita therapy (Reynolds, 1976) and to sensorimotor psychotherapy (Ogden et al., 2006; Ogden & Fisher, 2015; Chapter 14) are obvious.

Treatment through rest

As general procedures to strengthen the mental constitution, Janet suggested treatment through rest, isolation, and hypnotic sleep. Treatment through rest and isolation is self-evident and needs no further characterization. Janet wrote: "it simply consists in taking the patients away from their families, their ordinary social environment, and bring them immediately to a place wholly unknown to them" (1911, p. 642).

The basic idea is to remove the patients from their pathological milieu. Through isolation, the exhaustion caused by influences from the ordinary social environment of the patients can be reduced. Janet argued:

> The origin of their fixed ideas is to be found in their family, in the presence of particular persons, in conversations. These fixed ideas are incessantly activated and nurtured by everyday incidents and become stronger and stronger in the milieu where they originated.
>
> *(1911, p. 643)*

To distance the patient from the stressful environment, treatment through rest and isolation takes place in a sanatorium. To this extent, treatment through rest and isolation is another parallel to Morita therapy (Reynolds, 1976). However, the patients are not left to live for themselves but they enter a therapeutic milieu. Without doubt, the patients take their fixed ideas with them to the new environment, but while being there they do not think of them as much. Therefore, the fixed ideas are not incessantly activated by associations, and in a best-case scenario are forgotten. Additionally, isolation simplifies the patients' lives. This is no small advantage for patients whose ability for mental synthesis is impaired.

Last but not least, Janet recommended also treatment through rest by means of hypnotic sleep. He stated: "The hypnotic sleep is mainly used to make the subject express his persistent emotions, show their origins, and consent to exert efforts of the will and attention necessary to modify the cerebral equilibrium" (1911, p. 651).

Treatment through rest and isolation is but a first step. Another one has to follow.

Simplicity of life

Janet proposed simplicity of life (*simplicité de la vie*) as the most general goal for treating the basic disturbances of dissociative disorders. Yet, simplicity of life achieved by unspecific therapeutic procedures appropriate is not only for dissociative disorders but also for mental disorders in general, for instance, depression, schizophrenia, anxiety disorders, or some personality disorders. Procedures enhancing simplicity of life are even more important than ordinary treatment through rest and isolation because the faults and shortcomings of the conduct of one's life become particularly obvious in mental, psychosomatic, and even somatic disorders. They are symptoms of deeper-lying failings of the human constitution and, like measuring instruments, are appropriate and sensitive indicators of the deficiencies and shortcomings in lifestyle and the conduct of one's life. Janet stated:

> I sum up: In simple life, all difficulties with the family, love, religion, fortune, and happiness are reduced to a minimum. In it the daily struggle for life, the worries about the future, as well as other complications and confusions of life, are removed.
>
> *(1911, p. 677)*

Because patients often get stuck (*accrochés*) in seemingly hopeless situations, the basic principle of simplification of life is to reduce unnecessary stress and keep life as unaffected by it as possible. Patients have to be freed (*désaccrocher*) of their seemingly hopeless situations by solving as many of their mostly complex problems of life as possible. One means of achieving this goal is to organize and structure life. This kind of treatment is also carried out by psychagogic or psychotherapeutic counselling and instructions in strategies for problem solving. Sometimes, such a therapeutic approach becomes very difficult or even impossible, since therapists usually do not solve the problems of their patients, but can give hints about heuristics for problem solving.

Conclusion

Janet's impressive proposals for a multimodal treatment of dissociative disorders, well-founded on his pathopsychological concepts and his later theory of human conduct, can be seen as an early effort in achieving an evidence-based psychotherapy.

Moreover, Janet's approach, particularly realized in his three-volume study *Les Médications Psychologiques* (1919; English translation, *Psychological Healing*, 1925) and its summary *La Médecine Psychologique* (Janet 1923a; English translation *Principles of Psychotherapy*, 1924), reveals a profound design of the first real counter-conception to psychoanalysis. This was not actually seen for several decades, due to Janet's cautious theorizing according to his methodological orientation and his sceptical views, and above all because of the strong impact of the psychoanalytic movement in medicine and society. The breakthrough and progress of psychologically based psychotherapies during the last 50 years allows the recognition of the fundamental compatibility of his earlier concepts like dissociation, and fixed ideas, or his later resource-model of human agency and its concepts of tendency, force, tension, etc., with modern psychological theories. In the same way, Janet's discussions of interventions with respect to his demands of a differential therapy for psychological disturbances underlines the modernity and utility of his thinking for research and practice in psychotherapy.

Notes

1 Modified version of K. E. Bühler and G. Heim (2011), "Etiology, pathogenesis, and therapy according to Pierre Janet concerning dissociative disorders." *American Journal of Psychotherapy* 65, 2011: 190–200; by kind permission of the *Association for the Advancement of Psychotherapy*. The authors are grateful to Andrew Moskowitz for his comments.
2 For German translations of these two reports on Lucie, see: Janet, 2013, pp. 124–144, pp. 145–187.

14

ACTS OF TRIUMPH

An interpretation of Pierre Janet and the role of the body in trauma treatment

Pat Ogden

[handwritten: Janet was curious & independent rather than authoritarian & traditional]

> Psychotherapy is a totality of therapeutic procedures of all kinds, both physical and moral, applicable alike to bodily and to mental disorders, procedures determined by the consideration of psychological phenomena which have previously been studied, and above all by the consideration of the laws which regulate the development of these psychological phenomena and their association, whether with one another, or with physiological phenomena.
>
> *(Janet, 1925, p. 1208)*

Throughout his writings, Pierre Janet asserted that incorporating physical action in treatment might not only help to alleviate disorders of movement and body sensation, but also positively affect the workings of the mind. A careful and perceptive observer of human behaviour, Janet was dedicated to approaching psychology in a scientific manner with "curiosity and independence", instead of "authority and tradition" (Ellenberger, 1970). Through such observation, he recognized that the awkwardness and irregularities of his patients' movement patterns were related to their mental difficulties. He posed the following question, still relevant for clinical explorations of somatic approaches today:

[handwritten margin: he explores how body movements treated affect the mind]

> Does it not seem likely enough that a transformation of movements by means of a process of education may have an effect upon the totality of the patient's activities, and thus prove competent to prevent or remove the mental troubles?
>
> *(1925, p. 725)*

In the mid-1800s, a variety of body-oriented approaches were already being implemented in treatment (Janet, 1925). These approaches included training in posture and alignment of the spine, using rhythmical movements, incorporating massage and passive movement to help patients regain awareness of sensation, and teaching patients to "break up their movements into the component elements" (1925, p. 726).

Ellenberger (1970) remarked that "Janet stands at the threshold of all modern dynamic psychiatry. His ideas have become so widely known that their true origin is often unrecognized and attributed to others" (p. 406). The same can be said for Janet's contributions to somatic psychology. Janet's perspectives on somatic interventions for the treatment of trauma are the precursors of somatic psychotherapies conceptualized and applied throughout the last century and in recent times. David Boadella (2011) described Janet as the grandfather of body psychotherapy because he believed that one's ability to be present in the here and now was grounded in embodiment, which Janet called "corporality." Janet referred to his work as "psychological analysis," which was really a form of psycho-physical analysis that included behaviour and movement. This chapter will discuss and compare the somatic approaches Janet described with those of sensorimotor psychotherapy, focusing specifically on physical "acts of triumph" and the pleasure of the completed action (Ogden & Fisher, 2015; Ogden, Minton, & Pain, 2006).

Acts of triumph

The instinctive defensive actions that constitute an adaptive response to threat are often ineffective or interrupted, and thus left incomplete in its execution. For example, the sexual abuse survivor might have wanted to fight her perpetrator but was overpowered and could not successfully fight back, nor could she escape. Components of such instinctive defences, having been ineffective, often continue in distorted, exaggerated forms (Herman, 1992), such as muscles held in a chronically tightened pattern, the tendency to be triggered suddenly into aggression or flight, or a chronic lack of tone or sensation in a particular muscle group (Ogden, Minton, & Pain, 2006). Janet (1925) noticed that "[traumatized] patients ... are continuing the action, or rather the attempt at action, which began when the thing happened, and they exhaust themselves in these everlasting recommencements" (p. 663). For example, a victim of childhood beatings may react with uncontrolled aggression towards his own children when he feels threatened; a war veteran may feel the urge to run or withdraw whenever she feels even slightly anxious. Janet (1907b) described more extreme continuations of defence: "Certain patients plainly manifest anger; they strike, scratch, bite, and their cries are menacing ... [T]he movements of defense of the arms stretched forward, the drawing back of the body, are quite characteristic" (pp. 102–103). Other patients exhibited "contraction of the abductor muscles (the guardians of virginity) brought about by the memory of rape or by that of unwanted sexual relationships" (Janet, 1925, p. 592). The adaptive execution of a sequence of defensive actions remains truncated, incomplete, and dissatisfying to the individual. Although patients may recognize that these reactions are vestiges of the past, they are nevertheless unable to modify their responses though top-down cognitive means.

Janet recognized that a sense of pleasure and joy spontaneously emerges when an action is thoroughly executed to completion. When defensive actions are effective and danger is averted, feelings of mastery, victory over threat, and the sense of relief ensue. These "acts of triumph" would have been achieved through escape or fighting back, but as we have seen these actions remain incomplete. Janet (1925) lamented that those "suffering from traumatic memory have not been able to perform any of the actions characteristic of the stage of triumph" (p. 669). However, the impulse for these defensive reactions still lives within the body, and completing these actions can become a focus of therapy. Fully executing the physical actions that were evoked at the time of the original trauma often renders them more available as adaptive responses in current reality. Without treatment to complete the defensive actions, these tendencies may indefinitely prevent the capacity for adaptive responses in the present (Ogden & Fisher, 2015; Ogden, Minton, & Pain, 2006).

Restoring acts of triumph

Janet's approach is aligned with the philosophy of sensorimotor psychotherapy, a body-oriented talking therapy developed by this author in the 1980s, to resolve trauma and attachment failures. One focus of this method is on completing incomplete actions through direct work with the sensation and movement of the body itself. To illustrate, I will describe Tina's treatment. As a child, Tina was forced to submit to her father's sexual abuse, which she endured without resistance. In treatment with me, she discovered her forgotten, dormant impulse to push away, run away, and protect herself. As she remembered how she became frozen and did not resist her father during the abuse, she became aware of the tension in her arms and a feeling of energy in her legs indicating that her body had wanted to both fight and run. These physical impulses that she did not, could not, act upon at the time of the abuse appeared spontaneously as I helped her to became meticulously aware of her physical sensations and impulses for action while remembering the abuse.

Janet had a deep understanding of the complexities of actions, asserting that "an action is not only the simple physical or mental action itself, but incorporates and expresses a person's beliefs, reflections, and experiences" (1930a, p. 7). Indeed, Tina's lost impulses to resist had become encoded not only in praxis of submission, but also as a belief: "I don't deserve to defend myself." Over the course of therapy, Tina learned to observe her body – her movements, sensations, impulses, posture, and gestures – and eventually fully to execute the impulses of her body to complete actions. For example, she learned to harness the tension in her arms to push hard with her hands and arms against a pillow held by her therapist. Such incomplete defensive responses, when completed, foster a sense of mastery and "triumph" that Janet describes.

Sequential steps to restoring acts of triumph

In teaching new physical actions, the therapist must pursue two goals (Janet, 1925). First, the specific action must challenge the patient's integrative capacity. Second, the action must not exhaust or "de-resource" the patient. This twofold aim requires precise tracking of and attunement to the patient on the part of the therapist, who must "hold" the patient at the limits of his or her window of tolerance (Siegel, 1999), to expand his or her integrative capacity and catalyze new movements. Practicing new actions of incremental complexity is crucial to the success of the therapy because if a patient is assigned too great a task, he is likely to fail. Instead, the patient's capacity and confidence is built over time as the tasks required elicit success. The therapist's slow, gradual instruction in the execution of the action helps the patient to "make correct and automatic reactions which will spare him the loss that would be caused by failure, as well as the cost of agitation and emotion" (Janet, 1925, p. 737). Janet goes on to note:

> Every living being … acquires … new tendencies by the method of trial and error, and he fixes them by numerous repetitions. At first a protective agitation drives him to make all sorts of movements, good, bad, and indifferent. Little by little, he learns to discontinue the unsuccessful movements, and to repeat only the successful movements.
>
> (pp. 783–784)

The therapist must assess what actions are possible for a patient to complete successfully at any given time. Increasingly more difficult tasks over time can be assigned as success is achieved. At first, Tina became markedly uncomfortable when executing physical gestures of self-defence, which felt "awkward" and "unfamiliar." When she attempted such motions of pushing with her arms, she would "not be there." Her neck and spine were "frozen" with limited range of motion. Her arms would collapse lifelessly at her sides and she said she wanted to "give up." I then instructed her to experiment with unlocking her knees, a task she could successfully complete, which helped Tina feel more grounded and provided a somatic resource to help her stay in the here and now. She practiced this simple action for several weeks until it became familiar. At that point, a higher-level task was explored: the actions of moving her legs and running – symbolic of a "flight" response. Eventually, I asked Tina to experiment with following the spinal movements of turning and orienting, releasing the "frozen" movement. She began to feel that she was more and more present in current time. Only after several therapy sessions was Tina finally able to execute successfully the actions of pushing away with her arms without exacerbating her dissociative tendencies. By that time, she had completed many of the "mental actions" associated with previous actions of physical grounding, running, and orienting, and she literally experienced the support of her lower body and spine, as well as having her fight, flight, and submissive parts became more integrated and less autonomous, along with her feeling that she was better able to regulate reactive parts of herself.

Economy of movement

Conflicting movements, such as pushing away while simultaneously pulling back, are a hallmark of disorganized/disoriented attachment patterns. When an attachment figure is also a source of threat, simultaneous or sequential arousal of two behavioural, or action, systems are elicited: that of defence and that of attachment. The activation of the two systems is reflected in physical actions that are not synchronous or mobilized in a unified direction, as clearly demonstrated in the Strange Situation studies (Main & Solomon, 1986, 1990).

Using the concept of "economy" of movement to describe physical actions that are inefficient or not harmonious, Janet (1925) quotes his colleague, Cabot:

> Why is it that we contract all our muscles when the need is to contract a few and leave the rest slack? How come it is that when we sit down to write a letter, we write not with the fingers of one hand but with all the muscles of the right arm and shoulder, and not infrequently with our faces, our tongues, and our legs?
>
> *(p. 726)*

My patient Kelley, a 26-year-old survivor of childhood sexual and physical abuse by her father, first made the movements of pushing away against a pillow held by the therapist. Exhibiting conflicted movements, her body pulled back while her arms pushed forward, her spine collapsed, her head drooped, and she averted her gaze. She reported that pushing away meant that she would be alone, a statement reflecting the conflict of her childhood abusive relationship with her father. Her body demonstrated this conflict by contracting unnecessary muscles in the simple act of pushing. Her muscles were working against each other: she pulled back and pushed away simultaneously.

When patients first attempt to execute a previously conflicted, ineffective, impeded, or disabled action their movement is typically not economical. They use the body inefficiently, often at odds with conscious intent. Such inefficient and uneconomical movements can be noticed in various gestures and actions, corresponding to patients' issues. A patient who avoids intimacy collapses when she attempts to reach out to her therapist; another with anxious attachment history cannot let go without holding on somewhere else in her body; a woman with low self-esteem cannot lift her chest or breathe deeply without tightening her back. Janet (1925) states, "We must learn to guide our motor energies intelligently to correct these bad habits" (p. 726).

As Kelley explored executing an integrated movement of pushing away with her arms against a pillow held that I held, I encouraged her to lengthen her spine, lift her head, and make eye contact while pushing against the pillow. I helped her not only to push with her arms but also to engage her back and legs, thus involving her entire body in one focused, coordinated action. After performing this movement several times, with progressively more integration and efficiency in her movement, Kelley noted the unfamiliarity of the economical defensive action, reporting that this movement is "entirely new – it makes me wonder what's been happening all this time." She realized that while she said "no," her body had been saying both "yes" and "no," a leftover from childhood abuse and her conflict between attachment and defense in relationship to her father. After practicing this integrated movement of pushing away, and working simultaneously with the cognitive distortions of "I will always be alone if I push anyone away," Kelley experienced that she had clearer boundaries with others.

Division of the personality was extensively noted by Janet (1901) who wrote about the successive alternation of two "psychological existences": "In one he has sensations, remembrances, movements, which he has not in the other, and consequently he presents, in a manner more or less clear ... two characters, and in some sort two personalities" (p. 491). Thus, as in Kelley's treatment, as new, integrated actions are explored, the parts of the self that the old and new actions reflect are also explored and integrated. Without exploring the parts connected to particular action tendencies, therapists run the risk of overriding rather than integrating parts of the self.

The importance of pleasure

When incomplete actions are executed to their full capacity, and thus thoroughly completed, the patient has reached the "stage of triumph" (Janet, 1925, p. 669). These completed actions evoke a sense of mastery and pleasure and involve changing cognitive distortions, such as "I don't have a right to protect myself," often learned in the context of abuse, into "I do have a right to protect myself." Janet (1925) eloquently reports

> When an action is being functionally restored, and when improvements are taking place, we almost always notice at a certain moment that satisfaction reappears in one form or another, a sort of joy which gives interest to the action, and replaces the feelings of uselessness, absurdity, and futility which had formerly troubled the patient in connection with the action.
>
> (pp. 988–989)

Kelley was relieved and exuberant when she was finally able to execute the physically defensive movements she had been unable to complete during childhood sexual abuse. Her feelings of helplessness and hopelessness were transformed into feelings of empowerment and mastery, as evidenced not only by her experience of pleasure in therapy sessions but also by her increased ability to engage in social interactions and experience pleasure with others. She would spontaneously smile and sometimes even burst into laughter when speaking of her capacity to set appropriate boundaries. Janet (1925) states:

> In order to finish the action we must put an end to all the movements that have been connected with it. If the close of the action is to be definitive, we must demobilize, must disperse, the forces that participated in the action. It is this dispersal of the recuperated energies which produces the temporary excitation of joy ... and all the feelings of triumph. ... This joy and this triumph are ... present after every action that has been well completed.
>
> (p. 666)

The pleasure and joy of the completed action are also notably present when physical sensation is restored. Janet (1925) describes Paul Sollier's reports (Sollier being a doctor, psychologist and contemporary of Janet's, known for his work with memory):

> When the restoration of sensibility is complete, when the patient has been fully reawakened, he usually gives utterance to feeling of astonishment and joy, in such terms as ... 'It is strange how large everything is here; the furniture and the other objects in the room seem brighter, I can feel my heart beating ... .' These feelings of well-being make the patient laugh, and give him a general aspect of gaiety and health.
>
> (p. 808)

Similarly, the stage of triumph is also experienced in sensorimotor psychotherapy sessions as clients safely experience body sensations and the completion of actions described above. Similar to Sollier's description, clients often spontaneously report feelings of aliveness, physical pleasure, and satisfaction at reconnecting with sensation.

This stage of triumph and the pleasure it engenders may have more significance that a simple "feel good" experience. Panksepp (1998) states that, a

> general scientific definition of the ineffable concept we call pleasure can start with the supposition that pleasure indicates something is biologically useful. ... Useful stimuli are those that inform the brain of their potential to restore the body toward homeostatic equilibrium when it has deviated from its biologically dictated 'set-point level.'
>
> (p. 182)

Teaching, practice, and mindfulness

The task of the therapist in facilitating acts of triumph is complex. The therapist must "ask certain precisely what action is lacking ... and teach the subject how to perform this action correctly" (Janet, 1925, p. 739). The patient himself is typically incapable of assessing actions that are inadequate or incomplete, for movement habits are acquired over years of practice in response to internal and external stimuli. These action tendencies are adaptively created in response to the demands of the context within which one lives:

> Every living being placed in a new environment adapts itself, first, by creating new combinations of movements that respond appropriately to the new ways in which the environment affects it, and then, by fixing these combinations of movements and building up corresponding tendencies, that is, dispositions to produce such a reaction correctly, rapidly, and easily in an automatic fashion.
>
> *(Janet, 1923a, p. 208)*

These movements become automatic adaptations to one's environment, and when patients attempt to change them and execute new, unfamiliar movements, they may feel awkward, unfamiliar, emotionally evocative, and even "wrong." The patient experiences the familiar, habitual movement as the "right" one even though the current environment is different from the one in which the action tendency was formed. As Janet (1925) states, patients "cannot change an action, cannot stop an action when once it is begun, even if the circumstances which led to its inception have completely changed" (p. 680).

Although patients may attempt to execute new actions independently, these attempts are usually unsuccessful. Janet (1925) clarifies why this is so:

> The patient ... is not familiar with the mechanism of the action which he is trying to learn. He would not know how to decompose it into its elements; he would not be able to repeat the useful elements of the movement one by one or to eliminate the futile elements.
>
> *(p. 738)*

To remedy this, Janet suggests that the patient should practice new actions under the close tutelage of a therapist who "demonstrates in detail the action which is to be acquired" (1925, p. 739). Throughout Kelley's treatment, I repeatedly demonstrated lengthening my own spine, making eye contact, pushing in a relaxed but effective manner, and so forth, so that Kelley could observe me executing an integrated action.

Janet advises that awareness of the body and its functions must be re-taught to the patient through the therapeutic relationship: "We have to accustom the subject to resuming possession of the function whose control he has lost; we have to enable him to regain a knowledge of his limbs and their movements" (1925, p. 756) New physical actions, such as pushing away or reaching out, can evoke memory accompanied by sensations or painful emotions related to the times when that same action was met with abuse or rejection. The therapist must help the patient separate the past from the present, and identify, clarify, and process the reactions associated with the past. This work requires keen psychological attention and perseverance, of which the patient is incapable without help (Janet, 1925).

In order to train new movement skills to the point where they become auto-matic, repetition is necessary. Patients must repeat the actions over and over for an extended period of time, with feedback from the therapist. Janet (1925) states:

> At first these operations demand intense conscious effort, but through repetition, in virtue of the mechanism of habit, they are performed with increasing ease and quickness, so that, at long last, they can be executed correctly without attention and almost unawares. Education thus consists of the production and repetition of a new action performed in the presence of a competent witness, who supervises it, corrects it, and has it repeated until the action becomes, not merely correct, but automatic.
>
> *(p. 736)*

Although Breuer and Freud (1895) stated that new actions should be mental actions (thus the advent of the "talking cure"), without the ability to perform corresponding physical actions the mental actions might prove insufficient. For example, Sam talked about wanting to be closer to, and more vulnerable with, his wife, but the tension in his body prevented the proximity-seeking action of reaching out to connect with others, obstructing his capacity for intimacy.

As new actions are taught and practiced in therapy, patients gradually learn the mechanics of the action itself, deal with the uncomfortable sensations and emotions, and separate the past from the present. They are assigned incremental homework tasks to practice the action in their environment. Sam first practiced the simple physical action of reaching out, just as a physical exercise, until he could execute the motion in a relaxed, economical movement. His therapist observed the movement and helped Sam to perform the action efficiently with-out undue contraction. When this was easy for Sam, his therapist asked him to execute the action while imagining his wife standing before him. Then he was instructed to add the words, of Sam's construction: "I need to talk with you." Eventually, Sam was able actually to reach out to his wife and better express his feelings. The act of reaching out then emerged spontaneously in Sam's life. After months of therapy, he reported that when he returned for a visit to his childhood home to reconnect with his best childhood friend, who unbeknownst to Sam was an alcoholic, Sam found himself reaching out instead of tightening up and becoming aggressive. He talked to his friend and to his wife, and reported that he even cried a little with her. Sam attributed his newfound ability to reach out to others for support to the practice in therapy. He stated that he had talked about how he has difficulty acknowledging his needs and reaching out, but it did not change his behaviour like completing the action of reaching out in therapy did.

Conclusion

Janet did not believe that health could be restored through bottom-up, somatic methods alone, but through integrating them with top-down interventions: "Just as, in [somatic education], we dispel symptoms by helping the subject to perform the outwardly directed actions demanded by extant situations, so now we must help him to perform internal actions related to past happenings" (Janet 1925, p. 679). Janet believed that the main effect of somatic approaches was "achieved through the education of the subject. The patient must be compelled to look at what is being done, to feel the movements, to collaborate as far as he is able" (p. 757). As the therapist helps the patient make new physical actions, he simultaneously assists the patient to make new internal actions related to separating the past from the present.

In sensorimotor psychotherapy treatment, helping the patient make these new internal actions necessitates practicing mindfulness, a key to developing awareness of internal and physical action patterns, and to increasing integrative capacity (Ogden & Fisher, 2015; Ogden, Minton, & Pain, 2006). Through mindfulness of internal experience, top-down cognitive direction is harnessed to bring awareness to internal processes, particularly body sensation and impulses. Patients are taught to be mindful of the sensations, impulses, emotions, memories, and thoughts that emerge spontaneously as the movement is executed. As Janet suggests:

> We have to amend not [only] the movements of the body but the movements of the mind. We should exercise the mind itself [to] encourage the development of the faculties which seem to be lacking in the patient, the faculties which will enable him to make headway against his malady.
>
> *(1925, p. 728)*

Through the integration of top-down and bottom-up approaches, the patient gradually learns to be mindful of his internal experience, enabling increased choice over both internal and external action.

Janet believed that working with the body is integral to psychotherapy. He understood that who we are, what we feel, and what we believe are intrinsically connected to our bodies. He recognized that the body's patterns of movement, posture, and sensation reflect and perpetuate patients' difficulties and, therefore, that the body itself is a viable and beneficial target for therapeutic intervention, along with emotions and cognitive distortions. As Janet (1925) looks to the future, he states:

> Some day we may hope to learn how to distinguish clearly the symptoms for which, and the patients in whom, [somatic] education is applicable, and to note clearly what place this special form of treatment ought to occupy in the treatment as a whole. It will then be discovered that educational treatment is not all sufficing, but that it certainly has an important part to play.
>
> *(p. 787)*

Therapists today might consider heeding Janet's advice to integrate work with the body into their clinical practice so that they can better help patients to heal the wounds of the past, live more fully in the present, and envision a rich and fulfilling future.

EPILOGUE

Dissociation in the *DSM-5*: Your view, *S'il vous plaît, Docteur Janet?*[1]

Ellert R. S. Nijenhuis

There was a heat wave in Amsterdam this summer. Spending time at the nearby beaches seemed by far the best idea. Still, each day witnessed a lengthy queue waiting to enter the Van Gogh museum. Eager to admire Vincent's paintings, whose beauty and importance had completely escaped his contemporaries, the crowd endured the stinging midday sun. Geniuses live ahead of their time. Imagine they could visit the years they anticipated. What would it be like for Vincent to experience how he had finally reached the hearts of millions? What would happen to *his* artist's heart?

Similarly, what would it be like for brilliant intellects to see how their hard work fares over time, for better or worse? I imagine how Pierre Janet would read the *DSM-5* (APA, 2013). Would he be pleased, critical, or disappointed perhaps? What would he have to say to the authors of the section on the dissociative disorders, and of other references to dissociation in this influential classificatory system?

"*Mesdames, Messieurs,*" opened the brilliant Frenchman, "please accept my congratulations on the new version of the *DSM-5*, and on the dissociative disorders section in particular. I heard that some *collègues* wished to bury these diagnoses for once and for all. You have successfully resisted this unfortunate movement! Reviewing my life's work in 1930 (1930a, p. 127), I remarked that after the death of Charcot, hysterical patients seemed to disappear because they were now designated by other names. It was said that their tendency towards dissimulation and suggestibility made an examination dangerous and interpretations doubtful. I was and still am convinced that these criticisms were grossly exaggerated and based on prejudice and misapprehension. I was under the illusion that my early works were not in vain and that they had left some definite ideas.[2] Your work testifies that my hopes have come true.

"*Bien,* the term hysteria has disappeared, but not the disorders it captured. You may remember that the generic term hysteria as we used it in the nineteenth century covered more mental disorders than your classification of dissociative disorders. I thus was particularly keen to check if the forms of hysteria that were described in the *DSM-IV* as conversion disorder and acute (ASD) and posttraumatic stress disorder (PTSD) would still be classified separate of the dissociative disorders? *Oui, Mesdames et Messieurs,* in our view these disorders constituted forms of hysteria, and I have tried to demonstrate that what unites them is a dissociation of the personality as a whole system in two or more subsystems."

Janet's face grew concerned. "Please allow me to voice my mixed feelings regarding conversion symptoms and disorders. The continued recognition and classification of the involved symptoms and conditions are certainly important. When I began my clinical studies, it was felt that sensorimotor symptoms such as various hyperesthesias, anesthesias, analgesia, and paralyses were among the major symptoms of hysteria. For example, you might want to consult or reread Briquet's already old book on hysteria from 1859. Phenomena such as hysterical amnesias and mental intrusion symptoms such as reenactments of traumatic memories were originally not that clearly included. In fact, *mes collègues et moi* had to struggle to get recognition for hysteria's mental symptoms! So I wonder why you, like the authors of *DSM-IV,* do not regard conversion symptoms and disorders as dissociative symptoms and disorders? Why can loss of memory be a dissociative symptom, but not loss of bodily sensations? And why can intrusions such as hearing voices be dissociative, but not intrusions of bodily sensations or movements? If only by conceptual logic, I believe that your distinction does not completely hold.

"*Alors, je suis confus.* Moreover, there are strong empirical reasons for recognizing sensorimotor dissociative symptoms. In my age, already a long time ago, we did not have your exquisite methods of empirical research and statistical analyses at our disposal. Peeking at contemporary research, it strikes me that, consistent with our clinical observations, the classic sensorimotor hysterical symptoms are excellent predictors of the complex dissociative disorders that you recognize. In fact, they are as indicative of these disorders as the mental, or cognitive-emotional, dissociative symptoms that you describe in detail (e.g. Müller-Pfeiffer *et al.,* 2013). Let me say in passing that depersonalization disorder seems to be an exception in this regard, but then, the personality of most individuals with this condition does not encompass two or more different conscious and self-conscious subsystems. Considering that conversion symptoms are the characteristic of the complex dissociative disorders that the *DSM-5* lists, it seems very likely that these symptoms are in fact dissociative symptoms, *n'est ce pas?*"

Anticipating a rejoinder, Janet continued: "One could counter that the opening sentence of the *DSM-5* dissociative disorders section at page 291 clearly states that dissociative disorders can include a disruption of and/or discontinuity in the normal integration of body representation, motor control, and behaviour. *Bien sûr*, and this statement is certainly an improvement over the opening line of the dissociative disorders section in *DSM-IV*. That system did not include any reference to bodily functions as if all the work on hysterical sensorimotor symptoms and disorders that my nineteenth-century *collègues* and me did had lost all meaning. Thus, the new statement is a welcome correction. I also noticed that the 'A' criterion for dissociative identity disorder (DID) states that the implied disruption of identity involves discontinuities in sense of self and sense of agency that are accompanied by alterations in sensorimotor functioning. At page 293, you have detailed that individuals with this disorder may experience that their body is 'not mine' and/or 'not under my control.'

"Reading these lines, I must admit that I had hoped you would have brought *DSM-IV* conversion symptoms and disorder home to, *s'il vous me permettez l'expression*, hysteria. This integrative act would also bring the *DSM* and *ICD* more in line with each other. You are obviously aware that the *ICD-10* (WHO, 1992) includes dissociative disorders of movement and sensation. But I felt a little disappointment and puzzlement at page 297, where you use the label 'conversion disorder (functional neurological symptom disorder).'

"This label presents some problems. For example, what distinguishes sensorimotor dissociative symptoms from conversion symptoms? If the difference were only terminological, you would have said so, right? You must be committed to the view that there *are* real differences between the two concepts, or else your statement that '[d]issociative symptoms are common in individuals with conversion disorder' (p. 321) is clearly tautological.

"Another reason why I find it a bit difficult to follow your logic regarding dissociation and conversion is that you have left the concepts of conversion and functional neurological symptoms undefined. I also wonder why in your view bodily anaesthesia but not memory loss can involve a functional neurological symptom? Cognitive-emotional dissociative symptoms do have a particular functional neurological description. In this regard I am intrigued by the fascinating work of *Monsieur le professeur* Markowitsch (2003). In the old days I also conceded that any mental problem will (eventually) have a particular neurophysiological description – even if that description will never completely explain the phenomenon. Knowing patterns of neurophysiological activity is of little value if one does not know what an individual was trying to achieve, and what meaning his or her actions had for him or her, as *le philosophe* Arthur Schopenhauer[3] explained before me, and *le philosophe et biologiste* Francisco Varela (1996) after me. Schopenhauer (1958, Vol II, p. 13) emphasized that '[i]t is just as true that the knower is a product of matter as that matter is a mere idea of the knower; but it is also one-sided. For materialism is the philosophy of the subject who forgets to take account of himself.' In consonance with Schopenhauer, phenomenologists point out that the third-person perspective of 'objective science' presupposes the first-person perspective. Philosophical materialists overlook or ignore this important fact. In this spirit, Varela (1996, p. 334) emphasizes that '[t]he phenomenological approach starts from the irreducible nature of conscious experience. Lived experience is where we start from and where all must link back to, like a guiding thread.' A quite related problem is that a philosophy that, *tiens*, dissociates mind and body, I mean, that regards mind and the body as different substances, raises the riddle of how the two would communicate? Neither Descartes nor anyone else could solve it. *Le problème est insoluble! Pas de dualisme!*

"Why not follow Spinoza's philosophy, in which mind and matter are comprehended as two different attributes of a singularly existing substance? This substance – Spinoza called it *Dieu ou la nature* – probably has many more attributes than we know and can know. If we accept his philosophical monism, then any symptom and disorder that the *DSM-5* or any other classificatory system of mental disorders involves will have a mental (psychological/psychosocial) and functional neurological description (even if neither of the two provides a complete understanding). So, I ask, must the text on dissociation and conversion be read in terms of the elusive philosophical dualism? If so, how about the philosophical concerns regarding this persuasion, and if not, how could I understand your curious distinction between psychology and neurology? And if you still prefer conversion, what gets converted into what?"

Janet's face expressed his concerns regarding conversion and brought unpleasant intrusions of his struggles with Freud. Turning the subject, his eyes brightened up. "*Mesdames, Messieurs*, let me interrupt my little criticisms and focus on some other features of the *DSM-5* that, *à mon avis*, seem to involve a step ahead, and hold a promise.

"I am heading at two themes. The first is the statement at page 291 that '[i]n the DSM-5, the dissociative disorders are placed next to, but are not part of, the trauma- and stressor-related disorders, reflecting the close relationship between these diagnostic categories. Both acute stress disorder and posttraumatic stress disorder contain dissociative symptoms, such as amnesia, flashbacks, numbing, and depersonalization/derealization.' My reservations regarding the alleged dissociative nature of depersonalization and derealization aside, the text does not clearly describe 'the close relationship.' I presume it is twofold.

"One relationship is that stress disorders and dissociative disorders are both causally related to one or more adverse or otherwise stressful events (but there are also other causal factors). It is stimulating to hear that contemporary research basically supports my extensive clinical observations that there is a relationship between the severity of hysteria and the severity, duration, and repetition of adverse/stressful events, and that these events can have a causal role. I was not the first to document this connection. In his empirical study of hysteria (1859), *Monsieur* Briquet examined many cases and concluded that consistent with the clinical observations of predecessors such as *Messieurs* Sydenham, Whytt, Cheyne, and several others, hysteria is most commonly and causally related to *les passions de l'âme, et surtout les passions tristes*.[4] These emotions primarily involved maltreatment of children by their parents, and maltreatment of wives by their husbands. They could also relate to relational troubles or other stressful life events. Briquet also found that it is not the mere occurrence of these adversities and stressors, but that there are also predisposing factors such as a sensitive nervous system, female gender, and hereditary influences. As authors of the *DSM-5*, you clearly state that '[t]he dissociative disorders are frequently found in the aftermath of trauma, and many of the symptoms, including embarrassment and confusion about the symptoms or a desire to hide them, are influenced by the proximity to trauma.' Your explicit recognition that hysteria is causally related to adversities and stressors (in a context of other causal factors) is a fortunate development. It will certainly be useful to clinicians and thankfully received by the patients.

"Another relationship between stress disorders and dissociative disorders that the *DSM-5* clearly recognizes is the presence of dissociative symptoms in both disorders. In this regard, I am happy to see that you have recognized the existence of what you have called 'positive' and 'negative' dissociative symptoms. You write at page 291 that the positive symptoms involve 'unbidden intrusions into awareness,' whereas the negative symptoms pertain to 'inability to access information or to control mental functions that normally are readily amenable to access or control.' If I am not mistaken, you herewith return to my distinction between hysteria's mental stigmata (i.e. losses or negative dissociative symptoms) and mental accidents (i.e. intrusions or positive dissociative symptoms) (cf. Nijenhuis, 2004). However, it puzzles me that you regard depersonalization and derealization as positive symptoms. Don't they involve losses? Something – i.e. the actions of personification, and of realization regarding exteroceptions – is absent that should be present! Positive dissociative symptoms involve the presence of actions and contents that should be absent. Illustrations of this are intruding voices, hyperesthesias, and bodily movements."

Janet felt a need to balance his critique with well-deserved praise. "Returning to the theme that stress disorders and dissociative disorders both involve dissociative symptoms, I feel you hit the nail on the head in stating that PTSD and ASD involve dissociative symptoms. However, you also puzzle me. One trouble is your distinction between different kinds of intrusions (p. 271 and p. 281). Criterion B1 concerns intrusion symptoms in the sense of intruding 'recurrent, involuntary, and intrusive distressing memories of the traumatic event(s).' B2 reads 'recurrent distressing dreams in which the content and/or affect of the dream are related to the traumatic event(s).' You also list B3 that involves '[d]issociative reactions (e.g. flashbacks) in which the individual feels or acts as if the traumatic event(s) were recurring.' *Naturellement*, reenactments of traumatic experiences and events are positive dissociative symptoms. But why would the phenomena of Criteria B1 and B2 then not also be dissociative?"

Janet stood firm: "I say B1, 2, and 3 involve dissociative intrusions. They address mental and behavioural actions and contents that the individual has not been able or willing to integrate. The difference between them, I mean, B1, 2, and 3, strikes me as a matter of degree. They involve partial and more complete intrusions, not different qualities. Also, traumatic memories and nightmares are *someone*'s memories and dreams. They do not exist in an impersonal vacuum, but relate to what I have called 'dissociative subsystems of ideas and functions.'

Thus, there are in most cases of ASD and PTSD two dissociative subsystems of ideas and functions. One however rudimentary subsystem is fixed in the traumatic memory or memories, and another far more elaborate subsystem has not integrated the trauma-fixated subsystem(s). Each of these involves a certain sense of self and agency.

"To get well, individuals with ASD, PTSD, and *DSM-5* dissociative disorders must synthesize, personify, and presentify these different subsystems, including their traumatic memories. When they are unable or too scared to engage in these actions, their disorder continues with all implied symptoms. I thus value your remark, on p. 291, that the positive dissociative symptoms, the intrusions, are accompanied by losses. Indeed, when a trauma-fixated dissociative subsystem effectively intrudes into a trauma-avoidant subsystem in one way or another, the intruded subsystem experiences mental accidents or positive dissociative symptoms such as traumatic memories, hearing the intruding subsystem's voice, experiencing this subsystem's bodily and emotional feelings, and being controlled by its movements. The intruded dissociative subsystem will typically attempt to avoid or delimit the intrusions, particularly when they pertain to troublesome feelings, thoughts, and actions. This evasion shows in losses, that is, in mental stigmata or negative dissociative symptoms such as emotional and bodily numbing. In extreme cases, the intruded subsystem loses consciousness or deactivates itself so that the intruding dissociative subsystem exerts full executive control. It is in this context that positive and negative symptoms are dissociative: one action or set of actions and implied contents are not integrated with another set of actions and these actions' implied contents. And isn't this precisely why you write at p. 291 that intrusions are accompanied by losses?

"A related issue that confuses me a bit is why you do not apply the distinction between negative and positive dissociative symptoms to specify the kinds of symptoms that are involved in ASD and PTSD? I wonder why you followed this inconsistent path? Was it perhaps guided by your wish to distinguish a 'dissociative subtype of PTSD?' In this phrase, you delimit the concept of dissociation to two negative symptoms that, *à mon avis*, might not even be dissociative: depersonalization and derealization. This would imply that there are also 'nondissociative' subtypes of PTSD. But this does not work given your recognition of positive dissociative symptoms, as in Criterion B3, and my point regarding B1 and B2. Since intrusions of nonintegrated trauma-related actions and contents are dissociative per definition, *any* subtype of PTSD is dissociative.

"Given my various comments on dissociation in DSM-5, I suggest a return to a single category of trauma- and stress-related disorders. Each involves a dissociation of the personality, but in some it is more complex than in others. In this regard, there are many intermediate forms between simple PTSD and DID as the most complex type. These intermediates should receive far more recognition and attention, because, *j'insiste*, simple PTSD and complex DID are extremes on a dimension of complexity. Each dissociative disorder is characterized by a particular degree of positive as well as negative dissociative symptoms. All involve dissociative subsystems of ideas and functions, and each subsystem generates its own sense of 'I,' and its own 'I–Me,' 'I–You,' and 'I–Object' relations. If we agree that conversion symptoms are sensorimotor expressions of the existence of a dissociation of the patient's personality, than conversion disorder fits the single category as well. As I say this, you will obviously realize that my proposal leads us back to *l'hystérie*, to the nineteenth-century group of trauma- and stress-related disorders that accommodates the twenty-first century constructs of ASD, PTSD, conversion disorder, and dissociative disorders.

"*Ainsi, chers amis*, I am eagerly looking forward to meeting the authors of DSM-6. If they would find a little value in my considerations, then the rebirth of hysteria, albeit under a different name, might become a reality. *Je vous remerci pour votre attention! Au revoir!*"

Notes

1 Originally published in *Journal of Trauma & Dissociation*, 2014, 15, 245–253. I am indebted to Onno van der Hart for his helpful comments on a previous version of the text.
2 See Janet, 1930a.
3 Janet's first education was in philosophy, and he became a professor of philosophy in Le Havre at the age of 22 years. I therefore assume he was aware of Schopenhauer's main works (1958). Janet was certainly familiar with Spinoza's philosophy (e.g. *Ethics*, 1677). His uncle and philosopher Paul Janet, who had a major influence on his nephew (Ellenberger, 1970), wrote an introduction to Spinoza's work and translated one of his books. Pierre Janet may also have known the works of phenomenologists such as those of phenomenology's founding father Edmund Husserl, who lived from 1859–1938. See Husserl (1970). He was certainly aware of the work of Henri Bergson, who was his classmate and who had a major influence on phenomenologists such as Maurice Merleau-Ponty.
4 See Briquet, 1859, p. 196.

REFERENCES

Adler, A. (1912). *The Neurotic Constitution: Outlines of a Comparative Individualistic Psychology and Psychotherapy*. New York: Moffat, Yard and Company.

Adler, G., & Buie, D. (1979). Aloneness and borderline psychopathology: The possible relevance of child development issues. *International Journal of Psycho-Analysis, 60*: 83–96.

Ainsworth, M. D. (1989). Attachments beyond infancy. *American Psychologist, 44*: 709–716.

American Psychiatric Association (1980). *Diagnostic and Statistical Manual of Mental Disorders* (3rd ed.). Washington, DC: American Psychiatric Press.

American Psychiatric Association (1994). *Diagnostic and Statistical Manual of Mental Disorders* (4th ed.). Washington, DC: American Psychiatric Press.

American Psychiatric Association (2013). *Diagnostic and Statistical Manual of Mental Disorders* (5th ed.). Washington, DC: American Psychiatric Press.

Ansell, E. B., Rando, K., Tuit, K., Guarnaccia, J., & Sinha, R. (2012). Cumulative adversity and smaller gray matter volume in medial prefrontal, anterior cingulate, and insula regions. *Biological Psychiatry, 72*: 57–64.

Arnsten, A. F., Raskind, M. A., Fletcher, B. Taylor, F. B., & Connor, D. F. (2015). The effects of stress exposure on prefrontal cortex: Translating basic research into successful treatment of post-traumatic stress disorder. *Neurobiology of Stress, 1*: 89–99.

Atmansprachen, H., & Fuchs, C. A. (2014). Introduction: The Pauli-Jung Conjecture. In: H. Atmansprachen & A. F. Christopher (Eds.), *The Pauli-Jung Conjecture: And its Impact Today* (pp. 1–6). London: Imprint Academic

Babinski, J. (1901). Définition de l'hystérie. *Revue Neurologique, 9*: 1074–1080.

Babinski, J. (1909). Définition de l'hystérie traditionelle: Phitiathisme. *La Semaine Médicale, 59(1)*: 3–8.

Bailey, P. (1928). The psychology of human conduct. *American Journal of Psychiatry, 8*: 209–234.

Bandura, A. (1977). Self-efficacy. *Psychological Review, 84*: 191–215.

Barach, P. (1991). MPD as an attachment disorder. *Dissociation, 4*: 117–123.

Barrucand, D. (1967). *Histoire de Hypnotisme in France*. Paris: Presses Universitaires de France.

Baruk, H. (1960). Contributions to the celebration of the centenary of Pierre Janet's birth—in French. *Revue Philosophique, CL*: 283–288.

Bateman, A., & Fonagy, P. (2015). The role of mentalization in treatments for personality disorder. In: W. J. Livesley, G. Dimaggio, & J. F. Clarkin (Eds.), *Integrated Treatment for Personality Disorder: A Modular Approach* (pp. 148–172). New York, NY: Guilford Press.

Baynes, C. (1928). *Contribution to Analytical Psychology*. London: Kegan Paul.

Bemporad, J. R. (1989). Freud, Janet and evolution: Of statuettes and plants. *Journal of the American Academy of Psychoanalysis, 17*: 623–638.

Benhima, G. (2010). *Die Konzeptionen der Neurotischen, Hysterischen und Psychasthenischen Persönlichkeiten bei Pierre Janet* [Conceptions of neurotic, hysteric, and psychasthenic personality in Pierre Janet]. Medical Dissertation Julius-Maximilian University of Würzburg, Germany.

Bergson, H. (1913). *Creative Evolution*. New York: Henry Holt.

Berman, E. (1981). Multiple personality: Psychoanalytic perspectives. *International Journal of Psycho-Analysis, 62*: 283–300.

Berrios, G. E., & Dening, T. R. (1996). Pseudohallucinations: A conceptual history. *Psychological Medicine, 26(4)*: 753–763.

Binet, A. (1890). Book review of P. Janet, *L'Automatisme psychologique. Revue Philosophique, 29(1)*: 186–200.

Bliss, E. (1986). *Multiple Personality, Allied Disorders and Hypnosis*. New York: Oxford University Press.

Boadella, D. (1997). Awakening sensibility, recovering motility. Psycho-physical synthesis at the foundations of body-psychotherapy: The 100-year legacy of Pierre Janet (1856–1947). *International Journal of Psychotherapy, 2*: 45–56.

Boadella, D. (2011). Psycho-physical synthesis of the foundations of body psychotherapy: The 100-year legacy of Pierre Janet (1859–1947). In: C. Young (Ed.), *The Historical Basis of Body Psychotherapy* (pp. 49–66). Stow, UK: Body Psychotherapy Publications.

Boeker, H., Richter, A., Himmighoffen, E. J., Bohleber, L., Hofmann, E., Vetter, J., & Nortoff, G. (2013). Essentials of psychoanalytic process and change: How can we investigate the neural effects of psychodynamic psychotherapy in individualized neuro-imaging? *Frontiers in Human Neuroscience 7*: 1–18.

Bogousslavsky, J. (2011). Hysteria after Charcot: Back to the future. *Frontiers of Neurology and Neuroscience, 29*: 137–161.

Bokanowski, T. (1996). Freud and Ferenczi: Trauma and transference depression. *International Journal of Psycho-Analysis, 77*: 519–536.

Bonomi, C. (2017). *The Cornerstone of Psychoanalysis: Vol 2: Sigmund Freud and Sándor Ferenczi*. London: Karnac.

Boon, S., & Draijer, N. (1993). Multiple personality disorder in the Netherlands: A clinical investigation of 71 patients. *American Journal of Psychiatry, 150*: 459–463.

Borgogno, F. (2010). Presentation for the Mary Sigourney Ceremony. www.sigourneyaward.org.

Bornstein, R. F. (1995). Active dependency. *Journal of Nervous and Mental Disease, 183*: 64–77.

Bornstein, R. F. (1998). Dependency in the personality disorders: Intensity, insight, expression, and defense. *Journal of Clinical Psychology, 54*: 175–89.

Bornstein, R. F., & Bowen, R. F. (1995). Dependency in psychotherapy: Toward an integrated treatment approach. *Psychotherapy, 32*: 520–534.

Boston Change Process Study Group (BCPG) (2007). The foundational level of psychodynamic meaning: Implicit process in relation to conflict and the dynamic unconscious. *International Journal of Psycho-Analysis, 88*: 843–860.

Boston Change Process Study Group (BCPG) (2008). Forms of relational meaning. *Psychoanalytic Dialogues*, 18: 197–202.

Bowlby, J. (1969). *Attachment and Loss. Vol. 1: Attachment*. New York: Basic Books.

Bowlby, J. (1973). *Attachment and Loss, Vol. II: Separation*. New York: Basic Books.

Bowlby, J. (1988). *A Secure Base: Parent-child Attachment and Healthy Human Development*. New York: Basic Books.

Brady Brower, M. (2010). *Unruly Spirits: The Science of Psychic Phenomena in Modern France*. Urbana and Chicago: University of Illinois Press.

Brand, B. L., & Frewen, P. (2017). Dissociation as a trauma-related phenomenon. In S. N. Gold (Ed.), *APA Handbook of Trauma Psychology*, Vol. 1 (pp. 215–241). Washington, DC: American Psychological Association.

Braun, B. G. (1986a). Issues in the psychotherapy of multiple personality disorder. In: B. G. Braun, (Ed.), *Treatment of Multiple Personality Disorder* (pp. 1–28). Washington, DC: American Psychiatric Press.

Braun, B. G. (Ed.) (1986b). *Treatment of Multiple Personality Disorder*. Washington, DC: American Psychiatric Press.

Breger, L. (2000). *Freud. Darkness in the Midst of Vision*. New York: J. Wiley & Sons.

Breger, L. (2009). *A Dream of Undying Fame*. New York: Basic Books.

Bremner, J. D. (1999). Acute and chronic responses to psychological trauma: where do we go from here? *American Journal of Psychiatry, 156(3)*: 349–351.

Brende, J. O. (1984). An educational-therapeutic group for drug and alcohol abusing combat veterans. *Journal of Contemporary Psychotherapy*, 14, 122–136.

Breuer, J., & Freud, S. (1895). *Studies on Hysteria. S.E., 2: 19–305*. London: Hogarth.

Breukink, H. (1923). Over de behandeling van sommige psychosen door middel van een bijzondere vorm der kathartisch-hypnotische methode. *Nederlands Tijdschrift Geneeskunde, 67*: 1321–1328.

Brill, A. A. (1937). Introduction. In: J. Breuer and S. Breuer. *Freud Studies in Hysteria*, trans. A. A. Brill, New York: Nervous and Mental Disease Publishing.

Bringer, J.-C. (1989). *Conversations with Jean Piaget*. Chicago, IL and London: The University of Chicago Press.

Briquet, P. (1859). *Traité Clinique et Thérapeutique de l'Hystérie*, Tome I [Clinical and therapeutic treatise on hysteria]. Paris: J-B Baillière et Fils.

Bromberg, P. M. (1995). Psychoanalysis, dissociation, and personality organization. In: P. M. Bromberg, *Standing in the Spaces: Essays on Clinical Process, Trauma, and Dissociation* (pp. 119–136). Hillsdale, NJ: Analytic Press.

Bromberg, P. M. (1996). Hysteria, dissociation, and cure: Emmy von N revisited. *Psychoanalytic Dialogues, 6*: 55–71.

Bromberg, P. M. (1998). *Standing in the Spaces: Essays on Clinical Process, Trauma, and Dissociation*. Hillsdale, NJ: Analytic Press.

Bromberg, P. M. (2006). *Awakening the Dreamer: Clinical Journeys*. Hillsdale, NJ: Analytic Press.

Bromberg, P. M. (2011). *The Shadow of the Tsunami and the Growth of the Relational Mind*. New York: Routledge.

Brooks III, J. I. (1993). Philosophy and psychology at the Sorbonne, 1885–1913. *Journal of the History of the Behavioral Sciences, 29*: 123–145.

Brooks III, J. I. (1998). *The Eclectic Legacy. Academic Philosophy and the Human Sciences in Nineteenth-Century France*. Newark: University of Delaware Press.

Brooks-Brenneis, C. (1996). Memory systems and the psychoanalytic retrieval of memories of trauma. *Journal of American Psychoanalytic Association, 44*: 1165–1187.

Brown, D. P., & Elliott, D. S. (2016). *Attachment Disturbances in Adults: Treatment for Comprehensive Repair.* New York: Norton.

Brown, D. P., & Fromm, E. (1986). *Hypnotherapy and Hypnoanalysis.* Hillsdale, NJ: Lawrence Erlbaum Associates.

Brown, D. P., Scheflin, A. W., & Hammond, C. D. (1998). *Memory, Trauma Treatment, and the Law.* New York: Norton.

Brown, P. (1994). Pierre Janet and therapeutic rapport. Paper presented at the 29th Annual Congress of the RANZ College of Psychiatrists. Launcestor, Tasmania.

Bucci, W. (1997). *Psychoanalysis and Cognitive Science: A Multiple Code Theory.* New York: Guilford Press.

Bühler, K.-E. (2003). Foundations of clinical logagogy. *Medicine, Health Care, and Philosophy, 6*: 303–313.

Bühler, K.-E. (2015). *Gedankensprünge ins Freie: Eine Anthologie zur Logagogik.* [Mental Leaps to Well-Being: An Anthology of Logagogy]. München: Grin.

Bühler, K.-E., & Heim, G. (2001). General introduction to the psychotherapy of Pierre Janet. *American Journal of Psychotherapy, 55*: 74–91.

Bühler, K.-E., & Heim, G. (2009). Psychopathological approaches in Pierre Janet's conception of the subconscious. *Psychopathology, 42*: 190–200.

Bühler, K.-E., & Rother, K. (1999). Die Anthropologische Psychotherapie bei Victor Emil Freiherr von Gebsattel [Anthropological psychotherapy of Victor Emil Freiherr von Gebsattel]. *Fundamenta Psychiatrica, 13*: 1–8.

Carlson, E. A., & Sroufe, L. A. (1995). Contribution of attachment theory to developmental psychopathology. In: D. Cicchetti & D. J. Cohen (Eds.), *Developmental Psychopathology, Vol. 1: Theory and Methods* (pp. 581–617). Hoboken, NJ: John Wiley & Sons.

Carroy, J., Ohayon, A., & Plas, R. (2006). *Histoire de la Psychologie en France. XIXe–XXe siècles.* [History of Psychology in France. 19th and 20th Centuries]. Paris: La Découverte.

Cassidy, J., & Mohr, J. J. (2001). Unsolvable fear, trauma, and psychopathology: Theory, research, and clinical considerations related to disorganized attachment across the lifespan. *Clinical Psychology: Science and Practice, 8*: 275–298.

Cassullo, G. (2010). Back to the roots: The influence of Ian D. Suttie on British Psychoanalysis. *American Imago, 67*: 5–22.

Cassullo, G. (2014). Splitting in the history of psychoanalysis: From Janet and Freud to Fairbairn, passing through Ferenczi and Suttie. In: G. S. Clarke & D. E. Scharff (Eds.), *Fairbairn and the Object Relations Traditions* (pp. 49–58). London: Karnac.

Cassullo, G. (2018). Ferenczi before Freud. In: A. Dimitrijevic, G. Cassullo, & J. Frankel, *Ferenczi's Influence on Contemporary Psychoanalytic Traditions.* London: Karnac

Chadwick, P., Birchwood, M., & Trower, P. (1996). *Cognitive Therapy for Delusions, Voices and Paranoia.* London: Wiley Press.

Charcot, J.-M. (1882). Sur les divers états nerveux déterminés par l'hypnotisation chez les hystériques [On the various nervous states determined by the hypnotization of hysterics]. *Comptes Rendus. Académie des Sciences, 94.* 403–405.

Christodoulou, G. N. (1986). Role of depersonalization-derealization phenomena in the delusional misidentification syndromes. *Bibliotheca Psychiatrica, 164*: 99–104.

Chu, J. A. (2011). *Rebuilding Shattered Lives: The Responsible Treatment of Complex PTSD and Dissociative Disorders* (2nd ed.). New York: John Wiley & Sons.

Clarke, G. S. (2011). Suttie's influence on Fairbairn's object relations theory. *Journal of the American Psychoanalytic Association, 59*: 939–959.

Clarke, G. S. (2014). Fairbairn and Ferenczi. In: G. S. Clarke & D. E. Scharff (Eds.), *Fairbairn and the Object Relations Traditions* (pp. 333–342). London: Karnac.

Cloitre, M. (2016). Commentary on De Jongh et al.'s (2016) critique of ISTSS Complex PTSD guidelines: Finding the way forward. *Depression and Anxiety, 33*: 360–361.

Cloitre, M., Courtois, C. A., Ford, J. D., Green, B. L., Alexander, P., Briere, J., Herman, J. L., Lanius, R., Stolbach, B. C., Spinazzola, J., Van der Kolk, B. A., & van der Hart, O. (2012). The ISTSS Expert Consensus Treatment Guidelines for Complex PTSD in Adults. Retrieved from www.istss.org/

Cohen, C. P., & Sherwood, V. R. (1991). *Becoming a Constant Object in Psychotherapy with the Borderline Patient*. Northvale, NJ: Jason Aronson.

Cohen, J. (1985). Trauma and repression. *Psychoanalytic Inquiry, 5*: 164–189.

Cooley, C. H. (1902). *Human Nature and the Social Order*. New York: Scribner's.

Coons, P. M., & Milstein, V. (1986). Psychosexual disturbances in multiple personality: Characteristics, etiology, and treatment. *Journal of Clinical Psychiatry, 29*(2), 163–110.

Coons, P. M., & Milstein, V. (1992). Psychogenic amnesia: A clinical investigation of 25 cases. *Dissociation, 4*: 73–79.

Cortina, M., & Liotti, G. (2014). An evolutionary outlook on motivation: Implications for the clinical dialogue, *Psychoanalytic Inquiry, 34*: 864–899.

Courtois, C. A. (1999). *Recollections of Sexual Abuse: Treatment Principles and Guidelines*. New York: Norton.

Cozolino, L. (2002). *The Neuroscience of Psychotherapy: Healing the Social Brain*. New York: Norton.

Crabtree, A. (1993). *From Mesmer to Freud: Magnetic Sleep and the Roots of Psychological Healing*. New Haven, CT: Yale University Press.

Craparo, G. (2013). Addiction, dissociazione e inconscio non rimosso. Un contributo teorico secondo la prospettiva evolutivo-relazionale. *Ricerca Psicoanalitica, 24(2)*: 73–84.

Craparo, G. (2017a). Unrepressed unconscious and unsaid in addictive symptomatology. *Psychodynamic Practice, 23*: 282–292.

Craparo, G. (2017b). *L'enactment nella relazione terapeutica. Caratteristiche e funzioni*. Milano: Raffaello Cortina.

Craparo, G. (2018). *Inconscio non rimosso. Riflessioni per una nuova prassi clinica*. Milano: FrancoAngeli.

Craparo, G., & Mucci, C. (Eds.) (2016). *Unrepressed Unconscious, Implicit Memory, and Clinical Work*. London: Karnac.

Croq, L., & De Verbizier, J. (1989). Le traumatisme psychologique dans l'oeuvre de Pierre Janet. *Annales Médico-Psychologiques, 147*: 983–987.

Cutting, J., & Shephard, M. (Eds.) (1987). *The Clinical Roots of the Schizophrenia Concept: Translations of Seminal European Contributions on Schizophrenia*. Cambridge: Cambridge University Press

Dalenberg, C. J. (2000). *Countertransference and the Treatment of Trauma*. Washington, DC: American Psychological Association.

Damasio, A. R. (1994). *Descartes' Error: Emotions, Reason and the Human Brain*. New York: Avon Books.

Damasio, A. R. (2010). *Self Comes to Mind: Constructing the Conscious Brain*. New York: Pantheon Books.

Davies, J. (1998). Repression and dissociation—Freud and Janet: Fairbairn's new model of unconscious process. In: N. J. Skolnick & D. E. Scharff (Eds.), *Fairbairn Then and Now* (pp. 53–69). Hillsdale, NJ: Analytic Press.

Davies, J. M., & Frawley, M. F. (1994). *Treating the Adult Survivor of Childhood Sexual Abuse: A Psychoanalytic Perspective*. New York: Basic Books.

De Jongh, A., Resick, P. A., Zoellner, L. A., Van Minnen, A., Lee, C. W., Foa, E. B., Wheeler, K., ten Broeke, E., Feeny, N., Rauch, S. A. M., Chard, K. M., Mueser, K. T., Sloan, D. M., van der Gaag, M., Rothbaum, B. O., Neuner, F., de Roos, C., Hehenkamp, L. M. J., Rosner, R., & Bicanic, I. A. (2016). Critical analysis of the current treatment guidelines for Complex PTSD in adults. *Depression and Anxiety, 33*: 359–369.

Decker, H. S. (1986). The lure of nonmaterialism in materialistic Europe: Investigations of dissociative phenomena. In: J. M. Quen (Ed.), *Split Minds/Split Brains* (pp. 31–62). New York: New York University Press.

Deitz, J. (1992). Self-psychological approach to posttraumatic stress disorder: Neurobiological aspects of transmuting internalization. *Journal of the American Academy of Psychoanalysis, 20*: 277–293.

Delay, J. (1960). Pierre Janet et la tension psychologique. *Psychologie Française, 5*: 93–100.

Dell, P. (2009). *Understanding dissociation*. In: P. F. Dell & J. A. O'Neil (Eds.), *Dissociation and the Dissociative Disorders: DSM-V and Beyond* (pp.709–825). New York: Routledge.

Dell, P. F., & O'Neil, J. A. (Eds.) (2009). *Dissociation and the Dissociative Disorders: DSM-V and Beyond*. New York: Routledge.

Despine, A. (1840). *De l'Emploi du Magnétisme Animal et des Eaux Minérales, dans le Traitement des Maladies Nerveuses, suivi d'une Observation très curieuse de Guérison de Névropathie*. Paris: Germer Baillière.

Despine, P. (1880). *Le somnambulisme*. Paris: F. Savy.

Deutsch, H. (1942). Some forms of emotional disturbance and their relationship to schizophrenia. *Psychoanalytic Quarterly, 11*: 301–321.

Diamond, M. J. (1984). It takes two to tango: Some thoughts on the neglected importance of the hypnotist in an interactive hypnotherapeutic relationship. *American Journal of Clinical Hypnosis, 27*: 3–13.

Dimitrijevic, A., Cassullo, G., & Frankel, J. (Eds.) (2018). *Sandor Ferenczi's Influence on Contemporary Psychoanalytic Traditions*. London: Karnac.

Dozier, M., Stovall-McClough, K. C., & Albus, K. E. (2008). Attachment and psychopathology in adulthood. In: J. Cassidy & P. Shaver (Eds.), *Handbook of Attachment* (2nd Ed.) (pp. 718–744). New York: Guilford Press.

Dutra, L., Bureau, J., Holmes, B., Lyubchik, A., & Lyons-Ruth, K. (2009). Quality of early care and childhood trauma: A prospective study of developmental pathways to dissociation. *Journal of Nervous and Mental Disease, 197*: 383–390.

Ecker, W., & Gönner, S. (2008). Incompleteness and harm avoidance in OCD symptom dimensions. *Behaviour Research and Therapy, 46*: 895–904.

Eichelman, B. (1985). Hypnotic change in combat dreams of two veterans with PTSD. *American Journal of Psychiatry, 142*: 112–114.

Ellenberger, H. F. (1950). La psychothérapie de Janet. *L'Évolution Psychologique* (Special Pierre Janet issue): pp. 465–482.

Ellenberger, H. F. (1970). *The Discovery of the Unconscious*. New York: Basic Books.

Enskin, K., Bégin, M., Normandin, L., Godbout, N., & Fonagy, P. (2017). Mentalization and dissociation in the context of trauma. *Journal of Trauma and Dissociation, 18*: 11–30.

Erickson, M. E., & Rossi, E. L. (1979). *Hypnotherapy: An exploratory Casebook*. New York: Irvington.

Esquirol, J. E. D. (1832). Sur les illusions des sens chez aliénés [On the sensory illusions of the insane]. *Archives Generales de Medicine, 2*: 5–23.

Ey, H. (1968). Pierre Janet: The man and his work. In: B. B. Wolman (Ed.), *Historical Roots of Contemporary Psychology* (pp. 177–195). New York: Harper & Row.

Fairbairn, W. R. D. (1929). Dissociation and repression. In: E. D. Scharff & E. F. Birtles (Eds.), *From Instinct to Self. Selected Papers of W. R. D. Fairbairn. Volume II* (pp. 13–79). Northvale, NJ: Jason Aronson 1994.

Fairbairn, W. R. D. (1940). Schizoid factors in the personality. In: W. R. D. Fairbairn, *Psychoanalytic Studies of the Personality* (pp. 3–27). London: Tavistock, 1952.

Fairbairn, W. R. D. (1941). A revised psychopathology of the psychoses and psychoneuroses. In: W. R. D. Fairbairn, *Psychoanalytic Studies of the Personality* (pp. 28–58). London: Tavistock, 1952.

Fairbairn, W. R. D. (1946). Object-relationships and dynamic structure. In: W. R. D. Fairbairn, *Psychoanalytic Studies of the Personality* (pp. 137–151). London: Tavistock, 1952.

Fairbairn, W. R. D. (1952). Steps in the development of an object-relations theory of the personality. In: W. R. D. Fairbairn (Ed.), *Psychoanalytic Studies of the Personality* (pp. 152–161). London & Boston, MA: Routledge & Kegan Paul.

Fairbairn, W. R. D. (1953). Observations on the nature of hysterical states. In: E. D. Scharff & E. F. Birtles (Eds.), *From Instinct to Self. Selected Papers of W. R. D. Fairbairn* (Volume I) (pp. 74–92). Northvale, NJ: Jason Aronson, 1994.

Falzeder, E. (2007). The story of an ambivalent relationship: Sigmund Freud and Eugen Bleuler. *Journal of Analytical Psychology, 52*: 343–368.

Farber, B. A., Lippert, R. A., & Nevas, D. B. (1995). The therapist as attachment figure. *Psychotherapy: Theory, Research, Practice, Training, 32*: 204–212.

Farina, B., Speranza, A. M., Dittoni, S., Gnoni, V., Trentini, C., Maggiora-Vergano, C., Liotti, G., Brunetti, R., Testani, E., & Della Marca, G. (2013). Memories of attachment hamper EEG cortical connectivity in dissociative patients. *European Archives of Psychiatry and Clinical Neuroscience, 264*: 449–458.

Faure, H. (1983). Préface à la réédition de 1983. In: P. Janet, *L'État Mental des Hystériques* (2nd ed.). Marseille: Lafitte Reprints.

Felitti, V. J., & Anda, R. F. (1997). *The Adverse Childhood Experiences (ACE) Study*. United States: Centers for Disease Control and Prevention. Available from: www.cdc.gov/ace/index.htmhy

Felitti, V. J., & Anda, R. F. (2010). The relationship of adverse childhood experiences to adult health, well-being, social function, and health care. In: R. Lanius, E. Vermetten, & C. Pain (Eds.), *The Effects of Early Life Trauma on Health and Disease: The Hidden Epidemic* (pp. 77–87). Cambridge, UK: Cambridge University Press.

Felmingham, K., Kemp, A. H., Williams, L., Falconer, E., Olivieri, G., Peduto, A., & Bryant, R. (2008). Dissociative responses to conscious and non-conscious fear impact underlying brain function in post-traumatic stress disorder. *Psychological Medicine, 38*(12): 1771–1780.

Ferenczi, S. (1911). Exploring the unconscious. In: S. Ferenczi, *Final Contributions to the Problems and Methods of Psycho-Analysis* (pp. 308–313). London: Karnac.

Ferenczi, S. (1913). Il valore della psicoanalisi per la giustizia e la società [The value of psychoanalysis for justice and society]. In: *Opere* [Collected Works] (vol II) (pp. 1–10). Milano: Raffaello Cortina.

Ferenczi, S. (1914). Progressi nella teoria psicoanalitica delle nevrosi (1907–1913) [Advances in the psychoanalytic theory of neuroses]. In: *Opere* [Collected Works] (vol II) (pp. 133–143). Milano: Raffaello Cortina.

Ferenczi, S. (1919). An attempted explanation of some hysterical stigmata. In: S. Ferenczi, *Further Contributions to the Theory and Technique of Psycho-Analysis* (pp. 110–117). London: Karnac.

Ferenczi, S. (1932a). Confusion of the tongues between the adults and the child (The language of tenderness and of passion). *International Journal of Psycho-Analysis, 30*: 225–230.

Ferenczi, S. (1932b). *The Clinical Diary of Sandor Ferenczi*. Cambridge, MA: Harvard University Press.

Ferenczi, S. (1936). Breve corso di psicoanalisi [A short course on psychoanalysis]. In: *Opere* [Collected Works] (vol. IV) (pp. 110–153). Milano: Raffaello Cortina.

Fiedler, P. (2006). Ein Blick zurück in die Zukunft: Pierre Janet überholt Sigmund Freud [Looking Back to Future: Pierre Janet Overtakes Sigmund Freud]. In: P. Fiedler (Ed.), *Trauma, Dissoziation, Persönlichkeit. Pierre Janets Beiträge zur modernen Psychiatrie, Psychologie und Psychotherapie* (pp. 35–56) [Trauma, Dissociation, Personality. Pierre Janet's Contribution to Modern Psychiatry, Psychology, and Psychotherapy]. Lengerich: Pabst.

Fiedler, P. (2008). *Dissoziative Störungen und Konversion: Trauma und Traumabehandlung* [Dissociative Disorders and Conversion. Trauma and Treatment of Traumata]. Weinheim, Basel: Beltz PVU.

Fine, C. G. (1988). The work of Antoine Despine: The first scientific report on the diagnosis of a child with multiple personality disorder. *American Journal of Clinical Hypnosis, 31*: 33–39.

Fineman, J. (1988). "The Pais de Calais": Freud, the transference, and the sense of woman's humor. In: J. Culler (Ed.), *On Puns: The Foundation of Letters* (pp. 100–114). Oxford: Basil Blackwell.

Fitzgerald, M. (2017). Why did Sigmund Freud refuse to see Pierre Janet? Origins of psychoanalysis: Janet, Freud or both? *History of Psychiatry, 28*: 358–364.

Flam, J. (2003). *Matisse and Picasso: The Story of Their Rivalry and Friendship*. Cambridge, MA: Westview Press.

Flam, J. (2015). *Matisse on Art*. Berkeley, CA: University of California Press.

Flournoy, T. (1900). *From India to the Planet Mars*. New Hyde Park, NY: University Books, 1963.

Fonagy, P. (1999). Memory and therapeutic action. *International Journal of Psycho-Analysis, 80*: 215–223.

Fonagy, P., & Bateman, A. W. (2005). Attachment theory and mentalization-oriented model of borderline personality disorder. In: J. M. Oldman, A. E. Skodol, & D. S. Bender (Eds.), *Textbook of Personality Disorders* (pp. 187–207). Washington, DC: American Psychiatric Publishing.

Fonagy, P., & Target, M. (2003). *Psychoanalytic Theories: Perspectives from Developmental Psychology*. London, UK: Routledge.

Fonagy, P., Bateman, A. W., Lorenzini, N., & Campbell, C. (2014). Development, attachment, and childhood experiences. In: J. M. Oldman, A. E. Skodol, & D. S. Bender (Eds.), *Textbook of Personality Disorders* (pp. 55–78). Washington, DC: American Psychiatric Publishing.

Fonagy, P., & Target, M. (2006). The mentalization-focused approach to self-pathology. *Journal of Personality Disorders, 20*: 544–576.

Frank, J. (1973). *Persuasion and Healing*. Baltimore, MD: John Hopkins University Press.

Freud, S. (1888). Hysteria. *S. E., 1*: 37–59. London: Hogarth.

Freud, S. (1892). Sketches for the 'Preliminary communication' of 1893 (1940–41). *S. E., 1*: 147–151. London: Hogarth.

Freud, S. (1893). On the psychical mechanism of hysterical phenomena. *S. E., 3*: 27–39. London: Hogarth.

Freud, S. (1894). The neuro-psychoses of defence. *S. E., 24*: 43–61. London: Hogarth.

Freud, S. (1896). Further remarks on the neuro-psychoses of defence. *S. E., 3*: 157–185. London: Hogarth.

Freud, S. (1900). The interpretation of dreams. *S. E., 4–5*: 1–600. London: Hogarth.

Freud, S. (1907). Creative writers and day-dreaming. *S. E., 9*: 141–154. London: Hogarth.

Freud, S. (1909). Five lectures on psycho-analysis. *S. E., 11*: 1–56. London: Hogarth.

Freud, S. (1910). The psycho-analytic view of psychogenetic disturbance of vision. *S. E., 11*: 209–218. London: Hogarth.

Freud, S. (1911). Formulations on the two principles of mental functioning. *S. E., 12*: 218–226. London: Hogarth.

Freud, S. (1914). Remembering, repeating, and working through. *S. E., 12*: 147–156. London: Hogarth.

Freud, S. (1915). Repression. *S. E., 14*: 146–158. London: Hogarth.

Freud, S. (1916–17). Introductory lectures on psycho-analysis. *S. E., 15*: 1–240. London: Hogarth.

Freud, S. (1923). The Ego and the Id. *S. E., 19*: 1–66. London: Hogarth.

Freud, S. (1925). An autobiographical study. *S. E.*, 20: 1–74. London: Hogarth.

Freud, S. (1937). Analysis terminable and interminable. *S. E., 23*: 209–254. London: Hogarth.

Freud, S. (1938). Moses and Monotheism. *S. E., 23*: 3–137. London: Hogarth.

Friedman, B. (1988). *Triggering dissociation: Identifying triggers and making therapeutic interventions.* Paper presented at the Fifth International Conference on Multiple Personality/Dissociative States. Chicago, IL, October 6–9, 1988.

Frust, L. R. (2008). *Before Freud: Hysteria and Hypnosis in Later Nineteenth-Century Psychiatric Cases.* New York: Bucknell University Press.

Gabbard, G. O. (1995). Countertransference: The emerging common ground. *The International Journal of Psycho-Analysis, 76*: 475–485.

Garrabé, J. (1997). *Henri Ey et la Pensée Psychiatrique Contemporaine.* Le Plessis–Robinson: Institut Synthélabo.

Gervai, J. (2009). Environmental and genetic influences on early attachment. *Child and Adolescent Psychiatry and Mental Health, 3*: 1–12

Gilbert, P. (1989). *Human Nature and Suffering.* London: LEA.

Gill, M. M., & Brenman, M. M. (1959). *Hypnosis and Related States: Psychoanalytic Studies in Regression.* New York: International Universities Press.

Goetz, C. G., Bonduelle, M., & Gelfand, T. (1995). *Charcot: Constructing Neurology.* New York: Oxford University Press.

Graham, P., & Van Biene, L. (2007). *Hierarchy of Engagement. The Self in Conversation*, vol. VI. Sydney: ANZAP.

Grawe, K. (2002). *Psychological Therapy.* Ashland, OH: Hogrefe and Huber.

Greenacre, P. (1954). The role of transference. *Journal of the American Psychoanalytic Association, 2*: 671–684.

Greenberg, L. S. (2004). Emotion-focused therapy. *Clinical Psychology and Psychotherapy, 11*: 3–16.

Gullenstad, S. E. (2005). Who is 'who' in dissociation? A plea for psychodynamics in a time of trauma. *International Journal of Psycho-Analysis, 86*: 639–656.

Gunderson, J. G. (1996). The borderline patient's intolerance of aloneness: Insecure attachments and therapist availability. *American Journal of Psychiatry, 156*: 752–758.

Harms, E. (1959). Pierre M. F. Janet (Historical notes), *American Journal of Psychiatry, 115*: 1036–1037.

Hart, J. (1983). The clinical eclecticism of Pierre Janet. In: J. Hart, *Modern Eclectic Therapy* (pp. 43–58). New York: Plenum Press.

Harvey, M. R., & Herman, J. L. (1994). Amnesia, partial amnesia, and delayed recall among adult survivors of childhood trauma. *Consciousness and Cognition, 4*: 295–306.

Haule, J. R. (1984a). "Soul-making" in a schizophrenic saint. *Journal of Religion and Health, 23*: 70–80.

Haule, J. R. (1984b). From somnambulism to the archetypes: The French roots of Jung's split with Freud. *The Psychoanalytic Review, 71*(4): 635–659.

Haule, J. R. (1986). Pierre Janet and dissociation: The first transference theory and its origins in hypnosis. *American Journal of Clinical Hypnosis, 29*: 86–94.

Havens, L. L. (1966). Pierre Janet. *Journal of Nervous and Mental Disease, 143*: 383–398.

Heim, G., & Bühler, K.-E. (2003). Pierre Janet: Ein Fall für die moderne Verhaltenstherapie? [Pierre Janet: A case of modern behaviour therapy?]. *Verhaltenstherapie und Verhaltensmedizin, 24*: 205–224.

Heim, G., & Bühler, K.-E. (2006). Psychological trauma and fixed ideas in Pierre Janet's conception of dissociative disorders. *American Journal of Psychotherapy, 60*: 111–129.

Herman, J. L. (1992). *Trauma and Recovery*. New York: Basic Books.

Herman, J. L., & Schatzow, E. (1987). Recovery and verification of memories of childhood sexual trauma. *Psychoanalytic Psychology, 4*: 1–14.

Herzen, A. (1887). *Le cerveau et l'activité cérébrale*. Paris: J.-B. Baillière et Fils.

Hilgard, E. R. (1977). *Divided Consciousness: Multiple Controls in Human Thought and Action*. New York: Wiley.

Hill, E. L., Gold, S. N., & Bornstein, R. F. (2000). Interpersonal dependency among adult survivors of childhood sexual abuse in therapy. *Journal of Child Sexual Abuse, 9*: 71–86.

Hobson, J. A., Pace-Schott, E. F., & Stickgold, R., (2003). Dreaming and the brain: Towards a cognitive neuroscience of conscious states. In: E. F. Pace-Schott, M. Solms, F. Blagrove, & S. Harnad (Eds.), *Sleep and Dreaming: Scientific Advances and Reconsiderations* (pp. 1–50). Cambridge: Cambridge University Press

Hobson, R. F. (1985). *Forms of Feeling: The Heart of Psychotherapy*. Hove and New York: Brunner-Routledge.

Hoek, A. (1868). *Eenvoudige Mededelingen aangaande de Genezing van eene Krankzinnige door het Levens-Magnetismus*. 's Gravenhage: De Gebroeders Van Cleef.

Hoffmann, N. (1998). *Zwänge und Depressionen. Pierre Janet und die Verhaltenstherapie* [Compulsions and Depressions. Pierre Janet and Behavior Therapy]. Berlin: Springer.

Holmes, E. A., Brown, R. J., Mansell, W., Fearon, R. P., Hunter, E. C., Frasquilho, F., & Oakley, D. A. (2005). Are there two qualitatively distinct forms of dissociation? A review and some clinical implications. *Clinical Psychology Review, 25*(1): 1–23.

Holmes, J. (1993). Attachment theory: A biological basis for psychotherapy? *British Journal of Psychiatry, 163*: 430–438.

Horowitz, J., & Telch, M. J. (2007). Dissociation and pain perception: An experimental investigation. *Journal of Traumatic Stress, 20*: 597–609

Horton, W. M. (1924). The origin and psychological function of religion according to Pierre Janet. *American Journal of Psychology, 35(1)*: 16–53.

Horvath, T., & Meares, R. (1979). The sensory filter in schizophrenia: A study of habituation, arousal, and the dopamine hypothesis. *British Journal of Psychiatry, 134*, 39–45.

Horvath, T., Friedman, J., & Meares, R. (1980). Attention in hysteria: A study of Janet's hypothesis by means of habituation and arousal measures. *American Journal of Psychiatry, 137(2)*: 217–220.

Howell, E. F. (2005). *The Dissociative Mind*. New York: Routledge.

Howell, E. F. (2011). *Understanding and Treating Dissociative Identity Disorder: A Relational Approach*. New York: Routledge.

Howell, E. F., & Itzkowitz, S. (Eds.) (2016). *The Dissociative Mind in Psychoanalysis: Understanding and Working with Trauma*. New York: Routledge.

Husserl, E. (1970). *The Crisis of European Sciences and Transcendental Phenomenology: An Introduction to Phenomenological Philosophy*. Evanston: Northwestern University Press. Posthumous German publication *Die Krisis der europäischen Wissenschaften und die transzendentale Phänomenologie: Eine Einleitung in die phänomenologische Philosophie*, W. Biemel (Ed.). Martinus Nijhoff, The Hague, 1954. (Original publication 1936.)

International Society for the Study of Trauma and Dissociation [ISSTD] (2011). Guidelines for treating dissociative identity disorder in adults, third revision. *Journal of Trauma & Dissociation*, *12*: 115–187.

Jackson, J. H. (1887). Remarks on evolution and dissolution of the nervous system. In: J. Taylor (Ed.), *Selected Writings of Hughlings Jackson*, vol. 11 (pp. 92–118). (First published Medical Press of Circular, 1887.) New York: Basic Books, 1958.

Jackson, J. H. (1958). *Selected Writings of John Hughlings Jackson*. New York: Basic Books.

Jacobs, W. J., & Nadel, L. (1985). Stress-induced recovery of fears and phobias. *Psychological Review*, *92*: 512–531.

James, W. (1907). *The Energies of Men*. Classics in the History of Psychology – an internet resource developed by Christopher D. Green. Toronto, Ontario: York University.

James, W. (1909). To Theodore Flournoy. In James H. (ed.) *The Letters of William James*, Vol.II. Boston, MA: The Atlantic Monthly Press.

Janet, P. (1885). Note sur quelques phénomènes de somnambulisme. *Bulletin de la Société de Psychologie Physiologique*, *1:* 24–32. Also in: *Revue Philosophique*, 1886, *21(1):* 190–198.

Janet, P. (1886a). Les actes inconscients et le dédoublement de la personnalité pendant l'état somnambulisme provoqué. *Revue Philosophique*, *22(2):* 577–792.

Janet, P. (1886b). Deuxième note sur le sommeil provoqué à distance et la suggestion mental pendant l'état somnambulique. *Bulletin de la Société de Psychologie Physiologique*, *2:* 70–80. Also in: *Revue Philosophique*, 1886, *22(2):* 212–223.

Janet, P. (1887). L'anesthésie systematisée et la dissociation des phénomènes psychologiques. *Revue Philosophique*, *23(1):* 449–472.

Janet, P. (1888). Les actes inconscients et la mémoire pendant le somnambulisme. *Revue Philosophique*, *25(1):* 238–279.

Janet, P. (1889). *L'Automatisme Psychologique: Essai de Psychologie Expérimentale sur les Formes Inférieures de l'Activité Humaine*. Paris: Félix Alcan. Reprint: Paris: Société Pierre Janet, 1973. (Italian edition: *L'Automatismo Psicologico*. Milano: Raffaello Cortina, 2013.)

Janet, P. (1891). Étude sur un cas d'aboulie et d'idées fixes. *Revue Philosophique*, *331(1):* 258–287.

Janet, P. (1893a). *L'État Mental des Hystériques: Les Stigmates Mentaux*. Paris: Rueff & Cie. (English edition: The Mental State of Hystericals: *The Mental Stigmate*. New York: Putnam's Sons, 1901).

Janet, P. (1893b). *Contribution à l'Étude des Accidents Mentaux chez les Hystériques*. Paris: Rueff & Cie.

Janet, P. (1893c). L'amnésie continue. *Revue General des Sciences*, *4:* 167–179.

Janet, P. (1893d). Quelques définitions récentes de l'hystérie (I) [Some recent definitions of hysteria]. *Archives de Neurologie*, *25(76):* 417–438.

Janet, P. (1893e). Quelques définitions récentes de l'hystérie (II) [Some recent definitions of hysteria]. *Archives de Neurologie*, *26(77):* 1–29.

Janet, P. (1894/5). Un cas de possession et l'excorcisme moderne. *Bulletin des Travaux de l'Université de Lyon*, *8:* 41–57.

Janet, P. (1894a). *Manual du Baccalaureat de l'Enseignement Sécondaire Classique, Moderne, Philosophique*. Paris: Nony.

Janet, P. (1894b). *L'État Mental des Hystériques: Les Accidents Mentaux*. Paris: Rueff & Cie. (English edition: *The Mental State of Hystericals*. New York: Putnam's Sons, 1901).

Janet, P. (1894c). Histoire d'une idée fixe. *Revue Philosophique*, *37(1):* 121–163.

Janet, P. (1894d). Quelques définitions récentes de l'hystérie. [Some recent definitions of hysteria] *Archive de Neurologie*, *26:* 1–29.

Janet, P. (1895). Les idées fixes de forme hystérique. *Presse Medicale, 3*: 201–203.

Janet, P. (1897). L'influence somnambulique et le besoin de direction. *Revue Philosophique de la France et de L'Étranger, 43*: 113–143.

Janet, P. (1898a). *Névroses et Idées Fixes* (Vol. 1). Paris: Félix Alcan.

Janet, P. (1898b). Le traitement psychologique de l'hystérie. In: A. Robin (Ed.), *Traité de Thérapeutique Appliquée* (pp. 140–216). Paris: Rueff & Cie.

Janet, P. (1901). *The Mental State of Hystericals*. New York: Putnam's Sons.

Janet, P. (1903). *Les Obsessions et la Psychasthénie*. Paris: Félix Alcan.

Janet, P. (1904). L'Amnésie et la dissociation des souvenirs par l'émotion. *Journal de Psychologie, 1*: 417–453.

Janet, P. (1905). Les oscillations du niveau mental. *Revue des Idées, 2*: 729–755.

Janet, P. (1907a). Le problème du subconscient. *VIe Congrès International de Psychologie tenu à Genève du 2 au 7 Août 1909 sous la Présidence de Th. Flournoy*.

Janet, P. (1907b). *The Major Symptoms of Hysteria*. New York, London: Macmillan.

Janet, P. (1907c). A symposium on the subconscious. IV. *Journal of Abnormal Psychology, 2*: 58–67.

Janet, P. (1907d). L'analyse psychologique et la critique des méthodes de psychothérapie [Psychological analysis and the criticism of psychotherapeutic methods]. In: Pierre Janet (2004), *Leçons au Collège de France (1895–1934)* (pp. 53–54). [Lessons at the College de France (1895–1934)]. Paris: L'Harmattan.

Janet, P. (1909a). *Les Névroses*. Paris: Ernest Flammarion.

Janet, P. (1909b). Problèmes psychologiques de l'émotion. *Revue Neurologique, 17*: 1551–1687.

Janet, P. (1910a). Le subconscient. *Scientia, 4(7)*: 64–79.

Janet, P. (1910b). Une Félida artificielle. *Revue Philosophique, 69*: 329–357.

Janet, P. (1911). *L'État Mental des Hystériques* (2nd enlarged ed). Paris: Félix Alcan.

Janet, P. (1913). *Psycho-analysis: Report to the Section of Psychiatry, XVIIth International Congress of Medicine*. London: Hodder & Stoughton.

Janet, P. (1919). *Les Médications Psychologiques*. Paris: Félix Alcan. (English edition: *Psychological Healing*. New York: Macmillan, 1925).

Janet, P. (1920). La tension psychologique, ses degrés, ses oscillations. *British Journal of Psychology, 1*: 1–15.

Janet, P. (1921). La tension psychologique, ses degrés, ses oscillations. [Psychological tension, its degrees, its oscillations]. *British Journal of Psychology (Medical section), 1*: 209–224.

Janet, P. (1923a). *La médecine psychologique* [Psychological Medicine]. Paris: Flammarion. (English edition: *Principles of Psychotherapy*. London: Allen and Unwin, 1924).

Janet, P. (1923b). *La tension psychologique et ses oscillations*. In: G. Dumas (Ed.), *Nouveau Traité de Psychologie* (pp. 386–411). Paris: Félix Alcan.

Janet, P. (1924). *Principles of Psychotherapy*. London: Allen and Unwin.

Janet, P. (1925). *Psychological Healing*. New York: Macmillan.

Janet, P. (1926a). *De l'Angoisse à l'Extase, Vol 1: Un Délire Religieux, la Croyance*. Paris: Félix Alcan.

Janet, P. (1926b). *Les Stades de l'Évolution Psychologique et le Rôle de la Faiblesse dans le Fonctionnement de l'Esprit*. Paris: A. Chahine.

Janet, P. (1927a). *La Pensée Intérieure et ses Troubles*. Paris: A. Chahine.

Janet, P. (1927b). A propos de la schizophrénie (Concerning schizophrenia). *Journal de Psychologie Normale et Pathologique, 24* : 477–492.

Janet, P. (1928a). *De l'Angoisse à l'Extase, Vol 2: Les Sentiments Fondamentaux*. Paris: Félix Alcan.

Janet, P. (1928b). *L'Évolution de la Mémoire et de la Notion du Temps*. Paris: A. Chahine.

Janet, P. (1929a). *L'Évolution Psychologique de la Personnalité*. Paris: A. Chahine.

Janet, P. (1929b). *The Major Symptoms of Hysteria: Fifteen Lectures given in the Medical School of Harvard University*. New York: The MacMillan Company. (Original publication 1907)

Janet, P. (1930a). Autobiography. In: C. A. Murchinson (Ed.), A *History of Psychology in Autobiography* (pp. 123–133). Vol. 1. Worchester, Mass: Clark University Press. Also Autobiography of Pierre Janet. In: C. D. Christopher (Eds.), Classics in the History of Psychology: An internet resource. York University, Toronto, Ontario.

Janet, P. (1930b). L'analyse psychologique. [Psychological analysis]. In: C. A. Murchison (Ed.), *Psychologies of 1930* (pp. 369–373). Worchester, MA: Clark University

Janet, P. (1932a). *La Force et la Faiblesse Psychologiques*. Paris: Maloine.

Janet, P. (1932b). *L'Amour et la Haine*. Paris: Maloine.

Janet, P. (1932c). L'hallucination dans le délire de pérsecution. *Revue Philosophique*, *113(1)*: 61–98.

Janet, P. (1932d). Les croyances et les hallucinations. *Revue Philosophique, 113(1)*: 278–331.

Janet, P. (1932e). Les sentiments dans le délire de persecution. *Journal de Psychologie*, *29*:161–240.

Janet, P. (1934). *L'Intelligence avant le Langage*. Paris: Flammarion.

Janet, P. (1935a). *Les Débuts de l'Intelligence*. Paris: Flammarion.

Janet, P. (1935b). Réalisation et interprétation. *Annales Médico-Psychologiques, 93*: 329–366.

Janet, P. (1936a). Le langage intérieur dans l'hallucination psychique. *Annales Médico-Psychologiques, 94*: 377–386.

Janet, P. (1936b). Mémoires originaux – Le langage interieur dan l'hallucination (Internal language in the psychic hallucination). *Annales Médico-psychologiques*, Tome II (3): 377–386.

Janet, P. (1937). Psychological strength and weakness in mental diseases. In: *Factors Determining Human Behavior* (pp. 64–106). Cambridge, MA: Harvard University Press.

Janet, P. (1938). La psychologie de la conduite. In: H. Wallon (Ed.), *Encyclopédie Française*, Tome VIII (La vie mentale) (pp. 808–816). Paris: Société de Gestion de l'Encyclopédie Française.

Janet, P. (1945). La croyance délirante. *Schweizerische Zeitschrift für Psychologie, 4*: 173–187.

Janet, P. (1947a). Caractères de l'hallucination du persécuté. In: A. Michotte (Ed.), *Miscellanea Psychologica* (pp. 237–253). Paris: Albert Louvain.

Janet, P. (1947b). *Les Croyances Religieuses*. Unpublished manuscript.

Janet, P. (2008). *Les Névroses*. Paris: L'Harmattan.

Janet, P. (2013). *Die Psychologie des Glaubens und die Mystik nebst anderen Schriften*. Berlin: Matthes & Seitz.

Jung, C. G. (1902). On the psychology and pathology of so-called occult phenomena. *C.W., 1*: 3–88. Princeton, NJ: Princeton University Press.

Jung, C. G. (1907). *The Psychology of Dementia Praecox. C.W., 3*: 1–151. Princeton, NJ: Princeton University Press

Jung, C. G. (1914). The content of psychoses. *C.W., 3*: 153–178. Princeton, NJ: Princeton University Press.

Jung, C. G. (1916/–1948). General aspects of dream psychology. *C.W., 8*: 237–280. Princeton, NJ: Princeton University Press.

Jung, C. G. (1917a). *Collected Papers on Analytical Psychology*. New York: Moffat Yard and Company.

Jung, C. G. (1917b). The conception of the unconscious. In: C. G. Jung, *Collected Papers on Analytical Psychology* (pp. 445–448). New York: Moffat Yard and Company.

Jung, C. G. (1918). The role of the unconscious. *C.W.*, *10*: 3–28. Princeton, NJ: Princeton University Press.

Jung, C. G. (1921). Psychological types. *C.W.*, *6*. Princeton, NJ: Princeton University Press.

Jung, C. G. (1928). Mental disease and the psyche. *C.W.*, *3*: 226–232. Princeton, NJ: Princeton University Press.

Jung, C. G. (1934). A rejoinder to Dr. Bally. *C.W.*, *10*: 535–544. Princeton, NJ: Princeton University Press.

Jung, C. G. (1946). An Account of the transference phenomena based on the illustrations to the "Rosarium Philosophorum". *C.W.*, *16*: 203–323. Princeton, N.J: Princeton University Press.

Jung, C. G. (1948). General aspects of dream psychology. *C.W.*, *8*: 237–280. Princeton, NJ: Princeton University Press

Jung, C. G. (1952). *Symbols of Transformation*. *C.W.*, *5*. Princeton, NJ: Princeton University Press

Jung, C. G. (1957). Foreword to Jacobi: "Complex/Archetyoe/Symbol". *C.W.*, *18*: 532–533. Princeton, NJ: Princeton University Press.

Jung, C. G. (1973). *Experimental Researches, C.W., 2*. Princeton, NJ: Princeton University Press.

Jung, C. G. (1975). *The Structure and Dynamics of the Psyche. C.W., 8*. Princeton, NJ: Princeton University Press.

Jung, C. G. (1982). *The Psychogenesis of Mental Disease C.W., 3*. Princeton, NJ: Princeton University Press.

Jung, C. G. (2009). *The Red Book: Liber Novus* (Reading Edition). New York: Norton.

Jung, C. G., & Schimd-Guisan, H. (2013). *The Question of Psychological Types*. Princeton, NJ: Princeton University Press

Kanfer, F. H. (1991). *Self-management and Self-regulation*. Berlin: Springer.

Kast, V. (1992). *The Dynamic of Symbols: Fundamentals of Jungian Psychotherapy*. New York: Fromm Psychology.

Kennerley, H. (1996). Cognitive therapy of dissociative symptoms associated with trauma. *British Journal of Clinical Psychology*, *35*: 325–340.

Khan, M. M. (1963). The concept of cumulative trauma. *Psychoanalytic Study of the Child*, *18*: 151–158.

Klein, M. (1946). Notes on some schizoid mechanisms. *International Journal of Psycho-Analysis*, *27*: 99–110.

Klein, M. (1952). Notes on some schizoid mechanisms. In: M. Klein, P. Heimann, S. Isaacs, & J. Riviere (Eds.), *Developments in Psycho-Analysis* (pp. 292–320). London: Hogarth.

Kluft, R. P. (1987). An update on multiple personality disorder. *Hospital & Community Psychiatry*, *38(4)*: 363–373.

Kluft, R. P. (1994). Countertransference in the treatment of MPD. In: J. P. Wilson & J. D. Lindy (Eds.), *Countertransference in the Treatment of PTSD* (pp. 122–150). New York: Guilford Press.

Kluft, R. P., & Fine, C. G. (Eds.) (1993). *Clinical Perspectives on Multiple Personality Disorder*. Washington, DC: American Psychiatric Press.

Knox, J. (2003). *Archetype, Attachment, Analysis*. London: Routledge.

Kohut, H. (1966). Forms and transformations of narcissism. *Journal of the American Psychoanalytic Association*, *14*: 243–257.

Kravis, N. (1992). The "prehistory" of the idea of transference. *International Review of Psychoanalysis*, *19*: 9–22.

Krystal, H. (1988). *Integration and Self-healing: Affect, Trauma, Alexithymia*. New York: Norton.

Kubie, L. S., & Margolin, S. (1944). The process of hypnotism and the nature of the hypnotic state. *American Journal of Psychiatry, 100*: 611–622.

Lamb, C. S. (1982). Negative hypnotic imagery and fantasy: Application to two cases of "unfinished business". *American Journal of Clinical Hypnosis, 24*: 266–271.

Lamb, C. S. (1985). Hypnotically induced deconditioning: Reconstruction of memories in the treatment of phobias. *American Journal of Clinical Hypnosis, 24*: 56–62.

Lanius, R. A., Bluhm, R., Lanius, U., & Pain, C. (2006). A review of neuroimaging studies in PTSD: heterogeneity of response to symptom provocation. *Journal of Psychiatric Research, 40(8)*: 709–729.

Lanius, R. A., Williamson, P. C., Bluhm, R. L., Densmore, M., Boksman, K., Neufeld, R. W., Gati, J. S., & Menon, R. S. (2005). Functional connectivity of dissociative responses in posttraumatic stress disorder: A functional magnetic resonance imaging investigation. *Biological Psychiatry, 57*: 873–884.

Lanius, R. A., Williamson, P. C., Boksman, K., Densmore, M., Gupta, M., Neufeld, R. W., & Menon, R. S. (2002). Brain activation during script-driven imagery induced dissociative responses in PTSD: A functional magnetic resonance imaging investigation. *Biological Psychiatry, 52(4)*: 305–311.

Laub, D. (1992). An event without a witness: Truth, testimony and survival. In: S. Felman & D. Laub (Eds.). *Testimony: Crises of Witnessing in Literature, Psychoanalysis, and History* (pp. 75–92). London, UK: Routledge.

Laub, D., & Auerhahn, N. (1989). Failed empathy: A central theme in the survivor's holocaust experience. *Psychoanalytic Psychology, 6*: 377–400.

Levine, H. B., Reed, G. B., & Scarfone, D. (2013). *Unrepresented States and the Construction of Meaning: Clinical and Theoretical Contributions*. London: Karnac.

Levy, S., & Lemma, A. (2004). *The Perversion of Loss: Psychoanalytic Perspectives on Trauma*. London: Whurr.

Lewis, D. O., Yeager, C. A., Swica, Y., Pincus, J. H., & Lewis, M. (1997). Objective documentation of child abuse and dissociation in 12 murderers with dissociative identity disorder. *American Journal of Psychiatry, 154*: 1703–1710.

Lichtenberg, J. D. (1989). *Psychoanalysis and Motivation*. Hillsdale, NJ: The Analytic Press.

Linehan, M. M. (1993). *Cognitive-behavioral Treatment of Borderline Personality Disorder*. New York: Guilford Press.

Linehan, M. M. (2014). *DBT Skills Training Manual* (2nd. ed.). New York: Guilford.

Lingiardi, V. (2008). Playing with unreality: Transference and Computer. *International Journal of Psycho-Analysis, 89*: 111–126.

Lingiardi, V., & De Bei, F. (2011). Questioning the couch: Historical and clinical perspectives. *Psychoanalytic Psychology, 28*: 389–404.

Lingiardi, V., & McWilliams, N. (2015). The Psychodynamic Diagnostic Manual (2nd edition) (PDM-2). *World Psychiatry, 14(2)*: 237–239.

Lingiardi, V., & McWilliams, N. (Eds.) (2017). *The Psychodynamic Diagnostic Manual. Second Edition* (PDM-2). New York: Guilford Press.

Liotti, G. (1992). Disorganized/Disoriented attachment in the etiology of dissociative disorders. *Dissociation, 5*: 196–204.

Liotti, G. (1999). Disorganized attachment as a model for the understanding of dissociative psychopathology. In: J. Solomon & C. George (Eds.), *Disorganized Attachment as a Model for the Understanding of Dissociative Psychopathology* (pp. 291–317). New York: Guildford Press.

Liotti, G. (2000). Disorganized attachment, models of borderline states, and evolutionary psychotherapy. In: P. Gilbert & K. Bailey (Eds.), *Genes on the Couch: Essays in Evolutionary Psychotherapy* (pp. 232–256). Hove: Psychology Press.

Liotti, G. (2004). Trauma, dissociation and disorganized attachment: Three strands of a single braid. *Psychotherapy: Theory, Research, Practice and Training, 41*: 472–486.

Liotti, G. (2006). A model of dissociation based on attachment theory and research. *Journal of Trauma & Dissociation, 7*: 55–73.

Liotti, G. (2007). Internal working models of attachment in the therapeutic relationship. In: Gilbert, P. & Leahy, R. L. (Eds.), *The Therapeutic Relationship in the Cognitive-behavioral Psychotherapies* (pp. 143–161). London, UK: Routledge.

Liotti, G. (2009). Attachment and Dissociation. In: P. Dell & D. K. O'Neill (Eds.), *Dissociation and the Dissociative Disorders* (pp. 53–65). New York & London: Routledge.

Liotti, G. (2014a). Le critiche di Pierre Janet alla teoria di Sigmund Freud: Corrispondenze nella psicotraumatologia contemporanea. *Psichiatria e Psicoterapia, XXXVIII*, (1): 31–40.

Liotti, G. (2014b). Disorganized attachment in the pathogenesis and the psychotherapy of borderline personality disorder. In: A. N. Danquah & K. Berry (Eds.), *Theory in Adult Mental Health* (pp. 113–128). London, UK: Routledge.

Liotti, G. (2016). Infant attachment and the origins of dissociative processes: An approach based on the evolutionary theory of multiple motivational systems. *Attachment: New Directions in Psychotherapy and Relational Psychoanalysis, 10*: 20–36

Liotti, G., & Farina, B. (2011). *Sviluppi Traumatici: Eziopatogenesi, Clinica e Terapia della Dimensione Dissociativa* [Traumatic Developments: Etiology, Clinical Issues and Treatment of the Dissociative Dimension]. Milano: Raffaello Cortina.

Liotti, G., & Farina, B. (2013). La psicotraumatologia contemporanea e le teorie sui rapporti fra processi mentali coscienti e inconsci. *Sistemi Intelligenti, 25*: 553–564.

Liotti, G., & Gilbert, P. (2011). Mentalizing, motivation, and social mentalities: Theoretical considerations and implications for psychotherapy. *Psychology & Psychotherapy, 84*: 9–25.

Loewenstein, R. J. (1991). An office mental status examination for complex chronic dissociative symptoms and multiple personality disorder. *Psychiatric Clinics of North America, 14*: 567–604.

Loewenstein, R. J. (1993). Posttraumatic and dissociative aspects of transference and countertransference in the treatment of multiple personality disorder. In: R. P. Kluft & C.G. Fine (Eds.), *Clinical Perspectives on Multiple Personality Disorder* (pp. 51–85). Washington, DC: American Psychiatric Press.

Luijk, M., Roisman, G. I., Haltigan, J. D., Tiemeier, H., Booth-Laforce, C., Van IJzendoorn, M., Belsky, J., A. G., Uitterlinden, V. W. V., Jaddoe, A., Hofman, F. C., Verhulst, A., Tharner, M. J., & Bakermans-Kranenburg (2011). Dopaminergic, serotonergic, and oxytonergic candidate genes associated with infant attachment security and disorganization? In search of main and interaction effects. *Journal of Child Psychology & Psychiatry, 52*: 1295–1307.

Lyons-Ruth, K. (2003). Dissociation and the parent-infant dialogue: A longitudinal perspective from attachment research. *Journal of the American Psychoanalytic Association, 51*: 883–911.

Lyons-Ruth, K., & Jacobvitz, D. (2008). Attachment disorganization: Genetic factors, parenting contexts, and developmental transformation from infancy to adulthood. In: J. Cassidy & P. Shaver (Eds.), *Handbook of Attachment Theory, Research and Clinical Applications* (2nd ed.) (pp. 666–697). New York: Guilford Press.

Lyons-Ruth, K., Bronfman, E., & Parsons, E. (1999). Maternal frightened, frightening, or atypical behavior and disorganized infant attachment patterns. *Monographs of the Society for Research in Child Development, 64*: 67–96.

Lyons-Ruth, K., Repacholi, B., McLeod, S., & Silva, E. (1991). Disorganized attachment behavior in infancy: Short-term stability in maternal and infant correlates and risk related subtypes. *Development & Psychopathology, 4*: 377–396.

MacLean, P. (1990). *The Triune Brain in Evolution: Role in Paleocerebral Functions.* Toronto, ON: University of Toronto Press.

Main, M. (1995). Recent studies in attachment: Overview, with selected implications for clinical work. In: S. Goldberg, R. Muir, & J. Kerr (Eds.), *Attachment Theory: Social, Developmental, and Clinical Perspectives* (pp. 407–474). Hillsdale, NJ: Analytic Press.

Main, M., & Hesse, E. (1990). Parents' unresolved traumatic experiences are related to infant disorganized attachment status: Is frightened and/or frightening parental behavior the linking mechanism? In: M. Main & R. Goldwyn (Eds.), *Attachment in the Preschool Years: Theory, Research, and Intervention* (pp. 161–182). Chicago, IL: University of Chicago Press.

Main, M., & Morgan, H. (1996). Disorganization and disorientation in infant strange situation behavior: Phenotypic resemblance to dissociative states. In: L. K. Michelson & W. J. Ray (Eds.), *Handbook of Dissociation: Theoretical, Empirical, and Clinical Perspectives* (pp. 107–138). New York: Plenum Press.

Main, M., & Solomon, J. (1986). Discovery of a new, insecure-disorganized/disoriented attachment pattern. In: T. Brazelton & M. Yogman (Eds.), *Affective Development in Infancy* (pp. 95–124). Norwood, NJ: Ablex.

Main, M., & Solomon, J. (1990). Procedures for identifying infants as disorganized/disorientated during the Ainsworth Strange Situation. In: M. Greenberg, D. Cicchetti, & E. Cummings (Eds.), *Attachment in the Preschool Years: Theory, Research and Intervention* (pp. 121–160). Chicago, IL: University of Chicago Press.

Makari, G. J. (1992). A history of Freud's first concept of transference. *International Review of Psychoanalysis, 19*: 415–432.

Makari, G. J. (2008). *Revolution in Mind: The Creation of Psychoanalysis.* New York: Harper Collins.

Mancia, M. (2006). Implicit memory and early unrepressed unconscious: Their role in the therapeutic process (How the neurosciences can contribute to psychoanalysis). *International Journal of Psycho-Analysis, 87*: 83–103.

Markowitsch, H. J. (2003). Psychogenic amnesia. *Neuroimage, 20*: 132–138.

Mayo, E. (1948). *Some Notes on the Psychology of Pierre Janet.* Cambridge, MA: Harvard University Press.

McCann, I. L., & Pearlman, L. A. (1990). *Psychological Trauma and the Adult Survivor: Theory, Therapy and Transformation.* New York: Brunner/Mazel.

McGuire, W. (Ed.) (1974). *The Correspondence Between Sigmund Freud and C.G. Jung.* Princeton: Princeton University Press.

McGilchrist, I. (2009). *The Master and his Emissary: The Divided Brain and the Making of the Western World.* New Haven CT: Yale University Press.

McKeown, J. M., & Fine, C. G. (Eds.) (2008). *Despine and the Evolution of Psychology: Historical and Medical Perspectives on Dissociative Disorders.* New York: Palgrave MacMillan.

Meares, R. (1993). *The Metaphor of Play: Disruption and Restoration in the Borderline Experience.* Northvale, NJ: Jason Aronson.

Meares, R. (1998). The self in conversation: On narratives, chronicles and scripts. *Psychoanalytic Dialogues, 8*: 875–891.

Meares, R. (1999). The contribution of Hughlings Jackson to an understanding of dissociation. *American Journal of Psychiatry, 156(12)*: 1850–1855.

Meares, R. (2000). *Intimacy and Alienation: Memory, Trauma, and Personal Being.* London: Routledge.

Meares, R. (2004). The conversational model: An outline. *American Journal of Psychotherapy, 58(1)*: 51–66.

Meares, R. (2005). *The Metaphor of Play: Origin and Breakdown of Personal Being* (revised and enlarged edition). London: Routledge.

Meares, R. (2009). Episodic memory, trauma and the narrative of self. *Contemporary Psychoanalysis, 31*: 541–555.

Meares, R. (2012a). *A Dissociation Model of Borderline Personality Disorder.* New York: Norton.

Meares, R. (2012b). From hysteria to borderline: A brief history. In: R. Meares, *A Dissociation Model of Borderline Personality Disorder* (pp. 14–33). London & New York: Norton.

Meares, R. (2012c). A malady of representations: Dysautonomic aspects of Borderline Personality Disorder. In: R. Meares, *A Dissociation Model of Borderline Personality Disorder* (pp. 248–267). New York: Norton.

Meares, R. (2012d). Dissociation in Borderline Personality Disorder. In: R. Meares, *A Dissociation Model of Borderline Personality Disorder* (pp. 112–156). New York: Norton.

Meares, R. (2016). *The Poet's Voice in the Making of the Mind.* London: Routledge.

Meares, R., & Hobson, R. F. (1977). The persecutory therapist. *British Journal of Medical Psychology, 50(4)*: 349–359.

Meares, R., & Horvath, T. (1972). "Acute" and "chronic" hysteria. *British Journal of Psychiatry, 121*(565): 653–657.

Meares, R., & Orlay, W. (1988). On self-boundary: A study of the development of the concept of secrecy. *British Journal of Medical Psychology, 61*: 305–316.

Meares, R., Hampshire, R., Gordon, E., & Kraiuhin, C. (1985). Whose hysteria: Briquet's, Janet's or Freud's? *Australian and New Zealand Journal of Psychiatry, 19*: 356–263.

Meares, R., Melkonian, D., Gordon, E., & Williams, L. (2005). Distinct pattern of P3a event-related potential in borderline personality disorder. *NeuroReport, 16(3)*: 289–293.

Meares, R., Schore, A., & Melkonian, D. (2011). Is borderline personality a particularly right hemispheric disorder? A study of P3a using single trial analysis. *Australian and New Zealand Journal of Psychiatry, 45*: 131–139.

Meares, R., Stevenson, J., & Gordon, E. (1999). A Jacksonian and biopsychosocial hypothesis concerning borderline and related phenomena. *Australian and New Zealand Journal of Psychiatry, 33*: 831–840.

Meares, R., Bendit, N., Haliburn, J., Korner, A., Meares, D., & Butt, D. (Eds.) (2012). *Borderline Personality Disorder and the Conversational Model: A Clinician's Manual.* (Norton series on interpersonal neurobiology). New York: Norton.

Meltzoff, A. N., & Moore, M. K. (1977). Imitation of facial and manual gestures by human neonates. *Science, 198*: 74–78.

Miller, A. (1986). Brief reconstructive hypnotherapy for anxiety reactions: Three case reports. *American Journal of Clinical Hypnosis, 28*: 138–146.

Minkowski, E. (1927a). *La Schizophrénie.* Paris: Payot.

Minkowski, E. (1927b). The essential disorder underlying schizophrenia and schizophrenic thought. In: J. Cutting & M. Shepherd (Eds.), *The Clinical Roots of the*

Schizophrenia Concept: Translations of Seminal European Contributions on Schizophrenia (pp. 188–212). Cambridge: Cambridge University Press 1987.

Modell, A. (1963). Primitive object relationships and the predisposition to schizophrenia. *International Journal of Psycho-Analysis, 44*: 282–292.

Modell, A. (1990). *Other Times, Other Realities: Towards a Theory of Psychoanalytic Treatment.* Cambridge, MA: Harvard University Press.

Modestin, J. (1987). Counter-transference reactions contributing to completed suicide. *British Journal of Medical Psychology, 60*: 379–85.

Moreau de Tours, J. J. (1845). *Du Hachisch et de l'Aliénation Mentale: Études Psychologiques.* Paris: Fortin, Masson & Cie. English edition: *Hashish and Mental Illness.* New York: Raven Press.

Morrison, A. P., Haddock, G., & Tarrier, N. (1995). Intrusive thoughts and auditory hallucinations: A cognitive approach. *Behavioural and Cognitive Psychotherapy, 23*: 265–280.

Moskowitz, A., & Corstens, D. (2007). Auditory hallucinations: Psychotic symptom or dissociative experience? *Journal of Psychological Trauma, 6 (2/3)*: 35–63.

Moskowitz, A., & Heim, G. (2011). Eugen Bleuler's *Dementia Praecox or the Group of Schizophrenias* (1911). A centenary appreciation and reconsideration. *Schizophrenia Bulletin, 37*: 471–479.

Moskowitz, A., Barker-Collo, S., & Ellson, L. (2005). Replication of dissociation-psychoticism link in New Zealand students and inmates. *Journal of Nervous & Mental Disease, 193*: 722–727.

Moskowitz, A., Read, J., Farrelly, S., Rudegeair, T., & Williams, O. (2009). Are psychotic symptoms traumatic in origin and dissociative in kind? In: P. F. Dell & J. O'Neil (Eds.), *Dissociation and the Dissociative Disorders: DSM-V and Beyond* (pp. 523–534). New York: Routledge.

Mucci, C. (2008). *Il Dolore Estremo: Il Trauma da Freud alla Shoah* [The Extreme Pain. Trauma from Freud to the Shoah]. Rome, Italy: Borla.

Mucci, C. (2013). *Beyond Individual and Collective Trauma: Intergenerational Transmission, Psychoanalytic Treatment, and the Dynamics of Forgiveness.* London: Karnac.

Mucci, C. (2018). *Borderline Bodies. Affect Regulation Theraphy for Personality Disorders.* New York: Norton.

Müller-Pfeiffer, C., Rufibach, K., Wyss, D., Perron, N., Pitman, R., & Rufer, M. (2013). Screening for dissociative disorders in psychiatric out- and day care-patients. *Journal of Psychopathology and Behavioral Assessment, 35*: 592–602.

Myers, C. S. (1915). A contribution to the study of shell shock. *Lancet, 1*: 316–320.

Myers, C. S. (1940). *Shell Shock in France 1914–18.* Cambridge: Cambridge University Press.

Nemiah, J. C. (1979). Dissociative amnesia: A clinical and theoretical reconsideration. In: F. Kihlstrom & F. J. Evans (Eds.), *Functional Disorders of Memory* (pp. 303–323). Hillsdale, NJ: Lawrence Erlbaum.

Nemiah, J. C. (1980). Psychogenic amnesia, psychogenic fugue, and multiple personality. In: H. I. Kaplan, A. M. Freedman, & B. J. Sadock (Eds.), *Comprehensive Textbook of Psychiatry* (Vol. 2) (pp. 942–957). Baltimore: Williams & Wilkins.

Nemiah, J. C. (1984). The unconscious and psychopathology. In: K. S. Bowers & D. Meichenbaum (Eds.), *The Unconscious Reconsidered* (pp. 49–87). New York: Wiley.

Nemiah, J. C. (1989). Janet redivivus: The centenary of *L'Automatisme Psychologique.* *American Journal of Psychiatry, 146(12)*: 1527–1529.

Nicolas, S. (2002). *Histoire de la Psychologie Française.* Paris: Press Editions.

Nicolas, S., & Gounden, Y. (2017). Centenaire Ribot (deuxième partie). La réception de l'oeuvre de Théodule Ribot publiée chez l'éditeur Baillière (1874–1883) [Centenary of Ribot. Part 2. The reception of Théodule Ribot's works published by the editor Baillière]. *Bulletin de Psychologie, 70*: 179–195.

Nicolas, S., & Makowski, D. (2017). Centenaire Ribot (première partie). La réception de l'oeuvre de Théodule Ribot publiée chez l'éditeur Ladrange (1870–1873) [Centenary of Ribot. Part 1. The reception of Théodule Ribot's works published by the editor Ladrange]. *Bulletin de Psychologie, 70*: 163–178.

Nijenhuis, E. R. S. (2004). *Somatoform Dissociation: Phenomena, Measurement, & Theoretical Issues*. New York: Norton.

Nijenhuis, E. R. S. (2015). *The trinity of trauma: Ignorance, fragility, and control*. Göttingen: Vandenhoeck & Ruprecht.

Nijenhuis, E. R. S., & van der Hart, O. (1999). Forgetting and reexperiencing trauma: From anesthesia to pain. In: J. Goodwin & R. Attias (Eds.), *Splintered Reflections: Images of the Body in Trauma* (pp. 39–65). New York: Basic Books.

Nijenhuis, E. R. S., & van der Hart, O. (2011). Dissociation in trauma: A new definition and comparison with previous formulations. *Journal of Trauma & Dissociation, 12*(4), 416–445.

Nijenhuis, E. R. S., van der Hart, O., & Steele, K. (2002). The emerging psychobiology of trauma-related dissociation and dissociative disorders. In: H. D'haenen, J. A. den Boer, & P. Willner (Eds.), *Biological Psychiatry* (pp. 1079–1098). Chicester, New York: Wiley.

Nijenhuis, E. R. S., van der Hart, O., & Steele, K. (2004). Trauma-related structural dissociation of the personality. www.trauma-pages.com.

Ogawa, J. R., Sroufe, L. A., Weinfield., N. S., Carlson, E. A., & Egeland, B. (1997). Development and the fragmented self: Longitudinal study of dissociative symptomatology in a nonclinical sample. *Development and Psychopathology, 9*: 855–879.

Ogden, P., & Fisher, J. (2015). *Sensorimotor Psychotherapy: Interventions for Trauma and Attachment*. New York: Norton.

Ogden, P., Minton, K., & Pain, C. (2006). *Trauma and the Body*. New York: Norton.

Olio, K., & Cornell, W. (1993). The therapeutic relationship as the foundation for treatment of adult survivors of sexual abuse. *Psychotherapy, 30*: 512–523.

Ortu, F. (2013). Premessa all'edizione italiana. In: P. Janet, *L'Automatismo Psicologico* (pp. XI–XXIV). Milano: Raffaello Cortina.

Panksepp, J. (1998). *Affective Neuroscience: The Foundations of Human and Animal Emotions*. New York: Oxford University Press.

Panksepp, J., & Biven, L. (2012). *The Archaeology of Mind: Neuroevolutionary Origins of Human Emotions*. New York: Norton.

Parson, E. R. (1984). The reparation of self: Clinical and theoretical dimensions in the treatment of Vietnam combat veterans. *Journal of Contemporary Psychotherapy, 14*: 4–56.

Paskauskas R. A. (Ed.) (1993). *The Complete Correspondence of Sigmund Freud and Ernest Jones 1908–1939*. Cambridge: Harvard University Press.

Paulhan, F. (1889). *L'Activité Mentale et les Élements de l'Esprit*. http://archive.org/details/b28052511.

Peebles-Kleiger, M. J. (1989). Using countertransference in the hypnosis of trauma victims: A model for turning hazard into healing. *American Journal of Psychotherapy, 48*: 518–530.

Pérez-Rincón, H. (2012). Pierre Janet, Sigmund Freud and Charcot's psychological and psychiatric legacy. In: J. Bogousslavsky (Ed.), *Following Charcot: A Forgotten History of Neurology and Psychiatry* (pp. 115–124). Basel: Karger.

Perry, C. (1984). Dissociative phenomena of hypnosis. *Australian Journal of Clinical and Experimental Hypnosis, 12*: 71–84.

Perry, C., & Laurence, J. R. (1984). Mental processing outside of awareness: The contributions of Freud and Janet. In: K. S. Bowers & D. Meichenbaum (Eds.)*The Unconsciousness Reconsidered* (pp. 9–48). New York: Wiley.

Piaget, J. (1959). *The Language and Thought of the Child* (3rd ed.). London: Routledge & Kegan Paul.

Pichon-Janet, H. (1950). Pierre Janet: Quelques notes sur sa vie. *L'Evolution Psychiatrique: Hommage à Pierre Janet*, 345–355.

Pichot, P. (1996). *Une Siècle de Psychiatrie* [A Century of Psychiatry]. Le Plessis-Robinson: Synthélabo.

Pick, D. (1989). *Faces of Degeneration*. Cambridge: Cambridge University Press.

Pitman, R. K. (1984). Janet's *Obsessions and Psychasthenia*: A synopsis. *Psychiatric Quarterly, 56*: 291–314.

Pitman, R. K. (1987). Pierre Janet on obsessive-compulsive disorder (1903): Review and commentary. *Archives of General Psychiatry, 44*: 226–232.

Pope, H. G., Hudson, J. I., & Mialet, J. P. (1985). Bulimia in the late nineteenth century: the observations of Pierre Janet. *Psychological Medicine, 15*: 739–743.

Porges, S. W. (2007). The polyvagal perspective. *Biological Psychology, 74*: 116–143.

Porges, S. W. (2011). *The Polyvagal theory: Neurophysiological foundation of emotions, attachment, communication, and self-regulation*. New York: Norton.

Porges, S. W. (2016). *The Polyvagal Theory: Transformative Power of Feeling Safe*. Melbourne, Vic: Australian Childhood Foundation Conference.

Postel, J., & Quetel, C. (2004). *Nouvelle Histoire de la Psychiatrie* [New History of Psychiatry]. Paris: Dunod.

Prévost, C. M. (1973a). *Janet, Freud et la Psychologie Clinique* [Janet, Freud and Clinical Psychology]. Paris: Payot.

Prévost, C. M. (1973b). *La Psycho-Philosophy de Pierre Janet* Paris: Payot.

Putnam, F. W. (1989a). *Diagnosis and Treatment of Multiple Personality Disorder*. New York: Guilford.

Putnam, F. W. (1989b). Pierre Janet and modern views of dissociation. *Journal of Traumatic Stress, 2*: 413–429.

Putnam, F. W. (1992). Are alter personalities fragments or figments? *Psychoanalytic Inquire, 12*: 95–111.

Putnam, F. W. (1997). *Dissociation in Children and Adolescents: A Developmental Perspective*. New York: Guilford.

Putnam, F. W., Guroff, J. J., Silberman, E. K., Barban, L., & Post, R. M. (1986). The clinical phenomenology of multiple personality disorder. *Journal of Clinical Psychiatry, 47*: 285–293.

Rabinbach, A. (1990). *The Human Motor: Energy, Fatigue, and the Origins of Modernity*. New York: Basic Books.

Raymond, F., & Janet, P. (1898). *Névroses et Idées Fixes* (Vol. 2). Paris: Félix Alcan.

Read, J., & Argyle, N. (1999). Hallucinations, delusions, and thought disorder among adult psychiatric inpatients with a history of child abuse. *Psychiatric Services, 50*: 1467–1472.

Reite, M., & Fields, T. (Eds.) (1985). *The Psychobiology of Attachment and Separation*. Orlando, FL: Academic Press.

Reynolds, D. K. (1976). *Morita Psychotherapy*. Berkeley, CA: University of California Press.

Rolnik, E. J. (2012). *Freud in Zion*. London: Karnac.

Ross, C. A. (1989). *Multiple Personality Disorder: Diagnosis, Clinical Features, and Treatment.* New York: Wiley.

Ross, C. A. (1997). *Dissociative Identity Disorder: Diagnosis, Clinical Features and Treatment of Multiple Personality* (2nd ed.). New York: Wiley.

Ross, C. A., Anderson, G., & Clark, P. (1994). Childhood abuse and the positive symptoms of schizophrenia. *Hospital & Community Psychiatry, 45*: 489–491.

Rothschild, B. (2000). *The Body Remembers: The Psychophysiology of Trauma and Trauma Treatment.* New York: Norton.

Rycroft, C. (2004). Dissociation of the Personality. In: R. L. Gregory (Ed.), *The Oxford Companion to the Mind* (pp. 258–259). Oxford: Oxford University Press.

Sachs, R. G., Frischholz, E. J., & Wood, J. I. (1988). Marital and family therapy in the treatment of multiple personality disorder. *Journal of Marital and Family Therapy, 14,* 249–259.

Saillot, I. (2005). *Pierre Janet's Hierarchy: Stages or Styles?* Janetian studies online Vol. 2. http//pierre-janet.com/JSarticles/2005/hierar.doc.

Saillot, I. (2008). *La hiérarchie des tendances de Pierre Janet et sa confrontation à quelques expérimentations contemporaines.* Conférence au Congrès de la Société Française de Psychologie, Nantes, 13–15 September 2007. *Janetian Studies Vol. 5,* on line.

Sandler, J., & Fonagy, P. (Eds.) (2011). *Recovered Memories of Abuse: True or False?* London: Karnac.

Sapolsky, R. M., Krey, L. C., & McEwen, B. S. (1984). Glucocorticoid-sensitive hippocampal neurons are involved in terminating the adrenocortical stress response. *Proceedings of the National Academy of Sciences, 81*: 6174–6177.

Schopenhauer, A. (1958). *The World as Will and Representation,* Vol. I (1818) and Vol. II (1844). Clinton, MA: The Falcon's Wing Press. Original title: *Die Welt als Wille und Vorstellung.*

Schore, A. N. (1994). *Affect Regulation and the Origin of the Self.* Hillsdale, NJ: Erlbaum.

Schore, A. N. (2001). The effects of early relational trauma on right brain development, affect regulation, and infant mental health. *Infant Mental Health Journal, 22*: 201–269.

Schore, A. N. (2003). *Affect Regulation and the Repair of the Self.* New York: Norton.

Schore, A. N. (2009). Attachment trauma and the developing right brain: Origins of pathological dissociation. In: P. F. Dell & J. O'Neill (Eds.), *Dissociation and the Dissociative Disorders: DSM-V and Beyond* (pp. 107–141). London: Routledge.

Schore, A. N. (2011). Foreword. In: P. M. Bromberg, *The Shadow of the Tsunami and the Growth of the Relational Mind* (pp. ix–xxxi). New York: Routledge.

Schore, A. N. (2012). *The Science of the Art of Psychotherapy.* New York: Norton.

Schumpf, Y. R., Reinders, A. A. T. S., Nijenhuis, E. R. S., Luechinger, R., Van Osch, J. P., & Jäncke, L. (2014). Dissociative part-dependent resting-state activity in dissociative identity disorder: A controlled fMRI perfusion study. *PLoS ONE, 9(6)*: e98795.

Schwartz, L. (1951). *Die Neurosen and die Dynamische Psychologie von Pierre Janet.* Basel: B. Schwabe. French edition: *Les Névroses et la Psychologie Dynamique de Pierre Janet.* Paris: Presses Universitaires de France, 1955.

Shamdasani, S. (2003). *Jung and the Making of Modern Psychology.* London: Cambridge University Press.

Shamdasani, S. (2012). *C.G. Jung: A Biography in Books.* New York: Norton.

Shapiro, D. (1965). *Neurotic Styles.* New York: Basic Books.

Sherrington, C. S. (1906). *The Integrative Action of the Nervous System.* New Haven, CT: Yale University Press.

Sherrington, C. S. (1932). Inhibition as a co-ordinative factor. *Nobel Lectures, Physiology and Medicine 1922–1941.* Amsterdam: Elsevier.

Siegel, D. J. (1999). *The Developing Mind.* New York: Norton.

Sjövall, B. (1967). *Psychological Tension: An Analysis of Pierre Janet's Concept of "Tension Psychologique" together with an Historical Aspect.* Norstedts, Sweden: Svenska Bokförlaget.

Skodol, A. E., Gunderson, J. G., Pfohl, B., Widiger, T. A., Livesley, W. J., & Siever, L. J. (2002). The borderline diagnosis I: psychopathology, comorbidity, and personality structure. *Biological Psychiatry, 51*: 936–950.

Slater, E. (1965). Diagnosis of "Hysteria". *British Medical Journal, 1(5447)*: 1395–1399.

Smith, A. H. (1984). Sources of efficacy in the hypnotic relationship: An object relations approach. In: W. C. Wester & A. H. Smith (Eds.), *Clinical Hypnosis: A Multidisciplinary Approach* (pp. 85–114). Philadelphia: Lippincott.

Solms, M., & Turnbull, O. (2002). *The Brain and the Inner World.* London: Karnac.

Solomon, J., & George, C. (2011). Disorganization of maternal caregiving across two generations: The origins of caregiving helplessness. In: J. Solomon & C. George (Eds.), *Disorganized Attachment and Caregiving* (pp. 25–51). New York: Guilford Press.

Solomon, M., & Siegel, D. J. (2003). *Healing Trauma: Attachment, Mind, Body and Brain.* New York: Norton.

Spiegel, R. (1986). Freud's refutation of degenerationism: A contribution to humanism. *Contemporary Psychoanalysis, 22*: 4–24.

Spiegel, D. (1990). Hypnosis, trauma, and dissociation. In: R. P. Kluft (Ed.), *Incest Related Syndromes of Adult Psychopathology* (pp. 247–261). Washington, DC: American Psychiatric Press.

Spiegel, D., Hunt, T., & Dondershine, H. E. (1988). Dissociation and hypnotizability in posttraumatic stress disorder. *American Journal of Psychiatry, 145*: 301–305.

Spinoza, B. (1677/1996). *Ethics.* London: Penguin Books.

Spurling, H. (1998). *The Unknown Matisse* (Vol. 1). London: Hamish Hamilton.

Spurling, H. (2005). *Matisse: The Masters* (Vol. 2). London: Hamish Hamilton.

St. Aubyn, E. (2012). *The Patrick Melrose Novels.* London: Picador.

Stark, M. (1994). *Working with Resistance.* Northvale, NJ: Jason Aronson.

Steele, K., Boon, S., & van der Hart, O. (2017). *Treating Trauma-related Dissociation: A Practical, Integrative Approach.* New York: Norton.

Steele, K., van der Hart, O., & Nijenhuis, E. R. S. (2001). Dependency in the treatment of complex posttraumatic stress disorder and dissociative disorders. *Journal of Trauma and Dissociation, 2*(4): 79–116.

Stern, D. N. (1985). *The Interpersonal World of the Infant.* New York: Basic Books.

Stern, D. N., Sander, L.W., Nahum, J. P., Harrison, A. M., Lyons-Ruth, K., Morgan, A.C., Bruschweiler-Stern, N., & Tronick, E. Z. (1998). Non-interpretive mechanisms in psychoanalytic therapy: The "something more" than interpretation. *International Journal of Psycho-Analysis, 79*: 903–921.

Stone, L. (1967). The psychoanalytic situation and transference. *Journal of the American Psychoanalytic Association, 15*: 3–58.

Sullivan, H. S. (1953). *The Interpersonal Theory of Psychiatry.* New York: Norton.

Summit, R. (1987). The hidden child phenomenon: An atypical dissociative disorder. In: B. G. Braun (Ed.), *Dissociative Disorders 1987: Proceedings of the 4th International Conference of Multiple Personality/Dissociative States* (p. 6). Rush-Presbyterian St Luke's Medical Center, Chicago.

Suttie, I. D. (1935). *The Origins of Love and Hate.* London: Free Association Books.

Titchener, J. L. (1986). Post-traumatic decline: A consequence of unresolved destructive drives. In: C. Figley (Ed.), *Trauma and its Wake. II* (pp. 5–19). New York: Brunner/Mazel.

Tögel, C. (1999). 'My bad diagnostic error': Once more about Freud and Emmy v. N. (Fanny Moser). *International Journal of Psycho-Analysis, 80*: 1165–1173.

Trevarthen, C. (2014). The human nature of culture and education. *Cognitive Science, 5(2)*: 173–192.

Tronick, E. (2016). *The buffer/transduction model of risk, resource depletion and outcome: mutual regulation and reparation for good or ill*. Melbourne, Vic: Australian Childhood Foundation Conference.

Tulving, E. (1983). *Elements of Episodic Memory*. Oxford, UK: Clarendon Press.

Tulving, E. (1985). How many memory systems are there? *American Psychologist, 40*: 385–398.

Tulving, E., & Schacter, D. L. (1990). Priming and human memory systems. *Science, 247(4940)*: 301–306.

Tulving, E., & Thomson, D. M. (1973). Encoding specificity and retrieval processes in episodic memory. *Psychological Review, 80*: 352–373.

Udolf, J. (1987). *Handbook of Hypnosis for Professionals* (2nd ed.). New York: Van Nostrand Reinhold Company.

Van Buren, J., & Alhanati, S. (2010). *Primitive Mental States: A Psychoanalytic Exploration of the Origins of Meaning*. London: Routledge.

van der Hart, O. (Ed.) (1988). *Coping with Loss*. New York: Irvington.

van der Hart, O., & Dorahy, M. (2006). Pierre Janet and the concept of dissociation. *American Journal of Psychiatry, 163*(9), 1646; author reply 1646.

van der Hart, O., & Horst, R. (1989). The dissociation theory of Pierre Janet. *Journal of Traumatic Stress, 2*: 397–412.

van der Hart, O., & Van der Velden, K. (1987). The hypnotherapy of Dr. Andries Hoek: Uncovering hypnotherapy before Janet, Breuer and Freud. *American Journal of Clinical Hypnosis, 29*: 264–271.

van der Hart, O., Nijenhuis, E., & Steele, K. (2006). *The Haunted Self: Structural Dissociation and the Treatment of Chronic Traumatization*. New York: Norton.

van der Hart, O., Steele, K., Boon, S., & Brown, P. (1993). The treatment of traumatic memories: Synthesis, realization, and integration. *Dissociation, 6*: 162–180.

van der Hart, O., Van Dijke, A., Van Son, M., & Steele, K. (2000). Somatoform dissociation in traumatized World War I combat soldiers: A neglected clinical heritage. *Journal of Trauma and Dissociation, 1(4)*: 33–66.

van der Hart, O., Witztum, E., & Friedman, B. (1993). From hysterical psychosis to reactive dissociative psychosis. *Journal of Traumatic Stress, 6*: 43–64.

Van der Kolk, B. A. (1987). The separation cry and the trauma response: Developmental issues in the psychobiology of attachment and separation. In: B. A. Van der Kolk (Ed.), *Psychological Trauma* (pp. 31–62). Washington, DC: American Psychiatric Press.

Van der Kolk, B. A. (1989). The compulsion to repeat the trauma. *Psychiatric Clinics of North America, 12*, 389–411.

Van der Kolk, B. A. (1996). Trauma and memory. In: B. A. Van der Kolk, A. C. McFarlane, & L. Weisaeth (Eds.), *Traumatic Stress: The Effects of Overwhelming Experience on Mind, Body, and Society* (pp. 214–241). New York: Guilford.

Van der Kolk, B. A. (2014). *The Body Keeps the Score: Brain, Mind, and Body in the Healing of Trauma*. New York: Penguin Books.

Van der Kolk, B. A., & Ducey, C. P. (1989). The psychological processing of traumatic experience: Rorschach patterns in PTSD. *Journal of Traumatic Stress, 2*: 259–274.

Van der Kolk, B. A., & Fisler, R. E. (1994). Childhood abuse and neglect and loss of self-regulation. *Bulletin of the Menninger Clinic, 58*: 145–168.

Van der Kolk, B. A., & van der Hart, O. (1989). Pierre Janet and the breakdown of adaptation in psychological trauma. *American Journal of Psychiatry, 146*: 1530–1540.

Van der Kolk, B. A., & van der Hart, O. (1991). The intrusive past: The flexibility of memory and the engraving of trauma. *American Imago, 48:* 425–454. Also in: C. Caruth (Ed.) (1995), *Trauma: Explorations in Memory* (pp. 158–182). Baltimore: John Hopkins University Press.

Van der Kolk, B. A., Brown, P., & van der Hart, O. (1989). Pierre Janet on posttraumatic stress. *Journal of Traumatic Stress, 2*: 365–378.

Van der Kolk, B. A., van der Hart, O., & Marmar, C. (1996). Dissociation and information processing in posttraumatic stress disorder. In: B. A. Van der Kolk, A. McFarlane, & L. Weisaeth (Eds.), *Traumatic Stress* (pp. 303–327). New York: Guildford.

van der Hart, O., Van der Kolk, B. A., & Boon, S. (1998). The treatment of dissociative disorders. In: J. D. Bremner & C. R. Marmar (Eds.), *Trauma, Memory and Dissociation* (pp. 253–283). Washington, DC: American Psychiatric Press.

Van der Veer, R., & Valsiner, J. (1988). Lev Vygotsky and Pierre Janet: On the origin of the concept of sociogenesis. *Developmental Review, 8*: 52–65.

Van Sweden, R. C. (1994). *Regression to Dependence: A Second Opportunity for Ego Integration and Developmental Progression*. Northvale, NJ: Jason Aronson.

Varela, F. (1996). Neurophenomenology: A methodological remedy for the hard problem. *Journal of Consciousness Studies, 3*: 330–349.

Vezzoli, C., Bressi, C., Tricarico, G., & Boato, P. (2007). Methodological evolution and clinical application of C.G. Jung's Word Association Experiment. *Journal of Analytical Psychology, 52*: 89–108.

Walant, K. B. (1995). *Creating the Capacity for Attachment: Treating Addictions and the Alienated Self*. Northvale, NJ: Jason Aronson.

Walusinski, O. (2014). The girls of the Salpêtrière. In: J. Bogousslavsky (Ed.), *Hysteria: The Modern Birth of an Enigma* (pp. 1–11). Basel, Switzerland: Karger.

Watkins, J. G., & Watkins, H. H. (1997). *Ego-States: Theory and Therapy*. New York: Norton.

Waxman, D. (1982). *Hypnosis: A Guide for Patients and Practitioners*. London: George Allen & Unwin.

Wetterstrand, O. G. (1892). Über den künstlich verlängerten Schlaf, besonders bei Behandlung der Hysterie, Epilepsie und Hystero-Epilepsie. *Zeitschrift für Hypnotismus, 1*: 17–23.

Wimmer, H., & Perner, J. (1983). Beliefs about beliefs: Representation and constraining function of wrong beliefs in young children's understanding of deception. *Cognition, 13*: 103–128.

Woolf, V. (1950). *Mr Bennett and Mrs Brown - The Captains Death Bed and Other Essays* (pp. 90–111). London: Hogarth.

World Health Organization (1992). *ICD-10*. Geneva: WHO.

INDEX

Page numbers in *italic* refer to figures. Page numbers in **bold** refer to tables.